BEHAVIORAL NEUROLOGY

BEHAVIORAL NEUROLOGY

Fourth Edition

JONATHAN H. PINCUS, M.D.

Chief of Neurology
Veterans Administration Medical Center
Washington, D.C.

Professor of Neurology
Georgetown University School of Medicine

GARY J. TUCKER, M.D.

Professor Emeritus
Department of Psychiatry and Behavioral Sciences
University of Washington School of Medicine

OXFORD
UNIVERSITY PRESS
2003

OXFORD
UNIVERSITY PRESS

Oxford New York
Auckland Bangkok Buenos Aires Cape Town Chennai
Dar es Salaam Delhi Hong Kong Istanbul Karachi Kolkata
Kuala Lumpur Madrid Melbourne Mexico City Mumbai
Nairobi São Paulo Shanghai Taipei Tokyo Toronto

Published by Oxford University Press, Inc.
198 Madison Avenue, New York, New York 10016
http://www.oup-usa.org

Library of Congress Cataloging-in-Publication Data
Pincus, Jonathan H., 1935–
Behavioral neurology / Jonathan H. Pincus, Gary J. Tucker.—4th ed.
p. cm.
Includes bibliographical references and index.
ISBN 0-19-513781-7 (cloth)—ISBN 0-19-513782-5 (pbk.)
1. Neuropsychiatry. I. Tucker, Gary J., 1934– II. Title.
[DNLM: 1. Nervous System Diseases. 2. Mental Disorders. WL 140 P647b 2003]
RC341 .P56 2003
616.89—dc21 2002018383

9 8 7 6 5 4 3 2 1

Printed in the United States of America
on acid-free paper

"It ought to be generally known that the source of our pleasure, merriment, laughter, and amusement, as of our grief, pain, anxiety, and tears, is none other than the brain. It is specially the organ which enables us to think, see, and hear, and to distinguish the ugly and the beautiful, the bad and the good, pleasant and unpleasant. Sometimes we judge according to the perceptions of expediency. It is the brain too which is the seat of madness and delirium, of the fears and frights which assail us, often by night, but sometimes even by day; it is there where lies the cause of insomnia and sleep-walking, of thoughts that will not come, forgotten duties, and eccentricities. All such things result from an unhealthy condition of the brain."

Hippocrates

PREFACE

Psychiatry and neurology have undergone revolutionary changes since the last edition of this book was published in 1985. There are now many new medications, discussed here, for the control of epilepsy, depression, mania, schizophrenia, obsessive-compulsive disorder, anxiety, and movement disorders. The discovery that the selective serotonin reuptake inhibitors (SSRIs) could control not only depression but also the symptoms of obsessive-compulsive disorder, phobia, and panic disorder has brought hope and relief to the sufferers from these conditions and their families and, perhaps even more importantly, has brought these illnesses into the realm of neuroscience. No one could argue today, as they did in the past, that these conditions are purely "psychological neuroses," disorders of the mind not the brain.

New, atypical antipsychotic drugs have provided relief for many of the symptoms of schizophrenia. These drugs have a much lower rate of extra pyramidal side effects than the neuroleptics available in 1985, especially with regard to the risk of tardive movement disorders. We discuss these and their presumed mechanism of action.

The expanded understanding of Parkinson's disease, its etiology and treatment, has provided a paradigm for the understanding of the role of catecholamines and indoleamines in depression. It has also highlighted a flaw in the amine hypothesis of depression. The changes wrought by dopamine replacement therapy in Parkinson's are realized within minutes. The antidepressant drugs induce changes in brain amines within minutes, too, but the onset of their antidepressant effect is delayed for 2 to 3 weeks. The amine hypothesis and alternate hypotheses for depression are presented. The physiological effects of psychological stress on the brain may be mediated through steroids that damage and even kill neurons in the hippocampus and elsewhere.

Our understanding of reparative brain mechanisms is expanding and may apply to the recovery of brain cells from stress. The old idea that new neurons do not form during postnatal life has been challenged. There is strong and growing evidence that neurogenesis occurs in the adult human brain, especially in the hippocampus. Adult mice provided with enriched environmental living conditions grew 60 percent more granule cells in the dentate gyrus of the hippocampus than genetically identical controls and outperformed the controls in learning. There has been an astounding increase of our appreciation of the many links between the brain and behavior.

With the introduction of DSM-IV, the diagnostic criteria for psychiatric disease have sharpened. Clinical studies have become more focused and DSM-IV has broadened our understanding of mental illness. The new insights provided by DSM-IV are contrasted with some older ideas.

The newest categorization of epilepsy has abolished many imprecise, confusing terms that were in use a generation ago, such as *petit mal*, *psychomotor*, *minor*, *focal*, and *grand mal*. The new terminology is used in this edition. Many clinical studies have clarified the relationship of pseudoseizures to true epilepsy. It has proven very difficult to distinguish pseudoseizures from the behavioral abnormalities that are the manifestations of complex partial seizures that arise from the frontal and occipital lobes. We review these features and summarize the criteria that differentiate them.

There is increasing appreciation of the frequency with which dissociation occurs. It is the operative feature in many conversion reactions, including pseudoseizures. This insight has only recently emerged. As residents, we were taught that dissociation was rare. It is not rare. The role of child abuse, physical, sexual, or both, and the resulting dissociative defenses have been implicated in the development of many personality disorders (antisocial, borderline, hysterical, paranoid, multiple) and mood disorders. From the days of Freud until recently, the role of abuse in causing subsequent cognitive and behavioral abnormalities has been ignored, but now we know that abuse is an important factor in many of them. The focus of current approaches to this subject is turning toward understanding the brain mechanisms that are altered by abuse. The concept that abuse changes the brain has brought this experiential factor within the purview of neurology. The role of abuse in affecting the organization and the function of the brain is a new addition to this book.

Abuse, like any environmental factor that is remembered, changes the brain.

One of the important themes of the first three editions of this book was that mental illnesses were the clinical manifestations of brain disease, most of it inherited. In this edition we emphasize that the environment changes the brain, sometimes permanently. Experience and heredity, together, shape the lasting connections in the brain that determine behavior and thought. Violence provides an example of a symptom that results from the interplay of experience, neurological disorders, and hereditary mental illness.

The role of the frontal lobes of the brain in modulating behavior and thought has achieved a new currency. Dysfunction of the executive capacities that are mediated through the frontal lobes is important in most of the psychiatric diseases, many movement and gait disorders, and some odd disorders that are located on the border between neurology and psychiatry, such as Tourette's syndrome. Violence and attention-deficit hyperactivity disorder are two symptomatic conditions that were not especially linked to frontal lobe disease in the past but are now thought to result largely from the loss of frontal control mechanisms.

Chronic dementias in the past were pretty much identified as "Alzheimer's," but now many other dementias of clinical significance have been delineated. A sterile argument that regarded the diagnosis of Pick's disease as uncertain if rare inclusions called Pick bodies were not seen in the frontal and temporal cortex at autopsy has been sidestepped. The diagnosis of frontotemporal atrophy (read Pick's disease) is now common as tests that assess the executive and frontal-cortical functions are more widely used. Lewy body dementia, a "new" condition, has bridged a gap between Alzheimer's and Parkinson's diseases.

The importance of badly made proteins to the dementias is now emerging. The abnormal proteins that seem to play a role in Parkinson's disease, Lewy body dementia, Alzheimer's disease, fronto temporal atrophy, Huntington's disease, and Creutzfeld-Jakob disease are variants of normal neuronal proteins, sometimes only a single amino acid different from the normal cellular constituent. The role of vascular dementia caused by small vessel disease in the symptomatology of Alzheimer's disease was not appreciated before the famous Nun's study. We have updated our discussion of the pathogenesis of Alzheimer's disease and the other dementias.

The tools to investigate brain disorders have advanced dramatically. It is now possible to see the brain at work in health and disease! Position emission tomography (PET), single photon emission computed tomography (SPECT), functional magnetic resonance (MR), and nuclear magnetic resonance (NMR) advances that were not available in 1985 for the investigation of brain disorders have become new research tools. Some (PET and SPECT) utilize radioactive isotopes. Though each technique is developing diagnostic niches in the fields of epilepsy, dementia, and vascular disease as the result of clinical research, none is easy to arrange. Positron emission tomography is expensive and is only done in a few large medical centers. Single photon emission computed tomography is more available but the need for coordination of physicians, radiologists, psychologists, nurses, and technicians has made SPECT unwieldy for its use in epilepsy. The need for isotopes has limited PET and SPECT in the evaluation of behavioral disorders in children and women of childbearing age. These limitations are being addressed increasingly by reaching out to functional MR techniques for the study of the brain.

This is to say that the uses of MRI have gone far beyond the superior static images that this technique provides. Even static MRI was not generally available in 1985. With functional MR, it is now possible to investigate the brain at work in real time without the radiation exposure that a radioisotope produces. The location of brain deficits in dyslexia and other cognitive deficits have been explored by this technique.

As dazzling as these techniques are for the investigation of behavioral disorders and as important as they may become in psychiatric and neurological diagnosis, at present the older techniques of clinical examination and neuropsychological testing are still much more sensitive and specific in both psychiatry and neurology. Our understanding of the use of these older clinical techniques has also expanded. It is now clear that the standard mini-mental status examination (MMSE) and intelligence quotient (IQ) testing essentially ignore the anterior third of the brain. It is possible for a patient to become a social imbecile because of disease of his frontal lobes and still have a normal MMSE and IQ. How does a clinician assess the part of the frontal lobes that lie anterior to the motor strip? Calling this region prefrontal implies that it lies in front of the frontal lobes and that the frontal lobes end in the motor strip, their most posterior component. The clinical tools for investigation of this region are available and have been validated in adults (not in children). It is embarrassing that they are often unused by neurologists, psychiatrists, and psychologists who are investigating behavioral deviations. The clinical tests for assessing the frontal lobes and their connections are described in this edition in some detail.

At the time of this writing, we may be on the brink of exciting new advances in the diagnosis and therapy of some of humankind's oldest enemies. The concept that neurons do not multiply and cannot be replaced in the mature brain has been challenged by the finding that neurons in the hippocampus do multiply and stem cells (primitive, undifferentiated cells) exist in reservoirs either in the walls of the ventricles or among astrocytes a few cell layers away from the ventricular surface. These stem cells can become new neurons or glia and may become the vehicles for the repair of damaged myelin or systems that have suffered neuronal cell loss. The mechanisms that control the migration, growth, and differentiation of stem cells are now being studied. Stem cells have provided some repair in mice with a hereditary disease of myelin formation. The excitement that these advances engender must be tempered by acknowledgement that the tremendous advances in genetics over the last 15 years have not provided any treatment of genetic disorders of the brain, though some definitive genetic tests have become available, such as the one for Huntington's disease.

Until similar tests become available for the diagnosis of the major mental illnesses, the dementing disorders, the movement disorders, and many of the epilepsies, we must persist in using the clinical skills of history and physical examination and the nosology that has been based on them. In the fields of psychiatry and neurology, the clinician is still the main diagnostic instrument.

J.H.P.
G.J.T.

CONTENTS

1. Epilepsy and Behavior, 1
   Idiopathic versus Symptomatic Epilepsy, 2
   Clinical Genetic Studies, 3
   Complex Partial Seizures—Temporal Lobe Origin, 4
      Subjective Feelings, 5
      Automatisms, 6
   Complex Partial Seizures—Extratemporal Origin, 8
   Electroencephalography and the Diagnosis of Epilepsy, 9
   Abnormal Electroencephalogram without Epilepsy, 13
   Pseudoseizures, 13
   Therapy, 16
   Blood Levels, 17
   Surgery in Epilepsy, 22
   Epileptogenesis, Cognitive, and Behavioral Deterioration, 24
   Psychosis, 29
   Affective Disorders, 34
   Anxiety Disorders, 35
   Sexual Behavior, 36
   Personality Disturbance, 37
   Violence, the Temporal Lobes, and the Limbic System, 38
      Anatomy, 39

Physiological Psychology, 40
Aggression and Violence as an Epileptic-like Discharge of the Limbic System, 43
Episodic Dyscontrol, 45
Conclusion, 46

2. Violence and Neurobiology, 61
Brain Damage, 61
Antisocial Personality and the Frontal Lobe, 64
Neurotransmitters and Hormones, 65
Mental Illness, 66
Abuse, 67
Violence as a Complex Psycho-Social-Biologic Interaction, 69
Sociological Aspects of Violence, 72
Conclusion, 76

3. Schizophrenia, 85
Clinical Features, 89
Age at Onset and Gender, 92
Changing Diagnostic Criteria and Symptomatic Classifications, 93
Schizoaffective Disorder, 94
Personality Disorders and Schizophrenia, 95
Course and Natural History, 95
Differential Diagnosis, 97
Differentiating from Other Psychiatric Disorders, 97
Neurological Diseases, 98
Drug Reactions, 100
Sleep Disorders, 100
Biologic Basis of Schizophrenia, 100
Genetics, 100
Biochemical Findings, 103
Neurological Abnormalities in Schizophrenic Patients, 106
Minor, nonlocalizing neurological abnormalities, 106
Electroencephalographic data, 111
Neuroimaging, 112
Neuropathological findings, 115
Psychological Testing for Schizophrenia, 116
Arousal, 118
Treatment, 118
Conclusion, 119

4. Disorders of Cognitive Function, 133
Regional Syndromes, 135
Clinical Symptoms Associated with Frontal Lobe Dysfunction, 136
Clinical Symptoms Associated with Parietal Lobe Dysfunction, 139
Clinical Symptoms Associated with Temporal Lobe Dysfunction, 141
Other Symptoms of Cortical Dysfunction, 142
Aphasia, 142

Apraxia, 146
Agnosia, 146
Alexia and Agraphia, 146
Dysfunctions Associated with Severing the Corpus Callosum—Split Brains, 147
Diffuse Disorders of Cognitive Function—Delirium and Dementia, 150
Alzheimer's Disease, 154
Vascular Dementia, 157
Pick's Disease and Dementia of the Lewy Body Type, 157
Human Immunodeficiency Virus-1 Dementia, 158
Occult Hydrocephalus, 158
Cerebral White Matter Dysfunction and Cognitive Changes, 159
Depression in Dementia, 160
Neuropsychological Testing, 161
Cognitive Syndromes in Childhood, 161
Early Childhood Autism, 162
Attention-Deficit Hyperactivity Disorder, 164
Treatment, 166
Attention-deficit hyperactivity disorder in adults, 167
Conclusion, 167

5. Movement, Mood, and Obsessive-Compulsive Disorders, 177
Parkinson's Disease, 177
Pathogenesis, 181
L-dopa, 181
Stages of Parkinson's Disease, 182
Stage I—early dopamine deficiency—mildly symptomatic, 182
Stage II—moderate dopamine deficiency—wearing off—fluctuations of motor activity, 183
Stage III—end stage of dopamine deficiency, 184
Protein Redistribution Diet, 186
Pharmacological Treatment, 186
The balance theory, 187
Surgical Treatments, 188
Transplants, 188
Pallidotomy/thalamotomy, 188
Brain stimulation, 189
Psychiatric Symptoms in Parkinson's Disease, 189
Depression, 189
Anxiety versus akathisia, 190
Painful dystonia, 191
Psychosis, 191
Dementia, 192
Etiology of Neurodegenerative Disorders, 193
Acute Drug-Induced Movement Disorders, 195
Tardive Movement Disorders, 195

Dystonia, 197
Dystonia and Mental Illness, 200
Chorea, 200
Treatment, 202
Motor Tics, Tourette's Syndrome, and Obsessive-Compulsive Disorder, 203
Affective Disorders, 205
Biologic Changes in Affective Disorders, 207
Structural changes, 207
Hypothalamic changes, 208
Anxiety and arousal, 209
Sleep, 209
Neurotransmitter changes, 210
Immune responses, 211
Genetics, 211
Stress and negative life events, 211
Treatment, 213
Conclusion, 214

6. Distinguishing Neurological from Psychiatric Symptoms, 229
Commonality of Neurological and Psychiatric Symptoms, 230
Panic Disorder/Hyperventilation as a Cause of Common Neurological Symptoms, 231
Somatization Disorder, 232
Unexplained Symptoms, 233
Conversion Disorders, 234
Specific Classical Conversion Symptoms, 235
Headache, 242
Conclusion, 245

7. Clinical Evaluation, 249
The Importance of the Clinical History, 250
Neurological Conditions Commonly Associated with a High Incidence of Psychiatric Complications, 254
The Clinical Examination of the Brain, 255
Cortical Functions, 256
Cognitive Functions, 257
Behaviors Associated with the Frontal Lobes, 258
Evaluation of the Frontal Lobes, 259
Cognitive aspects of the frontal lobe evaluation, 262
Mental Status Examination, 263
Imaging, 264
Clinical Laboratory Tests, 265
Electroencephalography, 265
Conclusion, 266

Index, 269

BEHAVIORAL NEUROLOGY

Chapter One

EPILEPSY AND BEHAVIOR

Epilepsy is a recurring behavioral, sensory, or subjective experience caused by an abnormal electrical discharge in the brain. Though abnormal electrical changes accompany seizures of any kind, they may not be reflected in the electroencephalogram (EEG) between seizures and sometimes epileptic EEG discharges occur in the absence of clinically apparent seizures. Generalized seizures always cause a disturbance in consciousness and the EEG is virtually always abnormal during such seizures. Partial seizures may not be associated with unconsciousness, with any abnormal movement, or with an epileptiform, scalp-recorded EEG, even during the episode.

It may not always be clear how much of a patient's behavior can be attributed to epilepsy and there may be disagreement among competent neurologists as to the relation of abnormal behavior to the seizure state. In such cases, a therapeutic trial of anticonvulsants may appear to resolve the medical problem, but the pragmatic definition of epilepsy as abnormal thought and behavior that resolves with the use of antiepileptic medications is medically and scientifically weak. Mental symptoms in mania and other disorders can improve during therapy with antiepileptic drugs in patients who do not have epilepsy.

The deviations of thought and behavior that may occur in epileptics can be the result of electrical epileptic discharges, the cerebral response to abnormal discharges, the destruction of tissue that has led to the epileptic condition, the medication used to treat the epilepsy, the serendipitous concurrence of unrelated conditions, or some combination of these.

IDIOPATHIC VERSUS SYMPTOMATIC EPILEPSY

The term *symptomatic epilepsy* is applied to seizure disorders with an identifiable cause, such as encephalitis, tumor, trauma, or known metabolic disease. In these conditions, seizures are considered to be a symptom of another disease. The term *idiopathic* epilepsy literally means an epilepsy unto itself, without other disease of the nervous system. The concept of idiopathic epilepsy is artificial. The epilepsy is surely the result of a physiological dysfunction, but the biochemical or neuroanatomical locus of the abnormality is not yet known. A high proportion of the relatives of younger patients with idiopathic epilepsy have abnormal EEGs, yet most of these persons never have clinical seizures. *Idiopathic* in younger patients probably should refer to *inherited* epilepsy, which usually begins in childhood or adolescence; hence, using a positive family history to diagnose genetically transmitted epilepsy as phenotypic expression may be incomplete: history is helpful in making a reliable diagnosis. It is not essential to have a positive family history. The clinical course, seizure type, and EEG characteristics are sufficient for this diagnosis.

The assumption that the brains of patients with idiopathic epilepsy of childhood onset are normal, except for the epilepsy, may be incorrect. The thinking processes and behavior of children with idiopathic epilepsy may not be normal even when the seizures have completely stopped. Thirteen of 20 children diagnosed as having benign Rolandic epilepsy (focal seizures arising near the Rolandic fissure) showed language impairment with difficulties in 2 or more of 12 standardized language tests. Language dysfunction, as revealed by these tests, correlated with learning difficulties at school, though the overall intelligence quotient (IQ) was average (Staden et al., 1998).

Some patients who have a genetic tendency to epilepsy also show other symptoms of brain dysfunction and have a history of events known to be associated with brain damage. Acquired brain damage may promote expression of the genetic trait, and to the extent that it does, the resulting seizures are symptomatic of brain damage. It is also true that even in symptomatic epilepsy, the mechanism by which identifiable lesions cause seizures is not well understood. Whether epilepsy is idiopathic or symptomatic, caused by a gene or a tumor, the lesion, i.e., tumor or abnormal gene, is ever-present but seizures are intermittent. There are cerebral mechanisms that prevent the spread of discharges, among them hyperpolarization and inhibition around the focus. Inhibition can involve sites far removed from the epileptic focus, even in the opposite hemisphere. The inhibiting control mechanisms are varied and many have separate genetic determinants. The impact of this neurophysiologic inhibition surrounding the epileptic focus on human behavior has never been assessed but some of the behavioral–cognitive distortions that epileptics encounter may originate in the activation of such natural "epilepsy control mechanisms." When these "control" mechanisms fail, the epileptic activity spreads and a clinical seizure occurs.

CLINICAL GENETIC STUDIES

For certain forms of generalized epilepsy, EEG studies have demonstrated a dominant mode of inheritance with incomplete penetrance and expressivity (Lennox et al., 1940; Metrakos and Metrakos, 1961; Bray and Weiser, 1964). Until the late 1980s, genetic influences on partial seizures were thought to be of minimal importance. Since then it has become clear that inheritance plays a major role in the pathogenesis of partial, focal seizures. Criteria for benign partial seizures, include the absence of any evidence of brain dysfunction other than the seizures themselves (no cognitive, motor or sensory deficit), a family history of epilepsy, onset of seizures after 2 years of age, stereotyped brief seizures, frequent nocturnal occurrence, spontaneous remission in adolescence, and EEGs with spikes that have a distinctive morphology and localization on a normal background of electrical activity. The two most common of the benign, focal, partial epilepsies are Rolandic and occipital epilepsy (Holmes, 1993).

Benign Rolandic epilepsy of childhood with centrotemporal spikes is the most common partial epilepsy syndrome in children. The onset of seizures is between the ages of 3 and 13 years old. The typical presentation is a partial seizure with parasthesias and tonic or clonic activity of the lower face associated with drooling and dysarthria. Seizures occur commonly at night and may become secondarily generalized. They are usually infrequent and are easily controlled. The EEG shows characteristic high-voltage sharp waves in the centrotemporal regions, which are activated with drowsiness and sleep. Atypical cases are common. The long-term medical prognosis is excellent with essentially all children entering long-term remission by mid-adolescence (Wirrel, 1998).

Benign occipital epilepsy of childhood is a partial epilepsy syndrome with elementary visual symptomatology frequently associated with other ictal phenomena. Seizures are usually followed by postictal headache and are often associated with interictal occipital rhythmic paroxysmal EEG activity that appears only after eye closure. Early-onset benign occipital epilepsy may consist of brief, infrequent attacks and prolonged status epilepticus. There is ictal deviation of the eyes or head or both and vomiting, starting in children between the ages of 3 and 7 years old. The benign focal epilepsies are commonly associated with migraine (Andermann and Zifkin, 1998).

Mothers of epileptics are more frequently epileptic than fathers of epileptics

(Annegers et al., 1976). This may not reflect the influence of some sex-linked genetic trait but rather may stem from the adverse effect of epilepsy and anticonvulsant medications on the male libido and sexual performance. A similar situation exists among the parents of schizophrenics (see pp. 101–103).

Twin studies have buttressed the view of the dominant inheritance of idiopathic epilepsy (Lennox, 1951; Inouye, 1960; Marshall et al., 1962). The same studies indicate a role for brain damage as a factor in the expression of the epileptic gene.

No study has shown a concordance rate for seizures or even epileptiform electroencephalographic abnormalities in monozygotic twins greater than 85 percent. Why do monozygotic twins not have the theoretically expected concordance rate of 100 percent? Acquired brain damage in one twin might explain nonconcordance in some monozygotic pairs. This could lower the seizure threshold enough to allow expression of the inherited epileptic gene.

Acquired brain damage can give rise to epilepsy in patients who may or may not have a genetic tendency to express epilepsy. The rates of epilepsy vary among social groups. The high rate of epilepsy among African-Americans (Shamansky and Glaser, 1979) may reflect social factors that influence the prevalence of acquired brain damage. There appears to be a disproportionate number of preterm and low–birth weight infants among the poor black population, especially males. Contributory factors may include poor prenatal care, smoking, drinking and drug use, malnutrition, teenage pregnancy, low income, and low educational status (Reed and Staley, 1977). Fatal child abuse is more common among African-Americans (Herman-Giddens et al., 1999) and lead exposure has been demonstrated in up to 18 percent of African-American children in the recent past (Mahaffey et al., 1982; Farfel, 1985; Pirkle et al., 1998). Boys have more developmental brain problems in childhood than girls do (Rapin and Allen, 1988), including epilepsy (Gissler et al., 1999).

COMPLEX PARTIAL SEIZURES—TEMPORAL LOBE ORIGIN

Most commonly, the discharges that produce complex partial seizures originate in deep, medially placed limbic nuclei in the temporal lobe, which consists of the amygdala and hippocampus. They may also arise from virtually any other part of the limbic system, not all of which is located in the temporal lobe. In addition, other areas of the nervous system may be the source of these discharges; they may arise from frontal, occipital, parietal, diencephalic, or upper brain stem regions and then can spread through one or both temporal lobes. When electrical activity spreads to the temporal lobes, the characteristic elec-

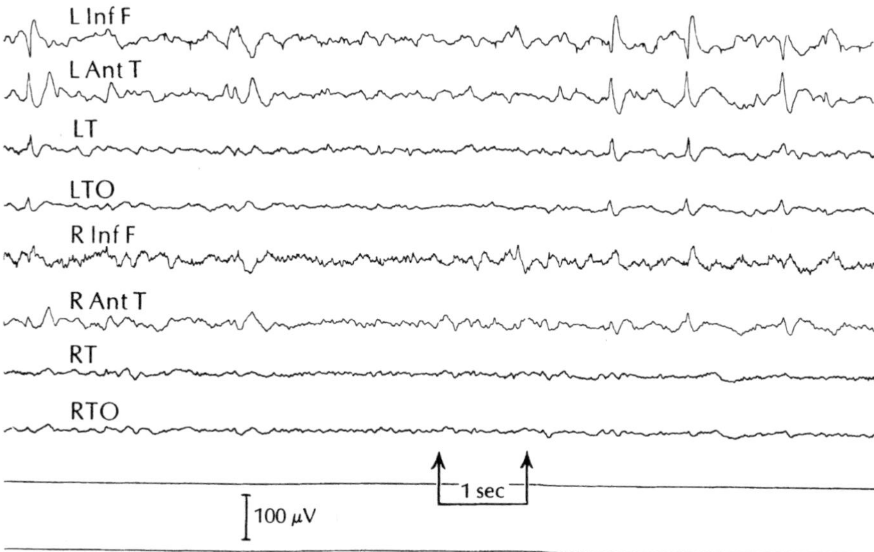

Figure 1–1 The EEG record of a 46-year-old man with psychomotor seizures. Note the well-localized, left anterior temporal spikes. *L Inf E*, left inferior frontal; *L Ant T*, left anterior temporal; *LT*, left temporal; *LTO*, left temporal occipital; *R Inf E*, right inferior frontal; *R Ant T*, right anterior temporal; *RT*, right temporal; *RTO*, right temporal occipital.

troencephalographic abnormality is temporal spiking (Fig. 1–1), unilaterally or bilaterally. There are no pathognomonic electroencephalographic configurations that make a diagnosis of complex partial seizures absolutely certain, and the resting EEG may be normal.

Subjective Feelings

Manifestations of complex partial seizures of temporal origin include subjective experiences, automatisms, and postural changes. The subjective feelings (cognitive, psychosensory, affective symptoms) include forced, repetitive, and disturbing thoughts, alterations of mood, sensations of impending disaster and anxiety, as well as inappropriate familiarity or unfamiliarity (déjà vu, jamais vu). Some patients have episodes of depersonalization, dream-like states, or sensations like those occurring in alcoholic intoxication. Metamorphopsias include visual distortions such as macropsia and micropsia. Auditory distortions, olfactory and gustatory hallucinations, and abdominal symptoms ("butterflies in the stomach," epigastric rising sensation) are some of the more common sensory experiences. Consciousness may be partially lost during complex partial seizures. To the extent that consciousness is impaired, the seizures are really generalized but the use of the term "partial" has been retained, perhaps inappropriately in some cases.

Automatisms

The automatisms of complex partial seizures are much more difficult to recognize as ictal events than the tonic–clonic stages of grand mal seizures. They tend to be repetitive and often consist of such oral activities as lip-smacking, chewing, gagging, retching, or swallowing. Some patients may perform a variety of complicated acts that seem to blend with normal behavior. Usually the behavior is inappropriate. The repetition of a phrase over and over again and the buttoning and unbuttoning of clothing are common. A few patients may assume bizarre positions resembling those of catatonic schizophrenia. These positions are held for varying periods of time. Some patients have fugue states. Fortunately, outbursts of directed, aggressive behavior are extremely rare, but when these outbursts lead to violence, they often present neurologists and psychiatrists with difficult medicolegal questions concerning the responsibility of an individual for his actions. Though the behavior of patients during complex partial seizures tends to be automatic, it may be influenced by environmental factors. Such an influence can be seen in the case of a patient who had a complex partial seizure while he was waiting in line at the hospital pharmacy to have his anticonvulsant prescription filled. It was a hot day and he was frustrated by the long wait. During the seizure, or possibly during the postictal confusional period following it, he shoved past the people who were in front of him until he came to the pharmacist's window where he stood, mumbling incoherently, until his wife led him away. After a minute or two of confusion, his sensorium cleared.

Sometimes it is quite difficult to distinguish behavior caused by complex partial seizures from episodic aberrations caused by postictal confusion, intoxication, dissociation, anxiety, obsessive-compulsive disorder, pavor nocturnus, narcolepsy, migraine, transient global amnesia, depression, panic disorder, delerium, postconcussion state, conversion disorder, or psychosis. To distinguish epilepsy from these, several questions regarding the patient's history are helpful: *(1)* Does the patient have a history of generalized seizures? *(2)* Is there a positive family history of epilepsy? *(3)* Is there a past history of events known to be associated with seizures such as brain injury? *(4)* Does the patient describe subjective alterations typical of complex partialseizures? *(5)* Has he been observed performing any of the characteristic automatisms? *(6)* Was he confused during the episode? *(7)* Is the patient's memory for events that occurred during the episode impaired? Though memory for the early events of the seizure may seem relatively well preserved, in epilepsy such memories are nearly always incomplete or incorrect. *(8)* Did the patient experience a postictal depression?

Though called *depression* the term describes the sensorium, not just the mood. Postictal depression is almost always present following a partial complex seizure of temporal lobe origin. It may be mild, and close questioning can be necessary to elicit a positive history. After the seizure, this depression may be manifest as only a brief period of fatigue, when the patient may wish to lie down, perhaps complaining of a headache or of not feeling quite normal. *(9)* Has he had other lapses during which he engaged in nearly identical behavior? Motor activity tends to be stereotyped in complex partial epilepsy. *(10)* Was the episode brief, lasting seconds to minutes? Although longer episodes can occur in epilepsy, they are unusual. In rare cases of complex partial epilepsy, there may be prolonged episodes of abnormal behavior lasting for hours or days, though epilepsy is very rarely manifested solely as a prolonged behavioral disturbance. When it is, it tends to be of frontal lobe origin. When considering episodic and especially patterned behavioral abnormalities, even when they are prolonged, the clinician should include some form of associated seizure disorder in his differential diagnosis. It can be extremely difficult to distinguish dissociative episodes from true complex partial seizures.

In addition to the preceding 10 features that may help in establishing a diagnosis of complex partial epilepsy, the EEG and the response to anticonvulsant therapy may be useful. The EEG may help to confirm the suspicion that an active seizure state exists. It also helps determine whether a disorder is diffuse, lateralized, or focal in origin. The characteristic interictal abnormality in complex partial seizures is an anterior temporal spike focus. Repeating the test during sleep or using nasopharyngeal or sphenoidal leads will reveal abnormalities in some patients, but the incidence of normal interictal records remains relatively high.

Depending on the criteria used for the diagnosis of epilepsy, normal sleep records may be seen in roughly one-third of epileptic patients. For this reason, activating agents such as metrazole and megimide have been used to induce electroencephalographic changes in patients suspected of being epileptic. Though this is often successful, results must be interpreted cautiously, given that these drugs, even in low doses, may induce epileptiform changes in some non-epileptic persons. These chemical activation methods are rarely used anymore.

If a normal interictal EEG does not rule out complex partial epilepsy, neither can the diagnosis of epilepsy be sustained merely on the basis of an abnormal record, given that 10 to 15 percent of the general population have abnormal EEGs. These abnormalities, however, are usually just slowing and are usually not of a paroxysmal or an epileptiform type (see pp. 265–266). Prolonged EEG recording is now widely used to try and capture a complex partial seizure (Bridges and Ebersole, 1985). If a seizure occurs during the recording and the seizure causes a change in the patient's state of consciousness, epileptiform abnormalities are almost always revealed. If no electrical epileptiform activity accompanies the episode, the episode is probably not epileptic and may be a pseudoseizure.

The use of a pharmacological response to establish a clinical diagnosis is difficult at best, and often impossible, yet a trial of anticonvulsant therapy, starting with phenytoin, carbamazepine, or valproic acid may sometimes provide useful diagnostic information. In such therapeutic trials, increasing doses should be given until either the seizures stop or signs of an overdose develop. The determination of the serum concentration of anticonvulsants is a useful guide to the adequacy of a therapeutic trial. Nystagmus is usually the first sign of toxicity with phenytoin but not always. Other signs of toxicity include slurred speech, ataxia, lethargy, difficulty concentrating, and dysmnesia.

COMPLEX PARTIAL SEIZURES—EXTRATEMPORAL ORIGIN

Complex partial seizures of extratemporal origin are even more frequently misdiagnosed than those of temporal origin. Common reasons for diagnostic errors are failure to recognize the epileptic origin of the attacks or to appreciate the localizing clinical seizure characteristics. Complex partial seizures of frontal lobe origin are brief, frequent attacks that begin and end suddenly. Complex motor automatisms may strongly suggest pseudoseizures. There may be kicking and thrashing, pelvic thrusting, masturbatory actions, raucous shouting, and verbalization. Episodes of complex partial frontal status epilepticus frequently develop during which the bizarre manifestations continue for hours and even days. The automatisms may be semipurposeful or purposeful. Interictal and sometimes ictal EEGs are often normal or nonspecifically abnormal. The stereotypy of the attacks suggests the diagnosis that may only be made with certainty in some cases by depth electrode study (Spencer, 1981, 1983; Spencer et al., 1982; Williamson and Spencer, 1985, 1986; Williamson et al., 1985a).

Thomas et al. (1999) observed 10 patients with nonconvulsive status epilepticus of frontal lobe origin. They noted that patients with unilateral foci manifested euphoria, disinhibition, distractability, and decreased word fluency. All these patients were alert and oriented even if they had a brief motor convulsion. In contrast, the patients with bilateral foci appeared confused and disoriented during the episode.

Occipital seizures can mimic those of temporal lobe origin. Scalp EEGs are often misleading. The initial clinical symptoms are the most important clue to correct diagnosis of occipital seizures and include elemental visual symptoms (e.g., colors, lights), visual loss, the sensation of the eyes being pulled or the sensations of movement in the absence of detectable movement, rapid forced eye blinking or eye flutter, and contralateral eye deviation (Williamson and Spencer, 1986; Williamson et al., 1992).

ELECTROENCEPHALOGRAPHY AND THE DIAGNOSIS OF EPILEPSY

The term *epileptiform* has been applied to any paroxysmal discharge recorded on EEG that contains spikes or sharp waves, either localized or generalized. Epileptiform discharges are usually associated with epilepsy, but it is also possible to have an epileptiform EEG and not have epilepsy (Peterson et al., 1968; Trojaborg, 1968; Zivin and Ajmone-Marsan, 1968).

If an epileptiform EEG cannot fully establish the diagnosis of epilepsy, neither does the finding of a normal interictal EEG rule out the possibility of epilepsy. Ajmone-Marsan and Zivin (1970) found epileptiform activity in only 56 percent of epileptics. In subsequent recordings an additional 26 percent of patients showed such activity. Fully 18 percent of the patients had at least three consecutively negative recordings and only 30 percent had epileptiform activity in all recordings.

The age of the patient at the time of the EEG and at the onset of seizures influenced the incidence of epileptiform tracings; these are much more common in children than adult epileptics. The type of epilepsy influenced the rate of positivity. Epileptiform EEGs were seen in almost 95 percent of patients with "absence" attacks. However, the authors of this important study failed to state how they established the diagnosis of epilepsy and this failure probably underlies one of their more surprising findings: that 98 percent of patients with complex partial seizures had an epileptiform EEG and, therefore, the authors claimed that complex partial seizures correlate better with the EEG than any other clinical seizure type! This conclusion is probably unwarranted.

Even though a high correlation between complex partial epilepsy and positive EEG has been confirmed many times (Gibbs and Gibbs, 1952; Glaser, 1967; Currie et al., 1971), this finding flies in the face of the common clinical experience that epileptiform EEG abnormalities in complex partial seizures are discovered less often than in patients with most other clinical types of epilepsy. Since the diagnosis of epilepsy is very much dependent on the EEG, the high correlation of epileptiform patterns with complex partial seizures in these reports may reflect the great difficulty that clinicians face in establishing this diagnosis solely on the basis of the history and observations. Clinicians are often dependent on the EEG for a positive diagnosis of complex partial epilepsy.

When consciousness is not impaired during a seizure, EEG abnormalities may not be present even during epileptic attacks, but the EEG provides a much better reflection of epileptic activity when the seizure impairs consciousness. While a patient is in an altered state of consciousness, the EEG provides the "gold standard" (albeit an imperfect standard) for differentiating true from pseudoseizures.

External scalp recordings *during the seizure* show epileptic activity in only 20 percent of the simple partial sensory seizures. In simple partial motor seizures, epileptic activity in scalp recordings *during the seizure* reveal epileptic abnormality in only 30 percent of the seizures (Devinsky et al., 1988). The site of origin of simple, partial seizures is the surface of the brain. Engel (1986) said, "In temporal lobe epilepsy patients in whom we have data from depth electrodes, probably 90 percent have no scalp or sphenoidal changes at a time when the depth electrodes show discharges restricted to one hippocampus and the patient may be having some experiential phenomena." Smells, tastes, and odd sensations are experiential phenomena. Confusion and loss of consciousness indicate a degree of epileptic spread that can virtually always be detected with an EEG.

Sphenoidal leads give essentially the same information that nasopharyngeal leads are supposed to provide, but with much less of a problem caused by artifactual activity. The difficulty of positioning the electrodes and the need for a surgical procedure to insert them has resulted in their use only in a few specialized clinics.

Sleep activation is least complicated in its interpretation when natural sleep is recorded. Many laboratories encourage a patient to drift off into sleep after obtaining an initial recording in the waking state. Most EEG activation occurs in the drowsiness or slow-wave phases during which it appears that there is enhanced synchrony that results from a lower cerebral resistance to the synaptic spread of convulsive potentials. Thus, in slow-wave sleep, discharges that are limited during wakefulness to deep structures such as the limbic structures now spread to cortical regions.

Sleep deprivation per se provides an additional degree of activation compared with sleep unrelated to deprivation (Mattson et al., 1965). For this reason sleep records are usually done after a period of sleep deprivation.

The sampling problem inherent in any standard electroencephalography lasting 45 to 60 minutes is obvious. For this reason 24-hour ambulatory cassette EEGs have been introduced. This is the EEG equivalent of Holter monitoring for cardiac arrhythmias; and it has proven to be quite useful, nearly doubling the incidence of epileptiform abnormalities as compared with standard EEGs in epileptic patients. In the initial tests of the cassette technique, the patients studied were known to have some epileptiform features by means of the much more elaborate cable telemetry with video recording of the patient and his EEG for 24 to 72 hours (Ebersole and Leroy, 1983a, b).

Liporace et al. (1998) compared the usefulness of a sleep deprived EEG of ordinary duration with a computer-assisted, 16-channel, 24-hour ambulatory

EEG in 46 patients with historical information consistent with epilepsy but whose initial screening EEG had been normal or nondiagnostic. Both the sleep deprived and ambulatory EEGs improved detection of epileptiform discharges by a similar amount (24% vs. 33%) but the ambulatory EEG was superior because it captured actual seizures in 15 percent of the patients that the sleep deprived EEG had missed.

Sedatives should not be used to induce sleep as a means of uncovering an epileptic focus. They introduce artifacts and some may suppress epileptic discharges.

The EEG manifestations of complex partial seizures may be minimal or not pathognomonic, and even with telemetry and cassette monitoring it may be difficult to distinguish seizures from pseudoseizures. The postictal elevation of serum prolactin promised to provide a biochemical marker of complex partial seizures as it does for generalized tonic–clonic seizures (Prichard et al., 1983, Lin et al., 1997) but the prolactin level does not rise following most complex partial seizures (Alving, 1998) and it may be elevated in some patients with pseudoseizures (Collins et al., 1983). Even when seizures elevate serum prolactin leads, the prolactin response attenuates with repeated seizures (Malkowicz et al., 1995). These considerations and the long delay in obtaining results have limited the usefulness of serum prolactin as a diagnostic tool in epilepsy.

A variety of new techniques have entered neurologic practice that can be useful as adjuncts to the EEG in the diagnosis of epilepsy. For the most part these techniques cannot establish or rule out the diagnosis of epilepsy if the EEG is normal but they can all be helpful in localizing the possible sites of origin of epileptic discharges. These include computerized tomography (CT), magnetic resonance imaging (MRI), and the dynamic, functional techniques: single photon emission computerized tomography (SPECT), positron emission tomography (PET), functional MRI (fMRI), and nuclear magnetic resonance (NMR) techniques.

Computerized tomography and MRI are static techniques. They provide information about the structure of the brain. Computerized tomography utilizes X-rays and is especially sensitive in identifying calcification and hemorrhage but is not sensitive for distinguishing tumors and scars from normal brain. Magnetic resonance imaging uses a magnet that energizes the hydrogen atoms in water and detects the wave of energy derived from them. The digitalization of the energy wave provides an image.

These two static techniques produce pictures of the brain as if it were a tomato that has been sliced and each slice is photographed. Magnetic resonance imaging is superior for identifying tumors, strokes, and scars and for this reason it is preferred for discovering the cause of epilepsy. For instance, MRI showed epileptogenic lesions in 38 of 300 consecutive patients with initial seizures, 17 of whom had tumors (King et al., 1998). Fifty of 250 patients who were evaluated for intractable partial seizures were shown to have space-occupying lesions with MRI, 35 of which were neoplastic (Boon et al., 1991). Volumetric analysis of MRI identified the atrophic, epileptic hippocampus in 17 of 110 cases of chronic temporal lobe epilepsy (Watson et al., 1997). Even in this specialized group of epileptics evaluated for surgery, 29 of 110 had primary generalized epilepsy. Magnetic resonance imaging findings in 26 percent of 341 patients with chronic, refractory epilepsy were normal (Li et al., 1995).

Without wishing to denigrate the important role of neuroimaging in diagnosing surgically treatable epilepsy, we want to emphasize the fact that epileptics, usually after their first seizure and often after years of intractable focal seizures, have normal MRI imaging studies. For this reason, dynamic imaging techniques have been tried to localize the site of origin of the epileptic discharges.

Of the techniques that provide an index of metabolic activity of the brain, two have proven to be clinically helpful in epilepsy: PET and SPECT. These have shown that during the interictal period there is a reduction in metabolic activity in the region of the focus. During ictus, metabolic activity becomes intense in the focus. A zone of interictal hypometabolism is commonly seen in patients with complex partial seizures of medial temporal origin but is less characteristic of seizures originating elsewhere in the brain. The epileptogenicity of hypometabolic zones must be proven electrographically. A hypometabolic zone on PET or SPECT without electroencephalographic definition does not support a diagnosis of epilepsy (Engel, 1991).

It is difficult to obtain PET scans and interpret the results during spontaneous partial seizures. Ictal scans can be more easily obtained with SPECT. Single photon emission computed tomography has been used during both intracranial and extracranial scalp EEG recording and has been found to be more accurate during than between seizures in localizing the source of epilepsy. During seizures, blood perfusion (measured by SPECT) increases. Between seizures, blood perfusion decreases focally (Boundy et al., 1996; Spanaki et al., 1999).

Abnormal increases and decreases in perfusion lack the specificity of EEG spikes. Not all focal changes in blood perfusion are caused by epilepsy. Regional increases and decreases in perfusion and cerebral activity can accompany the use of the brain.

Dynamic imaging tests have provided a means of studying neural systems that subserve a variety of cortical functions and show great promise for illuminating brain–behavior relationships. For example, dyslexics show deficient phonological task-related activity in the left posterior superior temporal gyrus, angular gyrus, and extrastriate cortex. These regions show increased activity during phonological activity in normals. Dyslexics show increased phonological task-related activity in the left inferior frontal gyrus, whereas normals do not. The increased activity in the frontal gyrus during testing in dyslexics may be a compensatory response to the failure of the more posterior areas (Shaywitz et al., 1998). Though such use-related hyperactivity in the frontal lobes in dyslexics is abnormal, it is not caused by epilepsy. Schorner et al. (1987), compared the clinical usefulness of MRI, PET, and SPECT techniques in localizing lesions.

ABNORMAL ELECTROENCEPHALOGRAM WITHOUT EPILEPSY

During the laboratory evaluation of a psychiatric patient, it is not uncommon to find an abnormal EEG when there is no evidence of overt seizures. As one might expect, the relationship between an abnormal EEG and behavior disturbance in nonepileptic patients can be difficult to define. All abnormal behavior comes from the brain. Disorders of behavior that are best handled by psychiatrists are generally not associated with EEG abnormalities. An abnormal EEG is generally a hallmark of a neurologic condition. Many conditions can cause abnormal EEGs besides epilepsy, but if the pattern of abnormality suggests epilepsy, how sure can a clinician be that a patient with a behavior disturbance and an abnormal EEG does not have a seizure disorder? The criteria for such a judgment are almost never explicitly stated.

The electroencephalographic abnormalities seen in some "psychopathic" patients with a history of aggressive behavior may possibly be secondary to the kind of brain damage that is properly the concern of neurologists. There is considerable evidence correlating electroencephalographic abnormalities with certain psychiatric symptoms (Tucker et al., 1965). This underscores the likelihood that neurological disease of the brain has behavioral consequences.

The incidence of EEG abnormality among "psychopaths" and children with serious behavior disorders is over 50 percent. In schizophrenic patients, the incidence is 24 to 40 percent (Ellingson, 1955; Hill, 1963; Williams, 1969). This indicates that there are neurologic components of these conditions. The diagnosis of epilepsy or psychosis cannot be made on the basis of electroencephalographic criteria alone, and the meaning of electroencephalographic abnormalities in the absence of seizures or clinical symptoms cannot always be determined.

PSEUDOSEIZURES

The differentiation of hysterical seizures and true epilepsy is very difficult. Despite common wisdom to the effect that tongue biting, incontinence, injuries, and seizures during sleep do not occur in pseudo-grand mal seizures, there are no firm clinical criteria for the diagnosis of hysterical seizures. Self-harm may occur with hysterical attacks (Ferriss, 1972; Rossen, 1974; Standage, 1975; Cohen and Suter, 1982) and urinary incontinence is common (Freud, 1949; Riley and Brannon, 1980).

Cohen and Suter (1982) found that of 51 patients with pseudoseizures, two reported self-injury, 13 reported urinary incontinence, 12 reported tongue lacerations, and 2 reported spells in sleep. The diagnosis of hysterical seizures was established by initiating and terminating an attack with suggestion and saline injection during EEG monitoring without any change in the record during the attack. This activation test induced urinary incontinence twice and tongue laceration once.

Using an EEG technique with suggestion to induce seizures, Lesser and his colleagues (1983) found that 50 of 79 patients referred to the Cleveland Clinic for differentiation between psychogenic and epileptic attacks had pseudoseizures. Five (10%) of these had both psychogenic seizures and true epilepsy. Eight patients had epileptiform records but either no psychogenic seizure was recorded or a definite decision could not be made. Among patients with known epilepsy, between 10 and 20 percent have experienced psychogenic seizures (Desai et al., 1979; Ramani et al., 1980; King et al., 1982).

Devinsky et al. (1996) found that of 387 consecutive admissions to an epilepsy center for evaluation, 25 percent of the patients had nonepileptic (pseudo) seizures and 20 percent of these patients had true epilepsy. In both the epileptics who had no pseudoseizures and the epileptics who had pseudoseizures, convulsive movements, staring, and automatisms were the most common manifestations. The nonepileptic seizure patients' convulsive movements lasted longer (5 min vs. 80 sec); they showed shaking without loss of consciousness, apparent blackouts, stiffening, and loss of consciousness without EEG changes; they were usually alert or slightly drowsy after the event whereas the epilepsy patients were usually more lethargic. The authors stressed that when a patient with a history of well-characterized seizure patterns begins to have different types of phenomena, one should suspect pseudoseizures but the EEG was the "gold standard" for diagnosis. The clinical state during ictus, the psychiatric state of the patient and/or the history of abuse in childhood fail to differentiate epileptic from pseudoseizures. The clinical neurologic observations (without EEG) during spells were often misleading. Several of the patients with pseudoseizures showed clinical characteristics that were identical to the epilepsy patients. Various provocative tests e.g., saline injection (Ney et al., 1996) or stress interviews (Cohen and Howard, 1991) have been used to diagnose pseudoseizures too, but, as with placebo interventions, there are always some false positives and some false negatives.

The history of sexual abuse in childhood is rife among patients with pseudoseizures but is also common among patients with true complex partial seizures (Alper et al., 1997). Physical and sexual abuse may be more likely to be directed at damaged children. Serious physical abuse of children that can cause brain damage and can generate epilepsy can start very early in life. It has been documented by videotape at 3 months of age (Southall et al., 1997). Thus, true epilepsy and the experience of child abuse can go together.

Arnold and Privitera (1996) confirmed that the history of early emotional trauma did not distinguish between true and pseudoseizures. They found no difference in DSM-IIIR diagnoses between patients with pseudoseizures and those with documented epilepsy. The main psychiatric diagnoses in both groups were major depression, post-traumatic stress disorder (PTSD), alcohol dependence, and panic disorder.

Total dependence on the EEG for differentiating pseudo- and true seizures has been criticized. Using long-term video EEG monitoring, Henry and Drury (1997) studied 145 epileptic patients, each of whom had interictal EEG spikes. There was no correlation between clinical seizure phenomena and epileptic EEG activity during what appeared to be real clinical seizures in 8 percent. The normal EEGs in these cases were false negatives.

Pseudoseizures are usually manifestations of dissociation. Dissociative disorders are under diagnosed. In prior editions of this book, for example, we did not even use the term *dissociation*. Yet dissociative disorders may comprise 10 percent of psychiatric populations (Coons, 1998). A very high proportion of patients with pseudoseizures attempt suicide (Roy, 1979), so the diagnosis of pseudoseizures should raise the question of depression. This possibility should be evaluated and depression treated, if present.

Because of the difficulty in establishing a diagnosis of dissociation, a number of questionnaires have been developed to identify dissociative episodes, one of which is the Dissociative Experiences Scale (DES). One hundred thirty-two patients with pseudoseizures were compared with sex and age-matched patients with complex partial seizures. The DES did not distinguish the two groups. The depersonalization/derealization factor of the DES was elevated in patients who reported childhood abuse. Though some of these had pseudoseizures, others had complex partial epilepsy (Alper et al., 1997).

Why do some abused children develop dissociative conversion reactions, including pseudoseizures, and others not? Good (1993) has pointed out that dissociative symptoms and disorders (amnesia, fugue, depersonalization, multiple personality, automatisms, and furors) can be induced by a variety of medications, drugs of abuse, medical illnesses, and other conditions that affect cerebral function. All of these are the result of abnormal cerebral activity. Past experiences, learning, and recall also affect cognition.

There may be a great similarity in the pathogenesis of dissociative symptoms related to abuse and epilepsy in that dissociative symptoms are the result of memories, permanently stored in the brain that "boil up" at times to recruit and dominate the functions of the cortex (Teicher et al., 1993). Similarly, but by a different electrophysiological mechanism, an epileptic focus spreads to recruit into its abnormal rhythms the activity of normal brain cells. Both epilepsy and dissociation result from permanent conditions of the brain that intermittently cause clinical syndromes. Though they are not identical disorders, anticonvulsant medications can have a stabilizing influence on both, especially when affective symptoms are also present (Tucker, 1998). Many anticonvulsants are excellent mood stabilizers. These include carbamazapine, valproic acid, lamotrigine, topiramate, and gabapentin (GHACMI, 1998). Yet lithium, the major mood stabilizer, must be used cautiously in epileptics as it can cause cognitive impairment, worsening of epilepsy, and aggressiveness (Schiff et al., 1982).

There is evidence that mood disorders, sexual abuse, and pseudoseizures are linked. Wyllie et al. (1999) performed psychiatric evaluation on 34 children with pseudoseizures (average age 14 years). Eleven (32%) had mood disorders and two others (11%) had psychosis. Eleven patients (32%) admitted to having suffered sexual abuse and this was especially frequent (64%) in the subgroup with mood disorders.

It is tempting to speculate that the sexual abuse of a child with a mood disorder is more likely to give rise to pseudoseizures. The special vulnerability of some abused children to the development of pseudoseizures could be explained if the experience of abuse and mood disorder interact to produce pseudoseizures. The beneficial effect of some anticonvulsant mood stabilizers on mood disorders would also explain why anticonvulsant mood stabilizers are beneficial in some patients with pseudoseizures.

THERAPY

The major principles of therapy for epilepsy are simple. Initially, a single drug should be used at a moderate dosage. The dosage should then be increased until either the seizures are controlled or signs of toxicity appear. If it is not possible to control seizures at nontoxic doses, a second drug should be added. When epilepsy is not controlled by two antiepileptic drugs (AEDs) prescribed together in therapeutic doses, it is very unlikely that any combination of AEDs will provide complete control. It is probably better to recognize this fact than to prescribe excessive numbers of AEDs at toxic doses (Kwan and Brodie, 2000).

The development and utilization of tests to determine the blood levels of the various medications, particularly phenytoin, carbamazapine, valproate, phenobarbital, primidone, and ethosuximide has mitigated this problem. The determination of serum levels has been of great help in determining whether a patient is taking his medicine as prescribed and whether more or less need be administered. Aside from the usual symptoms of toxicity with phenytoin (cerebellar symptoms, nystagmus, ataxia, sedation, euphoria) when the serum level of the drug is above 20 μg/ml, various psychiatric symptoms such as inattentiveness, confusion, depression, and psychosis may develop. In some instances, seizures increase in frequency. Milder behavioral symptoms that are commonly described by patients with high phenytoin blood levels include feelings of lower energy levels and initiative and decreased sociability and ability to concentrate.

Occasionally, complete seizure control is not possible without some degree of toxicity. In such cases, the functional capacity of the patient should determine what an acceptable degree of seizure control is. Among adult epileptics, grand mal seizures are generally the easiest to control, and complex partial seizures are the most difficult.

Between the introduction of phenytoin (Dilantin) in the 1930s and the 1980s, only a few new drugs, carbamazepine (Tegretol), valproic acid (Depakote), and clonazepam (Klonapin), became available for the treatment of generalized motor, focal, and complex partial seizures. (Smith et al., 1987) Carbamazepine has essentially the same spectrum of clinical usefulness as phenytoin, and it also has very similar side effects (Troupin, 1976). Dipropylacetate (valproic acid, Depakote) is a universally effective anticonvulsant, most useful for generalized seizures (mainly uncomplicated tonic–clonic spells, absence, and myoclonic). It has a long track record and has, during more than 2 decades of use, achieved a wide vogue as a first-line drug. (Delgado-Escueta et al., 1983; Wilder et al., 1983; Mattson et al., 1992).

Clonazepam, a benzodiazepine, is helpful in myoclonic seizures. It has broader efficacy, but sedation is common at therapeutic levels and therefore markedly limits its usefulness.

Several new anticonvulsants are now available. These include lamotrigine (Lamictal) (Ducac and Kamins, 1997), gabapentin (Neurontin), felbamate (Felbatol), topiramate (Topamax), and tiagabine (Gabatril). These are expensive drugs and marketing efforts have often emphasized that it is not necessary to obtain their blood levels, thus lowering the cost of their use.

The claim by pharmaceutical companies that their new anticonvulsants do not require blood level monitoring may be behind the fact that there are few published therapeutic ranges for the newer drugs. Without knowing the blood levels, it is not possible to determine if a patient with poor seizure control has taken his or her medication. The introduction of these agents has been a major advance in the control of epilepsy. However, the lack of blood level criteria and the cost of these drugs have been impediments to their use.

BLOOD LEVELS

Understanding of pharmacokinetics has tremendously improved our ability to use the older anticonvulsant drugs. This was of great practical value to the practicing physician. Buchthal et al. (1960) and other researchers demonstrated that a good correlation exists between serum levels of phenytoin and phenobarbital, seizure control, and symptoms of overdose. The capacity to determine serum levels of these older anticonvulsants represents, in our opinion, the single most important advance in seizure therapy since the introduction of phenytoin.

When serum phenytoin and phenobarbital levels were first measured in the Epilepsy Center at Yale, almost half of the patients had levels that were below the therapeutic range, though all patients were prescribed what was considered an adequate dose. Noncompliance was the main reason for this, but serial monitoring of serum levels was of great help in dealing with the problem. Over the course of 2 years, 48 patients followed at the Epilepsy Center experienced a steadily decreasing number of seizures when their anticonvulsant doses were adjusted to yield therapeutic levels in their sera, with the frequency of seizures per year in the group falling from 210 to 75 (McElligott, 1974).

In some instances, individual differences in drug metabolism explain an inadequate amount of medication. The standard dosage of phenytoin is usually 300 mg/day, but this is often too low. In rare cases, 500 mg is too low, and in two patients whom we have seen personally, 700 mg was necessary to produce serum levels of 10 to 20 μg/ml. In addition, other drugs can affect anticonvulsant blood levels; isoniazide, chloramphenicol, dicumerol, disulfiram, or sulthiame, for example, can markedly increase phenytoin levels (Goodman et al., 1990). Anticonvulsant agents such as carbamazepine and valproic acid can lower phenytoin serum levels (Mattson, 1976). Other anticonvulsants interact as well. Lamotrigine, for example, must be used cautiously with valproic acid as it can raise the blood levels of valproate to the toxic range.

It has been the practice of most physicians to prescribe anticonvulsants in divided doses, and patients have been advised to take their medications three and even four times a day. Pharmacokinetic analysis based on blood levels indicates that this is usually an irrational way of prescribing medication in adults (though children may require it) and often works to the detriment of seizure control given that patients are more likely to forget their medication when it must be taken so frequently (Cramer et al., 1989). In addition, midday doses can be inconvenient and embarrassing for adults at work and for children at school. The half-life of an anticonvulsant is the time it takes for the serum level of an anticonvulsant to drop to half its steady-state level after it has been discontinued (see Table 1–1). Drugs with half-lives of more than 20 hours seldom need to be given more than once a day. As can be seen in Table 1–1, phenytoin, phenobarbital, and ethosuximide have half-lives of over 24 hours. A long acting form of carbamazapine (Carbatrol) is available and can be given at 12-hour intervals. Gabapentin and valproic acid require more frequent dosing.

Anticonvulsants differ markedly in their effect on behavioral functions. There

Table 1–1 Commonly Used Anticonvulsants

DRUG	USUAL DAILY ADULT DOSE (MG)	THERA-PEUTIC BLOOD LEVEL (μG/ML)	DAYS TO ACHIEVE STEADY STATE (MAINTE-NANCE DOSE)	ADULT BLOOD HALF-LIFE (HOURS)	MAJOR INDICATIONS
Phenytoin (Diphenyl-hydantoin)	300–400	10–20	5–10	24–36	Generalized motor, focal motor and sensory, complex partial
Phenobarbital	90–120	15–30	14–21	96	Same
Primidone	750–1000	5–15	2–4	8	Same
Phenobarbital (derived)		15–30	14–21	96	
Carbamazepine	800–1000	4–8	2–4	12	Same
Ethosuximide	750–1000	40–100	5–6	60	Absence, myoclonic
Clonazepam	1–3	0.03–0.06	4–5	24	Myoclonic
Valproic acid	750–1000	50–90	1–3	8	Generalized motor, absence, myoclonic

Acetazolamide (Diamox) is a carbonic anhydrase inhibitor and may be effective in all seizure disorders, especially in myoclonic, atonic, akinetic seizures. High doses (30 mg/kg) are often necessary for seizure control.

Diazepam (Vadium) or *Lorazepam (Ativan)* has been effective in some minor motor seizure disorders when used orally, but it is most effective when used intravenously in the treatment of status epilepticus, where it has become the drug of choice, sometimes in combination with intravenous phenytoin.

Paraldehyde, choral hydrate, Amytal, and the short-acting barbiturates are sedatives and are used only in status epilepticus.

Steroids and *adrenocorticotropic hormone* are sometimes used in infantile spasms and juvenile minor motor seizures. In other types of seizures, and at other ages, they are epileptogenic.

are many anticonvulsants that are useful in psychiatric practice as mood stabilizers. Some of these approach the efficacy of lithium in treating affective psychosis. These drugs are preferred in patients who suffer both epilepsy and emotional disorders. Other anticonvulsants that can be extremely effective in controlling epilepsy have been reported to cause dysphoric states and even frank psychosis. These drugs are to be avoided in epileptics who have concomitant emotional disorders (Tables 1–2a and 1–2b).

Measurements of blood levels have also provided information on how to begin therapy rationally. For some time it has been known that, when phenytoin is started orally, it takes 5 to 10 days for the blood level to rise to the therapeutic

Table 1–2a Antiepileptic Drugs That May Be Helpful in Dysphoria/Psychosis

	USUAL MAINTENANCE (TOTAL DOSE/DAY)	USUAL DOSING FREQUENCY	HALF-LIFE (CHRONIC) IN HOURS	SEIZURE INDICATIONS	WATCH FOR
Carbamazepine (Post et al., 1996) (Tegretol; Carbatrol)	800–2400 mg	t.i.d.–b.i.d.	6–12	Generalized Tonic-Clonic Partial 2° Generalized	Macrolide antibiotics,[a] Birth control pills,[b] Lamotrigine,[c] IADH
Valproic acid (Post et al., 1996) (Depakote)	750–4000 mg	t.i.d–q.i.d.	8	Universal (but more effective in generalized than partial)	Lamictal,[c] birth defects, ovarian cysts, obesity, Alopecia,[d] Carnitine Deficiency[e]
Gabapentin (Ghaemi et al., 1998) (Neurontin)	900–4800 mg	t.i.d–q.i.d.	6	Partial 2° Generalized	
Lamotrigine (Walden et al., 1996) (Lamictal)	300–500 mg (Without valproic acid)	b.i.d–t.i.d.	20	Generalized Tonic-Clonic Partial 2° Generalized Myoclonic	Valproate[c] Carbamazepine[c]
Topiramate (Marcotte, 1998) (Topamax)	200–600 mg	b.i.d.–t.i.d	8	Partial 2° Generalized	Kidney stones, weight loss
Phenytoin (Fenwick, 1992) (Dilantin)	300–400 mg	q.d., b.i.d.	20	Generalized Tonic-clonic Partial 2° Generalized	Birth control pills[b], Pregnancy (Scolnik et al., 1994)

[a] Erythromycin and similar antibiotics can double carbamazapine levels.
[b] Reduces birth control pills' efficacy.
[c] Valproate levels raised by lamotrigine; carbamazepine levels lowered by lamotrigine.
[d] Valproate causes spinal bifida as a teratogenic effect (Ardinger et al., 1988), polycystic ovaries, alopecia, obesity, intention tremor.
[e] Severe liver damage.

Table 1–2b Antiepileptic Drugs That May Worsen or Cause Dysphoria/Psychosis

	USUAL MAINTENANCE (TOTAL DOSE/DAY)	USUAL DOSING FREQUENCY	HALF-LIFE (CHRONIC) IN HOURS	SEIZURE INDICATIONS
Phenobarbital (Brent et al., 1990)	60–240 mg	q.d.	72	Generalized Tonic-Clonic Partial 2° Generalized
Primidone (Brent et al., 1990)	250–1000 mg	t.i.d.–q.i.d.	72 as Phenobarbital; 8 as Primidone	Generalized Tonic-Clonic Partial 2° Generalized
Ethosuccimide (Fischer et al., 1965) (Zarontin)	500–1500 mg	q.i.d.	60	Absence Myoclonic
Felbamate (McConnell et al., 1996) (Felbatol)	1200–3600 mg	b.i.d.–t.i.d.	20	Atypical absence (Lennox-Gastaut) Partial 2° Generalized Generalized Tonic-Clonic
Tiagabine (Adkins and Noble, 1998) (Gabatril)	32–56 mg	b.i.d. q.i.d.	8	Partial 2° Generalized
Vigabatrin (Ferrie et al., 1996; Hancock and Osborn, 1999; Koo, 1999)	100 mg/kg/day	q.d.		West Syndrome (Ito, 1998)
(Sabril—not approved in the U.S.A.)	1–4 g	b.i.d.	12	

range. When a patient is given 1 to 2 mg/kg of phenobarbital orally, it takes almost 3 weeks to achieve steady-state levels in the therapeutic range. This takes 4 days when double the ordinary dose is given (Aird and Woodbury, 1974). To achieve therapeutic levels even more rapidly, 10 mg/kg of phenytoin or phenobarbital administered orally results in levels of 15 to 30 μg/ml within a few hours. Given intravenously it takes minutes. Though all anticonvulsant drugs may cause some degree of sedation at therapeutic levels, only the barbiturates and clonazepam regularly induce it.

SURGERY IN EPILEPSY

There are very few seizure disorders that will not respond to some combination of medications, but a small number of unfortunate individuals suffer from severe seizures that cannot be controlled by medical therapy. For such cases, there are several major surgical approaches, and they all seem to be effective in certain cases. Engel (1996) reported on the surgical results for refractory, partial epilepsy on 3579 patients from 100 specialized surgery-epilepsy centers (1986–1990) 69 percent were seizure free and 22 percent were improved after anterior temporal lobectomy.

Anterior temporal lobectomy usually involves removing the amygdala, anterior part of the hippocampus, entorhinal cortex, and a small portion of the temporal pole, leaving the lateral temporal cortex intact. Although other types of surgery for epilepsy are less frequent, the success rates for lesionectomy (n = 293) and hemispherectomy (n = 190) were similar. Corpus callosal sections (n = 563) led to improvement in 60 percent but only 7.6 percent became seizure free. Callosal section was particularly effective for drop attacks but not for generalized or partial seizures.

In general, epilepsy surgery has produced impressive results and it represents an important intervention for a small number of patients who have not responded to anticonvulsants. With the growth of specialized multidisciplinary centers for the treatment and study of epilepsy has come an increasing sophistication in the evaluation and selection of appropriate patients for surgery. Routinely, the evaluation for surgery now includes the following very costly testing: continuous video/EEG monitoring, MRI, often specialized MRI studies and volumetric analysis, PET and ictal SPECT, neuropsychological testing, and carotid amobarbital injection to determine hemispheric dominance (Polkey, 1993).

The reason for such extensive testing is that the site of origin of the seizures is difficult to pinpoint. Berkovic et al. (1995) claimed that if the MRI scan showed a visible lesion, removing the lesion provided good control of epilepsy. Careful EEG, SPECT, and other studies might not be necessary. The MRI cannot be relied upon exclusively, however, because seizures do not always arise in or immediately adjacent to the lesion. Still, patients with a discrete lesion are the most likely to benefit from surgical intervention.

Another surgical approach proposes performing en bloc anterior temporal lobectomy as seizures so frequently seem to either arise there or spread to the anterior temporal region (including the hippocampus) before a complex partial seizure is clinically apparent. Recent results for anterior temporal lobectomy indicate an 80 percent reduction of seizure frequency (Sperling, 1996). Engel (1996) described a syndrome of Mesial Temporal-Lobe epilepsy, which consists of early age of onset, increased incidence of febrile convulsion, and an increased incidence of Wada test memory asymmetries. Hermann et al. (1997) studied 107 patients with mesial temporal sclerosis and found that they showed generalized cognitive impairment. Verbal memory was impaired in those with left side lesions, but attention and executive functions remained intact.

It is clear that the more discrete the lesion, the better the outcome from surgery. Eliashav (1997) studied 60 patients who had anterior temporal lobe resection for intractable seizures because of glial tumors, hamartomas, or vascular malformations (followed for a mean period of 8.4 years). Of the patients, 80 percent became seizure free. Only three patients had a late recurrence of seizures. A prolonged history of seizures was associated with a poorer outcome. The tumor reoccurrence rate was only 3.3 percent. At follow-up, 67 percent were working but 59 percent noted some form of psychosocial improvement. Similar good results have been reported for resection of discrete frontal lobe lesions with a 67 percent seizure-free rate following surgery (Laskowitz et al., 1995). If the seizure focus is not localized, surgery is less successful. There are few contraindications to surgery though some centers are unwilling to operate on patients with a history of psychosis or low IQ. Most of the reports of excellent results represent the conclusions of the groups who have performed the evaluations that preceded surgery, but a recent randomized case-controlled study of 80 patients with intractable partial seizures was reported. Half of the patients had surgery, the other half were followed for 1 year with only medical treatment. Fifty-eight percent of the operated patients were seizure-free as compared with only 8 percent in the medical group at the end of a year (Wiebe and Blume, 2001).

Surprisingly little attention has been given to the psychiatric status of patients following epilepsy surgery. Blumer and his colleagues (1998) found that after surgery, 39 percent of 44 patients experienced either de novo psychiatric complications (6 psychotic, 6 dysphoric, 2 depressed) or exacerbation of a preoperative dysphoria (3 patients). This exceptional psychiatric morbidity had not been reported previously. Cognitive functioning assessed before and after surgery with neuropsychological testing is no substitute for psychiatric evaluation. More than half the readmissions to hospitals following epilepsy surgery are for psychiatric disorders (Wilson et al., 1999).

Alternative procedures may provide new therapeutic avenues for epileptics who have been unresponsive to medical therapy and for whom resective surgery is not feasible. These include bilateral stimulation of the centromedian thalamic nuclei (Velasco et al., 1995) and stimulation of the vagus nerve (Multicenter Study, 1995). Both of these procedures have improved generalized and partial seizures but the role of each in epilepsy control has yet to be fully explored. In the distant past, there were claims for cerebellar stimulation for the purpose of seizure control. Though some dramatic cases of improvement were reported (Cooper et al., 1973), overall results were not favorable and cerebellar stimulation has been abandoned.

EPILEPTOGENESIS, COGNITIVE, AND BEHAVIORAL DETERIORATION

Epilepsy has been inaccurately blamed for many of the problems that can develop in epileptics, including dementia. It is true that epilepsy can cause deterioration somewhat indirectly: traumatic brain injuries sustained during major motor seizures can cause intellectual losses (Trimble and Cull, 1989) and the drugs that are used to treat epilepsy can depress cognitive function, usually reversibly. Neither of these is especially common. Postictal depression can look like dementia if it occurs often enough. This form of cognitive decline is linked to seizure frequency and responds to seizure control as does nonconvulsive status epilepticus, a rare form of temporary confusion.

There is strong clinical evidence that seizures themselves do not cause deterioration: febrile seizures and electroconvulsive therapy (ECT) are benign. Even though Schiottz-Christensen and Bruhn (1973) showed that there was a performance IQ difference of 7 points on the Wechsler Intelligence Scale between the febrile seizure and control groups, in such a study, it is difficult to determine if brain damage is a cause or a result of a febrile seizure. All the evidence that seems to support the hypothesis that febrile seizures are harmful to the development of the brain do not distinguish preexistant brain damage as the cause of epilepsy and intellectual deficit from epilepsy as the cause of intellectual deficit and brain damage.

There is overwhelming evidence that febrile seizures are benign. Hauser et al. (1977) followed 657 patients with fever-induced seizures for more than 8000 person-years to assess risks for subsequent afebrile seizures. When patients with profound, preexisting neurological deficits were excluded, only 3 percent of the remaining 632 patients developed recurrent afebrile seizures. The characteristics of the febrile seizures that increased the risk of subsequent afebrile seizures were those that suggest that brain damage had preceded the initial febrile seizure: the presence of focal features and the prolonged duration of the seizure.

Thus, this study casts doubt upon the epileptogenicity of brief, generalized febrile seizures that occur in children who are otherwise normal.

Nelson and Ellenberg (1976) reported that recurrent nonfebrile epileptic seizures had occurred by 7 years of age in only 2 percent of 1706 children who had experienced at least one febrile seizure. Of those whose prior neurologic or developmental status was abnormal and whose first seizure was longer than 15 minutes, multiple or focal epilepsy developed at a rate of 9.2 percent as compared with 0.5 percent in a control group without febrile seizures. Of those whose preseizure neurological status was normal, epilepsy developed in only 1.1 percent, which is only slightly greater than that for children with no febrile seizures. Farwell, et al. (1994) and Berg et al. (1997) have reemphasized the benignity of uncomplicated febrile seizures.

The overwhelming evidence that febrile seizures do not cause cognitive or behavioral problems (Nelson and Ellenberg, 1977), must be added to those reports that question the harmful effect of febrile seizures on inducing subsequent nonfebrile seizures (epilepsy).

Behavioral disturbances and learning disorders in epileptic children may occur, not from seizures but from the use of antiepileptic medications. Farwell et al. (1990) have indicated that these disturbances may not be reversible. The question of whether, when, and how to treat febrile seizures remains unsettled. Why use potentially harmful drugs for a benign condition (Bourgeois, 1998)?

Repeated cerebral stimulation in animals can change the brain (Goddard et al., 1969) and provides a theoretical rationale for attempting prompt and complete seizure control to prevent further epilepsy. Animals with electrodes implanted in their brains were stimulated briefly each day with subconvulsant currents. During the first week there was no behavioral change or EEG after-discharge but during the second week, stimulation produced minimal focal seizures and during the third week, bilateral seizures. Some animals developed spontaneous seizures. This is the *kindling phenomenon* and is thought to underlie the development of independent "mirror" foci on the previously normal side of the brain opposite the primary focus, though not by everyone (Goldensohn, 1984).

The closest clinical approach to kindling is the use of ECT in mental illnesses. Epilepsy seldom begins after ECT (114 per 100,000). Although this rate is greater than in an age-adjusted nonpsychiatric cohort, it probably can be explained by individual vulnerabilities in the psychiatric population and cannot be attributed to ECT (Devinsky and Duchowny, 1983).

There are benign forms of epilepsy that children "outgrow" whether or not they are treated with AEDs (Astradsson et al., 1998) and some of these seizures are focal (Holmes, 1993). Epilepsy is not a long-term problem in these familial conditions, thus proving that seizures may not be epileptogenic.

In summary, febrile seizures, ECT, and familial forms of focal epilepsy in humans are not epileptogenic. There is little proof that the phenomenon of kindling exists in humans despite its demonstration in animals and the occasional development of a mirror focus in humans. Perhaps the cause of epilepsy and the status of the brain in which it occurs are more important than the seizure itself in determining future epileptogenicity.

A loss of neurons and glial scarring in the hippocampus, particularly Ammon's horn, has been described in the brains of epileptics. This has been related to anoxia and to a variety of behavioral and cognitive abnormalities in epileptics (Margierson and Corsellis, 1966; Ounstead et al., 1966). If epilepsy gives rise to such lesions, why do not all epileptics demonstrate them? Most brains of epileptics are normal, microscopically.

To measure intellectual deterioration in epileptics it would be necessary to control many factors, such as the age of the patient at onset of seizures, the duration of epilepsy, the clinical form of epilepsy (including the etiology and presence or absence of brain damage), the presence of other diseases, the social class and intelligence of the patient before disease onset, the drug used, its dosage and the blood level, the frequency of seizures, the length of time between the last seizure and the utilization of tests that reflect the functions of the patient that appear to have been affected. It hardly need be said that the perfect study has yet to be done.

A prospective study of the stability of IQ in 72 epileptic children tested within 2 weeks of the initial diagnosis and yearly for 4 years revealed no overall differences over time or in comparison with nonepileptic siblings. Eleven percent of the patients did experience a persistent drop in IQ of 10 points or more. In these, an early age of onset of seizures and the number of drugs to which the patient became toxic best predicted changes in IQ. This suggested that total seizure control, especially in younger children, should not be achieved at the price of repeated episodes of drug toxicity (Bourgeois et al., 1983).

The importance of AED toxicity in the pathogenesis of behavioral disorders and poor seizure control in patients with intractable epilepsy was highlighted by a study of 69 such patients of whom more than half were benefitted by withdrawal of sedative-hypnotic AEDs with respect to symptoms of drug toxicity and seizure control (Theodore and Porter, 1983). The improvement of patients with intractable epilepsy on tests of cognitive, perceptual, motor, and memory functions has been specifically related to withdrawal of barbiturates and an overall reduction in the number of AEDs but not to reduction of seizure frequency (Giordani et al., 1983). Armon et al. (1996) reported some disturbing but reversible cognitive changes in patients taking valproate for more than a year. Martin et al. (1999) reported that topiramate caused significant declines in attention and word fluency, but gabapentin and lamotrigine did not. One problem in assessing the harmful effects of AEDs on cognition is that IQ tests do not assay frontally mediated functions and the batteries of psychological tests used to establish the cognitive capacity of epileptics usually feature the IQ and omit all tests of frontal function, except word fluency, which is often depressed.

On the Wechsler Adult Intelligence Scale (WAIS), most epileptic patients have scores in the normal range, but the scores do tend to cluster around the lower end of the range (Rodin, 1968). Epilepsy often occurs in adults and children with learning disorders (Branford et al., 1998a, b). In most cases, epilepsy and learning disorders arise independently from a brain lesion such as congenital cerebral dysgenesis (micro-or macroscopic) (Gressen, 1998). The seizures that derive from such static lesions can worsen over the years and may be resistant to AEDs (Branford et al., 1998a, b); however, the learning disorder is not attributable to epilepsy but to the brain condition that caused epilepsy.

The etiology of cognitive dysfunction in patients with seizure disorders will vary. It is also apparent that ordinary cognitive tests such as measures of IQ are not the best measures of function and quality of life for seizure disorder patients. Perrine, et al. (1995) developed a quality of life scale for patients with seizure disorders and tested 257 patients. The patient's mood was the strongest predictor of the patient's quality of life, explaining 47 percent of the variance. Other factors that were pertinent, but not as important, were psychomotor speed, verbal memory, and language ability. The comprehensive evaluation and treatment of the patient with seizure disorders must take into account the patient's executive functioning and his emotional state.

There is no doubt that in a minority of epileptic patients, deterioration of intellect does occur. It is most often encountered in patients with incompletely controlled seizures (Chaudry and Pond, 1961; Rodin, 1968) but there is no convincing evidence that epilepsy per se causes deterioration. When it occurs, it is reasonable to assume that deterioration reflects progression of the condition that causes epilepsy the toxic effects of AEDs, or both (Trimble, 1987). In some cases the postictal depressions of patients with frequent seizures produce reversible pseudodementia.

Anoxia has been frequently suggested as the basic mechanism in epileptic deterioration, assuming that deterioration in epileptics is the result of epilepsy. There is no doubt that tissue anoxia can occur in all forms of epilepsy, and it could be an important factor in deterioration. One would expect anoxia to be especially important in generalized motor seizures, as opposed to complex partial seizures because in generalized motor seizures excessive muscular activity and apnea coincide with a generalized increase in neuronal firing rate, which creates a cerebral metabolic demand for oxygen that cannot be met. Guerrant et al. (1962) observed the opposite. Complex partial seizures were more likely to precede dementia and psychosis than grand mal seizures. Caplan et al. (1998) also failed to demonstrate more psychopathology or deterioration in patients who had generalized epilepsy.

Epileptic deterioration may not be caused by epilepsy at all. Seizures of temporal origin have often masqueraded as the cause of a syndrome: seizures increase, hemiparesis advancement and emotional deterioration, and intellectual decline. The existence of this syndrome has been one of the most substantial supports for the theory that seizures themselves, especially complex partial seizures of temporal lobe origin, damage the brain. This syndrome is actually caused by a focal inflammation in the temporal lobe. The origin of the inflammation is mysterious and may be autoimmune (Andrews et al., 1997). Seizures and cognitive decline are both the result of the inflammation. Seizures do not cause the intractability of seizures in that condition nor do seizures cause the dementia and hemiparesis. Yet it may appear as though seizures themselves have caused more seizures, hemiparesis, and cognitive decline. When the electrical focus is surgically removed and examined by neuropathologists, the characteristic subacute inflammation secures the diagnosis of Rasmussen's encephalitis. There is no other manner of establishing that diagnosis with certainty.

The diagnosis of epileptic deterioration, that is, deterioration caused by epilepsy, has often been misapplied. The dementia of cerebral dygenesis, brain tumors, or degenerative diseases that cause both epilepsy and dementia do not recover if epilepsy is controlled as both epilepsy and dementia are the resulting symptoms of the primary condition (Hart et al., 1998).

The impairment of recent memory that follows electroconvulsive therapy (ECT) occurs even when muscular activity during the ECT-induced seizure is abolished with succinycholine and oxygenation is artificially maintained. Yet there is no good evidence that this transient deficit induced by ECT can become permanent. There is no evidence that ECT induces any type of brain damage as shown by autopsy, CT/MRI, and neuropsychological studies of patients who had received ECT (Devanand et al., 1994). In fact, all the changes that ECT causes are transient: cognitive changes and spotty memory loss for events around the time of ECT administration. Devanand and his colleagues also looked at animal studies of electroconvulsant stimulation. These also showed no neuronal loss consequent to seizures; (there was neuronal loss after 1.5–2 hours of continuous seizure activity in primates, but this could be prevented with appropriate oxygenation and the use of muscle relaxants). This indicates that brain damage in prolonged status epilepticus is the result of an imbalance between cerebral oxygen need and the ability of the body to provide it. When muscles are paralyzed they do not engage in convulsive activity and consume less oxygen, leaving more for the brain. There is only some evidence from animal studies (Meldrum, 1978) that the mere passage of electricity or the transient disruption of the blood–brain barrier associated with seizures causes any type of brain damage.

In conclusion, there is little evidence that epilepsy causes dementia. When increasing seizures, dementia, or both occur in epileptic patients, some other etiology is likely. Therefore, any epileptic with cognitive decline is likely to have *(1)* a deterioration of the condition that causes his epilepsy; *(2)* anticonvulsant toxicity; or *(3)* frequent seizures. Investigation should include MRI, anticonvulsant blood levels, and EEG.

PSYCHOSIS

There is an increased incidence of serious psychopathology in patients with seizure disorders that ranges from 20 to 40 percent (Trimble, 1991). Conversely, seizure disorders are 3 to 7 times more common in groups of chronically hospitalized psychotic patients than in the general population (McKenna et al., 1985; Diehl, 1989). Dodrill and Batzel (1986) reviewed the literature of the association of psychopathology and epilepsy and concluded that there is a positive relation between the two. The advent of DSM-III in 1980 led to many advances in standardizing the diagnosis of psychiatric disorders. Victaroff (1994) used a standardized interview to assess the DSM-IIIR lifetime diagnoses of 60 patients with complex partial seizures. Thirteen percent had a history of psychosis.

In an older study designed to test the hypothesis that patients with complex partial seizures have more psychiatric disorders than have patients with grand mal epilepsy or general medical chronic illnesses, Guerrant et al. (1962) found that psychosis was present in 20 percent of patients with complex partial epilepsy but in only 4 percent of those with grand mal. The incidence of psychosis in the general population is about 1 percent (Srole et al., 1962).

Standard psychometric testing by Guerrant's group failed to confirm greater abnormality in patients with complex partial seizures. This discrepancy between the clinical impression of psychosis on the one hand, and conventional psychological test results, on the other, has been observed by several other investigators (Small et al., 1962; Stevens, 1966). It is likely that the standard psychological tests (IQ) assess aspects of cognitive functions that are different from the psychotic features that were uncovered during the clinical interviews.

Rodin et al. (1976) reported the greatest prevalence of serious behavioral abnormalities in temporal lobe seizure patients with more than one clinical seizure type. Patients with only CPE were not different from other seizure patients with respect to psychotic tendencies.

Though there had been many anecdotal reports linking schizophrenia and epilepsy (and occasionally even indicating their nonassociation), it was not until publication of a large study by Slater and Beard (1963) that a clear relationship between a psychosis resembling schizophrenia and epilepsy was established. Of 69 psychotic epileptics in this study, 80 percent showed evidence of temporal lobe dysfunction on the basis of a history of complex partial seizures or temporal lobe spiking on the EEG or both. The mean age of onset of psychosis was 30 years. The mean duration of the onset of the epilepsy before the onset of psychosis was 14 years. Seizures varied from rare to frequent and there was no relationship between psychosis and the dosage of anticonvulsant drugs. The low incidence of schizophrenia in the first-degree relatives of these patients strongly indicated that they were suffering from something other than classic schizophrenia. Though this group did show, at various times, all the cardinal features of schizophrenia, the psychoses in the epileptics deviated from norms for schizophrenia in some respects. Affective responsiveness was often preserved to an extent unusual in schizophrenia. In the later stages of the development of psychosis, the patient's personality was sometimes left essentially undamaged, which is rarely the case in the later stages of schizophrenia.

Bredkjaer et al. (1998) confirmed Slater and Beard's findings. The prevalence of schizophrenia-like psychoses was significantly higher in both male and female epileptics than in the general Danish population. These authors used a national patient register and the Danish Psychiatric Register for a record-linkage study of 67,116 people with epilepsy. The relationship between epilepsy and psychosis was evident even after people with learning disability or substance abuse were excluded as subjects. This study impressively supported the notion of an association between epilepsy and subsequent schizophrenia-like psychosis.

It may be extremely difficult for a clinician to distinguish ordinary schizophrenia from the schizophrenia-like psychosis of epilepsy. In both conditions, the psychosis may begin in the second or third decade, and the course varies. Remission may occur in either, though both tend to be chronic. Personality and affect tend to be less abnormal in epileptic psychosis, but symptomatically the two psychotic conditions may be virtually indistinguishable. The family history and a positive medical history of epilepsy aids in the diagnosis. In ordinary schizophrenia there is a high incidence of serious psychopathology in the immediate family of affected patients, with 10 to 15 percent of the first-degree relatives diagnosed as schizophrenic. By contrast, the incidence of schizophrenia in the families of patients with epileptic psychosis does not exceed that of the general population (Slater and Glithero, 1963). A history of epilepsy is, of course, the main distinguishing feature, being positive in epileptic psychosis and negative in ordinary schizophrenia.

The EEG may be of some help in the differential diagnosis, given that electroencephalographic abnormalities, particularly those related to the anterior temporal regions, are implicated in epileptic psychosis. There is an increase in frequency of abnormal EEGs in schizophrenics, but normal EEGs are not unusual in epileptic psychotics. Indeed, the phenomenon of *forced normalization* (normalized EEG in a psychotic epileptic) emphasizes the inverse relationship between the manifestations of epilepsy and psychosis. Some authors have commented on the tendency of some patients to become psychotic when seizures are controlled and vice versa. This is the clinical equivalent of the EEG phenomenon called forced normalization (Pond, 1957; Flor-Henry, 1969; Mignone, et al., 1970; Reynolds, 1971; Standage and Fenton, 1975; Pakalnis, 1987; Trimble, 1989; Krishnamoorthy and Trimble, 1999).

Epilepsy and psychosis could be related in at least three ways. They could vary inversely, psychosis appearing as seizures are controlled. Psychosis and seizures could be completely unrelated to each other, both independent manifestations of the same brain damage. They could vary directly, both psychosis and seizures worsening and clearing in parallel. Each of these situations seems to obtain in some cases.

There are two theories that could explain an inverse relationship between seizures and psychosis. *(1)* schizophrenia-like psychosis may result from the suppression of the epileptic focus and *(2)* AEDs may cause psychosis.

1. Physiologic neuronal inhibition occurs around an epileptic focus that even extends to the opposite side of the brain (Bruehl and Witte, 1995). Inhibition is expressed as neuronal hyperpolarization and hypometabolism that occurs during the interictal period. This inhibition of neurons is presumably what prevents a discrete epileptic focus from spreading over the brain during the interictal periods and prevents epileptic patients from having seizures continuously. When the surrounding inhibition fails, there is spread of the abnormal electrical activity generated by the focus. In patients with CPE, the spread of abnormal electrical discharge results in a complex partial seizure with secondary generalization. Although the phenomenon of inhibition is helpful in the sense that it limits the spread of epileptic discharges, it may have adverse behavioral effects, including psychosis, and what has been termed "the interictal state." This is a fluctuating disorder of cerebral functioning, with "fluidity of thought processes, loss of trains of associations, word finding difficulties, and faulty cognitive functioning" (Glaser et al., 1963; Glaser, 1964). These features suggest frontal lobe dysfunction, perhaps related to the general inhibition of neurons around the epileptic focus. Interictal cognitive disturbances are occasionally difficult to distinguish from affective disorders or psychosis. They may persist for days, weeks, or months; they may not be associated with a clear-cut seizure, though at times they may lead to one. When this is the case a major (grand mal) seizure may seem to clear up the interictal state, and the patient may return to a more normal mental condition, at least temporarily, perhaps because of the loss of inhibition that had suppressed the epileptic focus. During the interictal state, the EEG may show unmodified rhythms, desynchronization, or *forced normalization,* a term denoting the disappearance of abnormal discharges (Glaser, 1964).

2. When psychosis emerges as seizures are controlled, there may be a role of AEDs in causing it (Reynolds, 1971; Reynolds and Travers, 1974; Matsuura, 1999). Ethosuximide, a drug used almost exclusively in children, can rapidly precipitate a reversible schizophrenia-like psychosis in adults (and rarely in children). The mechanism involved is unknown, but predisposition to psychosis does not appear to be a factor (Fischer et al., 1965). Other anticonvulsant drugs that are well known to cause psychosis include vigabatrin, tiagabine, felbamate, bromides, tridione and phenurone.

Lesions in the temporal lobe and its limbic projections probably predispose an individual to a schizophrenia-like psychosis. This hypothesis has been supported by other studies performed over the past 50 years of psychotic epileptics (Pond, 1957; Glaser et al., 1963; Flor-Henry, 1969, 1972). Andermann et al. (1999) related psychosis in epileptics to brain pathology. Kanemoto et al. (1996) related epileptic psychosis to hippocampal sclerosis visible on the MRI, and Sachdev (1998) concluded that structural brain abnormalities such as cortical dysgenesis underly both psychosis and epilepsy in patients with both disorders. The presence of tissue pathology in the temporal lobe even seemed to explain transient postictal psychosis in a group of epileptic patients (Devinsky et al., 1995). Tumors in the temporal lobe can cause psychosis even without epilepsy (Malamud, 1967) as can encephalitis. The temporal lobes are likely to cause psychosis when they are damaged, whether or not the lesions give rise to epilepsy. When temporal lobe disease causes epilepsy, it is most likely to cause complex partial seizures (CPE) of temporal lobe type, hence the clinical association of CPE and psychosis.

Psychosis could be the direct result of epilepsy through the mechanism of kindling. Kindling occurs in animals. Repetitive subthreshold stimuli, particularly to areas of the limbic system, eventually lead to actual seizures; prior to these kindled seizures there are often marked behavioral changes. Kindling has never been documented in humans but the idea that an epileptic focus could "kindle" a psychosis has remained an attractive hypothesis to explain the occurrence of psychosis in patients with seizure disorders (Adamec, 1990). Kindling has also served as an attractive hypothesis for speculation about bipolar disorder and its relation to seizure disorders. Post (1992), drawing from the animal studies, speculated that there is a similar kindling process that goes on early in the course of bipolar disorder that then sensitizes other parts of the brain and particularly the temporal lobes that create not only symptoms similar to temporal lobe epilepsy, but make the bipolar disorder amenable to treatment with anticonvulsant drugs (Post, 1992, 1996; Atre-Vaidya, 1997).

Psychosis that occurs after a seizure is part of the postictal state and as such is a direct outgrowth of epilepsy. In specialized epilepsy monitoring units (Blumer et al., 1995; Kanner, 1996), it is customary to lower or stop anticonvulsants while the patient is being clinically and electroencephalographically studied. Kanner et al. (1996) noted postictal psychiatric events in 13 patients, 10 of whom had psychotic episodes of short duration (meantime, 66.5 hours) that disappeared either spontaneously or responded to psychotropic medication. The patients who continued to have seizures after the studies, even when the AED was resumed, also continued to have postictal psychiatric events. Ketter et al.

(1994) noted similar phenomena when withdrawing patients' AEDs for a drug trial of a new anticonvulsant medications.

These studies indicating that at least some of the psychotic episodes suffered by epileptics are postictal events that are directly related to the previous seizure provide some clues to the treatment of psychosis in epileptics. One of the first efforts should be directed to the most effective seizure control possible with antiepileptic medications. Clinically, this often means raising the anticonvulsant blood levels to the upper limits of the therapeutic window and, at times, even beyond. If the effective use of one anticonvulsant does not diminish the psychosis, the anticonvulsant should be changed. Persistance of psychosis indicates adding an antipsychotic neuroleptic. To date, there have been no large-scale studies of the use of neuroleptic medications to control psychotic symptoms associated with seizures (McConnell, 1998). Most of the reports are anecdotal, but there is now considerable experience in the use of neuroleptic medications in combination with anticonvulsants.

The older phenothiazines, butyrophenones, thioxanthenes, and pimozide have all been used in small doses for this purpose. Patients with seizure disorders can be very sensitive to medication changes and there may be an initial worsening of the mental or epileptic condition when psychotropic medications are introduced, changed, or increased. Consequently, most changes in medication should be made slowly. The new antipsychotic medications that are called atypical agents such as clozapine, quetiapine, rispiradone, olanzapine, and sertindole, have all induced clinical improvement. All seem to have very little tendency to lower the seizure threshold, except for clozapine (McConnell, 1998).

The evidence is strong that links limbic tissue dysfunction (unrelated to epilepsy) to psychosis and affective disturbance. There is some evidence that disease in the dominant hemisphere is more likely to produce psychosis than disease in the nondominant hemisphere (Flor-Henry, 1969; Taylor, 1975). We are unconvinced. The evidence that the dominant hemisphere is the source of psychological problems has been challenged by a careful psychological study of 27 children with either pure left (13) or pure right hemisphere (14) temporal lobe epilepsy. This study revealed no left–right differences in WISC, Halstead-Reitan, Achievement Test, and Personal Inventory scores. Cognitive, personality, and school problems were encountered in 10 (5 with left and 5 with right foci) and those showed lower neuropsychological test functioning than did the normally adjusted children (Camfield et al., 1984).

In conclusion, the evidence supports the notion that there is a schizophrenia-like psychosis in epilepsy that affects a minority of epileptics. Most of these have complex partial seizures. The postictal state, anticonvulsant use, the lesion in the brain that is causing epilepsy, and the neurophysiological response to a discharging focus in the brain may all cause or contribute to the development of a schizophrenia-like psychosis in epileptics.

AFFECTIVE DISORDERS

Although much of the literature on behavior disturbance in seizure disorders focuses on psychosis, it has become evident that affective disturbances are much more common (Schmitz et al., 1999). Many disorders of the brain have an affective component that is more than an emotional reaction to the illness (Silver, 1990; Popkin and Tucker, 1994; Blumer et al., 1995). Depressive symptoms can occur as a manifestation of an ictal event, during the postictal phase of a seizure (Robertson, 1998), as a medication effect, and probably as a manifestation of brain injury.

Blumer et al. (1995) described an interictal mood disorder that consists of labile depressive symptoms (depressed mood, anergia, insomnia, and pain), labile affective symptoms (fear, anxiety), and paroxysmal irritability and euphoric moods. Blumer's report needs to be confirmed by others but his emphasis on the high prevalence of depression and manic-like symptoms in epilepsy is supported by other data.

The suicide rate is very high in epilepsy (Gehlert, 1994), and suicide attempts are also more common (Matthew, 1981). Barraclough (1987) reported a 25-fold increase in suicide risk for patients with temporal lobe epilepsy. A higher incidence of every sort of psychopathology is usually found in university hospital populations and specialized epilepsy study centers as patients in these settings are usually highly selected and tend to be the more difficult and unusual cases. Lower incidence figures are usually associated with community surveys of normally distributed populations. Even so, the relationship between epilepsy and depression seems real.

Patients with seizure disorders and comorbid depression show high levels of hostility, guilt, and self-criticism as well as greater impairment of function (Guze, 1994; Robertson, 1994). The relationship to type of epilepsy or epilepsy syndrome is unclear and some have noted a preponderance of depressive symptoms with left-sided lesions (Mendez et al., 1994; Victoroff, 1994). Others have associated the depressive symptoms with partial seizures, male gender, and left epileptogenic focus (Strauss, 1992; Septien, 1993; Altshuler, 1999). To explain depression some have invoked the anticonvulsant therapy itself. Phenobarbital, vigabatrin, and combinations of other anticonvulsants have all been associated with depressive feelings (Brent et al., 1990; Mendez, 1993; Bauer, 1995) (see Tables 1–4a and 1–4b).

In a large epilepsy care center, Blumer (1997) found that half of all patients with chronic epilepsy experience an intermittent and polysymptomatic affective disorder. In comparison, fewer than 10 percent suffered from psychosis and these were the very patients who had the most severe affective disorders. Could the schizophrenia-like psychosis of epilepsy actually be a form of affective psychosis? Altschuler et al. (1999) did a 10-year follow-up study of 49 patients who had undergone surgery for refractory temporal lobe seizures. The incidence of affective disorder in these patients was quite high: 77 percent had a prior history of depression; 10 percent developed depression for the first time after surgery; and 50 percent showed complete remission of depression after surgery. Forty-seven percent had no recurrence of depression during the post-surgery follow-up.

Using a combination of tricyclic antidepressant and selective serotonin reuptake inhibitor, Blumer (1997) reported a good or excellent response in 15 of 22 refractory cases of psychosis with epilepsy. The affective disorders associated with seizures responded to antidepressant treatment though smaller doses and slower titrations were felt to be necessary. The reason for being cautious in using antidepressants is that they all lower seizure threshold to some degree. Even in patients without previous seizure disorders the tricyclic antidepressants and monamine oxidase inhibitors can lower the seizure threshold (Trimble, 1978). Bupropion, maprotiline, clomipramine, and amoxapine cause approximately 2–3 percent of patients to have seizures; maprotiline induces seizures in 15 percent. Venlafaxine causes seizures in only 0.2 percent and the SSRIs in approximately 0.1 percent (Maxmen, 1995). There seems to be no evidence in favor of one antidepressant over another with relation to efficacy of antidepressant effect, but the low potential of the new SSRIs to lower the seizure threshold would make them seem to be a logical first step in the treatment of depression in epileptics (Bryan et al., 1983).

As data on the effects of antidepressants on the hepatic cytochrome p450 system that is responsible for metabolizing many drugs emerge, the question of drug interactions is an important consideration in using anticonvulsants and antidepressants. One can potentially raise the blood level of the other. Some of the antidepressant drugs also may actually have a direct anticonvulsant effect in some cases. Favale et al. (1995) treated 17 patients with complex partial seizures with fluoxetine as an adjunct to their anticonvulsants and noted the complete cessation of seizures in six of the patients and a 30 percent decrease in seizure frequency in the rest. This has also been reported with some of the older antidepressants as well. Some patients with affective disorders and seizures may respond to treatment with carbamazepine alone for both conditions (Carrieri, 1993; Varney et al., 1993). Several studies have observed that psychotherapeutic and psychological efforts have been helpful in reducing seizure frequency as well as increasing coping skills and compliance with treatment (Fenwick, 1992; Mathers, 1992; Regan, 1993).

ANXIETY DISORDERS

Seizure disorders and anxiety disorders have many similarities, particularly panic attacks. Both are paroxysmal, sudden in onset, often with no precipitants, with marked feelings of fear, anxiety, or both, as well as autonomic and physical symptoms. Both result from abnormalities of the brain, and both conditions can respond to benzodiazepines. One of the most frequent sources of neuropsychiatric consultation by another physician is the patient who has episodic anxiety attacks with some depersonalization but who has not responded to initial treatment. Could such a patient have epilepsy? Many have postulated that there is a subgroup of panic attacks that are related to epilepsy and particularly to temporal lobe pathology (Dantendorfer et al., 1995). Others have postulated a relationship between dysfunction of parietal-frontal lobes and panic attacks (McNamara et al., 1990; Alemayehu et al., 1995). In epidemiological studies, Neubgebauer et al. (1993) noted a suggestive overlap between seizures and anxiety disorders, but Spitz (1991) found no relation between complex partial seizures and anxiety disorders. Seizures can cause repetitive obsessive thoughts and anxiety thus presenting as an atypical obsessive-compulsive disorder.

Seizure disorders can also cause recurrent memories, flashbacks, etc. that can mimic many of the features of post-traumatic stress disorder; and some patients with seizure disorder can develop agrophobic symptoms during seizures. However, patients with panic disorder usually do not manifest a disturbance of consciousness; there is usually a positive family history of panic disorder; there are no automatisms in panic disorder. However, the differential diagnosis can be difficult and diagnosis usually relies on a careful history and clinical examination and findings. To capture an episode on EEG, prolonged recording may be necessary. Weilburg et al. (1995) studied patients with atypical panic attacks with ambulatory EEG monitoring and found a significant number who showed focal paroxysmal EEG changes. Some of these patients had normal standard EEGs.

The treatment of anxiety symptoms in patients with seizure disorders is similar to the treatment of anxiety disorders in clinical practice. The symptoms often respond to psychological treatments, benzodiazepines, and antidepressants.

SEXUAL BEHAVIOR

Some have denied that there is any change in the sexual functioning of epileptics (Jensen et al., 1990; Duncan et al., 1997). Others have found hyposexuality in men (Murialdo, 1995) and some have described hyposexuality in women (Demerdash, 1991). Hyposexuality has been ascribed to the effects of epilepsy, resolving with successful anticonvulsant treatment (Silveira et al., 2001), to the effects of the brain damage that causes epilepsy, and to the medications used to treat epilepsy (Bergan et al., 1992; Isojarvi et al., 1995). Gastaut and Collomb (1954) reported hyposexuality in two-thirds of 36 male temporal lobe epileptics but found that hyposexuality was infrequent in patients with other types of epilepsy. A striking feature of this hyposexuality was poverty of sexual drive rather than impotence. The condition seemed to follow the onset of seizures.

In general, male sexual drive does not develop in complex partial epilepsy that begins in childhood, and sexual interest diminishes after the onset of complex partial epilepsy in adults. A study by Taylor (1969) of 100 complex partial epileptics before and after temporal lobectomy confirmed the findings of Gastaut and Collomb. Only 14 patients had a satisfactory sexual adjustment, preoperatively. Postoperatively, the sexual adjustment in these 14 was still normal; it improved in 22 other patients; and worsened in another 14. Fifty patients maintained the same poor adjustment. Those patients who improved also experienced the greatest relief from seizures. Since virtually every AED can cause impotence, the improved sexual function of those patrients with the best surgical results may simply reflect the benefit of a reduction in AED dosage.

The relationship between epilepsy and impotence has also been studied. Hierons and Saunders (1966) reported 15 cases of impotence unrelated to diminished libido in patients with temporal lobe lesions. It is not clear whether their report reflected the selection of patients studied or accurately represented the psychosexual adjustment of all patients with temporal lobe epilepsy.

It is not uncommon for sexual problems to appear in any chronically ill patient. But the experimental evidence that relates sexual function to the limbic system is a further reason to expect some sort of sexual dysfunction in complex partial epilepsy. Destructive lesions in the amygdala have given rise to indiscriminate hypersexuality (Kluver and Bucy, 1939) and stimulation of limbic structures has given rise to erections (MacLean and Ploog, 1962). "Sexual seizures" have been noted in temporal lobe epileptics but are quite rare (Currier et al., 1971). Sexual automatisms have more recently been identified with frontal foci (Spencer et al., 1983).

PERSONALITY DISTURBANCE

Many have postulated a specific epileptic personality. Such traits and behaviors as preoccupation with philosophical and religious concerns, dependency, humorlessness, circumstantially, hypergraphia, hyposexuality, viscosity, and paranoia have all been cited as typical of the epileptic personality (Waxman, 1975; Bear, 1977; Hermann, 1981). These observations rest on case reports. When large groups of epileptics are surveyed with standardized instruments, these specific traits do not seem to hold up well (Stevens, 1975; Menges, 1982; Stark-Adamec, 1985). With regard to specific personality type, one systematic study has been done by Mendez (1993) who found a wide range of personality disorders in an epilepsy clinic. These included borderline, explosive, and dependent. When these patients were compared to epileptic patients without a personality disorder, the former had more auras with psychic symptoms (fear, depersonalization, etc.) and fewer generalized tonic-clonic convulsions. Others have postulated a relationship to types of borderline personality disorder also (Andrulonis, 1982; Gunderson, 1989), as well as to increased episodic and impulsive behavior.

VIOLENCE, THE TEMPORAL LOBES, AND THE LIMBIC SYSTEM

One behavior that has often been thought to arise from an epileptic disorder of the brain, particularly the limbic system, is explosive rage and violence. This idea stems in part from animal studies where sites in the limbic system are stimulated and the animal either has a rage attack or becomes aggressive. As many epileptic patients have temporal lobe foci, it has been postulated that there may be an association of epilepsy and violence. Studies of prison populations have also shown a high incidence of EEG abnormality (Gunn and Bonn, 1971). Nonetheless, violence and aggression are very complex behaviors; the vast majority of epileptics are not violent, and the vast majority of criminals are neither epileptic nor excessively violent. Explanations that attribute violence or aggressive behavior to a specific anatomical site or disease are overly simplistic.

The limbic system is in constant interaction with the frontal lobes, striatum, thalamus, and the hypothalamus, as well as the neuroendocrine and immune systems (Mesulam, 2000). This constant interplay with other brain regions complicates the relationship between the limbic system and violent behavior and must be kept in mind throughout this chapter.

The term *limbic system* refers to the ring of deep, centrally located nerve cells of gray matter and connections between the hemispheres in the medial portions of the brain that play a role in emotions. Phylogenetically, many of the areas designated as the limbic system are among the oldest portions of the cortex; in lower creatures these structures largely subserve smell and have traditionally been called the rhinencephalon. But since all regions designated "limbic" are not related to olfaction, and since other brain regions in addition to the limbic system play a role in emotional functioning, the term has been criticized (Brodal, 1981).

Papez (1937) first pointed out that the limbic system was related to emotion and behavior and visceral reactivity in humans. He predicted that following stimulation of the hippocampus, there could be prolonged active electrical discharges, which resulted in very little spread to neocortical areas on the surface of the brain that would spread between and among the limbic system's other components. He predicted that these *reverberating circuits* of discharge within the limbic system would produce marked alterations in the subjective emotional life of an individual. In effect, Papez proposed an anatomical and physiological substrate for the intense affective reactions and instincts that are customarily the domain of much psychiatric theory and research.

At the time Papez published his paper on the limbic system, Freudian theory was in wide vogue. The idea of a phylogenetically ancient, deep, central portion of the nervous system that influenced behavior and thought not under conscious, neocortical control was consistent with some Freudian concepts of instinctual drive. The reasoning went something like this: The sense of smell in lower animals seems to be closely associated with memory, instinct, and emotion, for it is often smell that alerts an animal to danger and provokes fear, flight, or fighting, as well as sexual arousal and mating. Smell and memory in such animals must be related functions given that it is important for lower animals to remember the associations of particular smells. The autonomic nervous system must be closely related to the limbic system because such autonomic responses as pupillary dilation, piloerection, increased heart rate, and increased blood flow to skeletal muscles occur in response to environmental circumstances in which an animal must fight or flee or prepare for mating. Though the sense of smell is no longer as important to human life, the limbic system in man is still involved with emotions and memory, and disturbances of the limbic system disrupt them.

Anatomy

The gray matter components encompassed by the term *limbic system* include those in the anterior and medial portions of the temporal lobe and those outside the temporal lobe. Limbic components in the temporal lobe include the amygdala, hippocampus (both the gyrus hippocampus and its medial portion, the hippocampal formation, which is sometimes called Ammon's horn), and the uncus. Limbic components outside the temporal lobe include the mamillary bodies, anterior nucleus of the thalamus, gyrus cingulus, nuclei of the septum, portions of the midbrain tegmentum, and supracallosal gyri. The major tracts interconnecting these regions include the fimbria, fornix, mamillothalamic tract, anterior commissure, stria terminalis, stria medullaris, median forebrain bundle, and diagonal band of Broca (see Figs. 1–2 and 1–3). In order to conceptualize this system, it may be helpful to recall that many of the medial structures of the brain have the shape of a large "C"—with one end in the anterior temporal lobe and the other in or near the septal region. Among the limbic components that have this form are: *(1)* the gyrus cingulus; *(2)* the fimbria-fornix-mamillary body pathway; *(3)* the stria terminalis, which connects the amygdala and the septal area; and *(4)* the supracallosal gyrus and longitudinal striae, which connect the hippocampus region with the septal region. Other tracts with a curved shape are the media forebrain bundle, which connects the septal nuclei with the midbrain tegmentun, and the stria medullaris, which connects the septal region with the

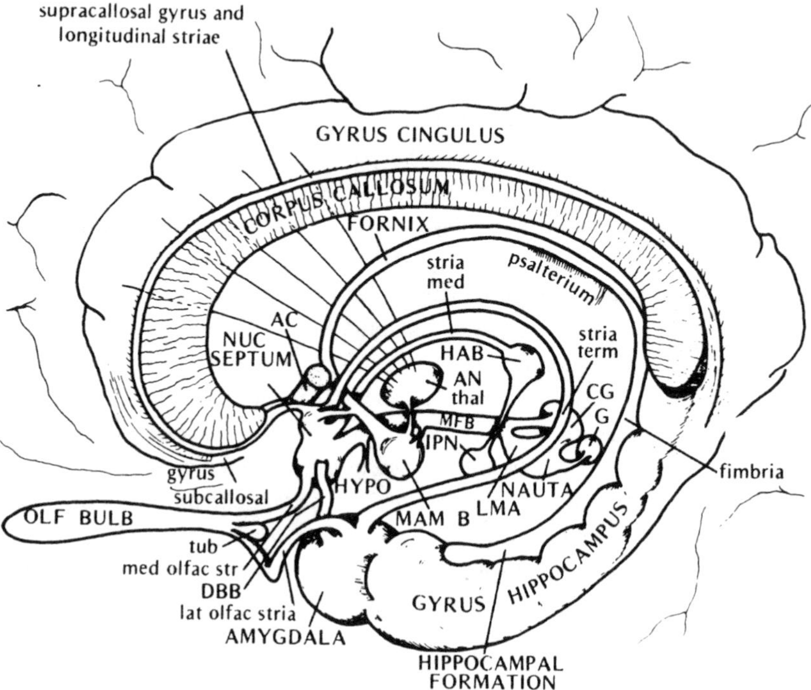

Figure 1–2 The limbic system. *AC*, anterior commissure; *ANthal*, anterior nucleus of the thalamus; *CG*, central gray matter of the midbrain; *DBB*, diagonal band of broca; *G*, Gudden's deep tegmental nucleus; *HAB*, habenula; *HYPO*, hypothalamus; *IPN*, interpeduncular nucleus; *LMA NAUTA*, lateral midbrain area of nauta; *lat olf stria*, lateral olfactory stria; *med olfac str*, medial olfactory stria; *MFB*, median forebrain bundle; *MAM B*, mamillary bodies; *stria med*, stria medullaris; *stria term*, stria terminalis; *tub*, tuber cinereum; *OLF BULB*, olfactory bulb; *NUC SEPTUM*, Septum.

habenula (Fig. 1–2). The anterior commissure is a tract that laterally connects the right and left amygdala. The diagonal band of Broca also runs laterally to connect the septum with the amygdala. The tracts that connect the gray matter of the limbic system generally contain both afferent and efferent fibers (Figs. 1–2, 1–3, 1–4). The richness of interconnections among regions of the limbic system can only partly be appreciated by the account above; actually not all the interconnections are known.

Physiological Psychology

There are rich interconnections between the frontal lobes and the limbic system. In general, the frontal lobe inhibits the limbic system (Porrino et al., 1981; Goldman-Rakic et al., 1984; Jay et al., 1995; Thierry et al., 2000). Lesions in

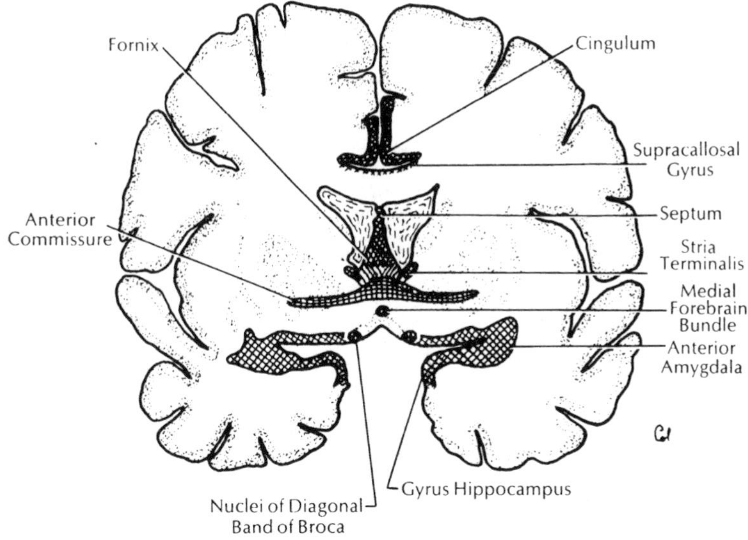

Figure 1–3 The limbic system: anterior coronal section.

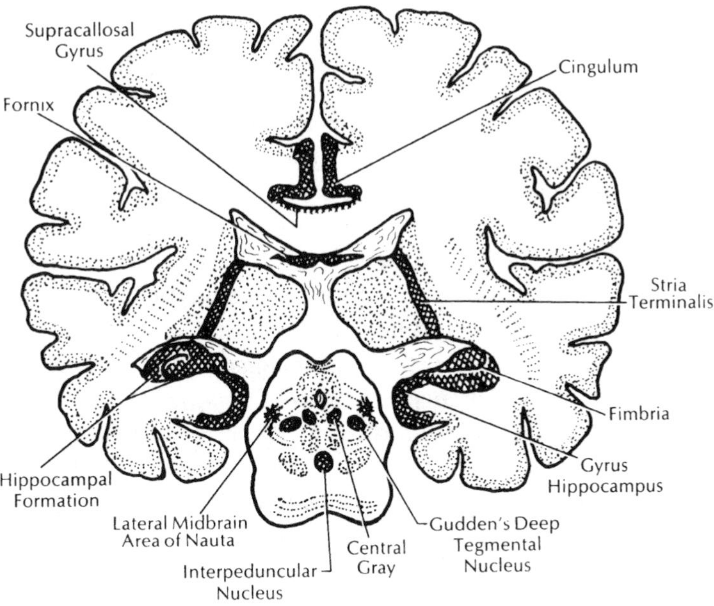

Figure 1–4 The limbic system: posterior coronal section.

either the frontal lobe or in the fibers that link frontal and limbic regions would tend to disinhibit the limbic system, permitting the expression of some primitive thoughts and behaviors.

Efforts to determine the function of the various components of the limbic system have involved stimulation and ablation studies in animals and to some extent in man. These have yielded evidence that these components influence memory, learning, emotional states (including anxiety, rage, placidity, and alertness), visceral and endocrine responses, and behavior (particularly aggressive), oral, and sexual activity. It is not possible to define the function of each of the components of the limbic system because none of them acts as a center for a particular function. All of the limbic system is more or less associated with all of the functions listed above. As Papez predicted, there is a strong tendency after electrical stimulation of any of the limbic components for prolonged electrical discharges to persist and to spread throughout the limbic system with comparatively little involvement of the neocortex (MacLean, 1952, 1954).

The specific aspects of behavior elicited by stimulation and ablation studies in the limbic system are of strong theoretical interest to both psychiatrists and neurologists given that the behavioral and cognitive alterations produced by experiments in animals closely resemble human responses that involve cognition and behavior. Stimulation of the hippocampus of cats results in apparent bewilderment and anxiety together with intense attention to something the animal seems to sense in the environment. Such phenomena have been considered alerting and defensive reactions, resulting perhaps from hallucinations induced by the stimulation. Amygdalar stimulation may produce similar reactions. Bilateral hippocampal destruction leads to recent memory loss with prevention of new learning in both animals and man. Destruction of other components of the limbic system also produces deficits in recent memory. Bilateral ablation of the anterior gyrus cingulus and bilateral division of the fornices produce similar deficits.

Stimulation of portions of the limbic system produces rage reactions in animals. Similar reactions have been seen after stimulation of the midbrain gray matter or the placement of destructive lesions in the septum. Stimulation of the amygdala in animals has provoked reactions that have been interpreted as reflecting feelings of fear. Sensations of fear have also been described in conscious human beings while this region was stimulated during surgery. Chewing, gagging, licking, retching, swallowing, bladder contractions, respiratory, pulse, and blood pressure increases, and increased secretion of adrenocorticotropic hormone (ACTH) have all been produced by amygdalar stimulation, as well as stimulation elsewhere in the limbic system. Such phenomena are quite similar to the manifestations of certain forms of epilepsy. This clinical similarity and the characteristic anterior temporal spikes seen in the EEG of patients with complex partial epilepsy led some clinicians to apply the term *limbic epilepsy* to such seizures (Fulton, 1953). The bizarre behavioral alterations (e.g., docility, loss of natural fear, compulsive oral activity, and heightened indiscriminate sexual activity) noted by Kluver and Bucy (1939) after bilateral removal of the anterior temporal lobe, amygdaloid nuclei, and overlying hippocampal cortex provided further evidence for the limbic system's role in these functions. Similar changes have been noted in man after bilateral temporal lobectomies, which, if performed somewhat caudal to the amygdala, also produce profound memory loss, particularly for recent events.

Considering the relationship between the limbic system and emotions, it might be predicted that diseases involving limbic components would cause emotional disorders. It also seems to be so in other conditions that involve limbic components (Gibbs, 1952; Malamud, 1967; Glaser and Pincus, 1969; Himmelhoch et al., 1970).

In patients being examined for epilepsy, electrical stimulation of the amygdala and the hippocampus after placement of chronic, implanted electrodes has produced brief alterations that mimic complex partial seizures and persist only during the passage of current and the limited after-discharge (Stevens et al., 1969). After such stimulation, however, mood and thought disturbances of psychotic proportions may persist for hours.

Aggression and Violence as an Epileptic-like Discharge of the Limbic System

A wide range of behaviors have been related to the limbic system, but perhaps aggression, and particularly aggression in epileptics, has received the most attention (Fenwick, 1986). The syndrome of episodic dyscontrol manifested by irrational or unprovoked expressions of rage presumably reflects epileptic-like discharges in the limbic system (Drake et al., 1992; van Elst et al., 2000). DSM-IV has included a category similar to episodic dyscontrol called Intermittent Explosive Disorder, and although this condition has been related to affective disorder, it does respond to anticonvulsant drugs (McElroy, 1999). Though some violence may result from epileptic-like discharges in the limbic system, this is rare. Many varied sources of violence in patients with seizures have been reported:

1. *An episode of directed violence could be the automatism of a complex partial seizure* (Mark and Ervin, 1970; Ashford, 1980; St. Hilaire, 1980). Delgado-Escueta et al. (1981) reported seven patients who demonstrated aggression toward inanimate objects or another person during seizures recorded with scalp electrodes. One report of three excessively violent male patients, one of whom had experienced grand mal seizures, utilized depth electrodes implanted in and around the amygdala with continual recordings for 3 to 7 weeks. This study conclusively demonstrated that the episodic rage attacks of all three men were associated with spiking discharges in the amygdala and that the behavior could be reproduced by stimulation. In only one patient was there a clear indication of an ictal basis of violent behavior from the surface EEG recordings (Smith, 1980).

2. *Directed violence could be an outgowth of the encephalopathy associated with a seizure or the postictal state* (Sommerville and Bruni, 1973; Gunn, 1978; Gunn, 1982). Kanemoto and his colleagues (1999) studied 57 episodes of postictal and 62 episodes of acute interictal behavioral disturbance in patients who, combined, had 134 complex partial seizures. Well-directed violent behavior against others and suicide attempts were more prevalent during the postictal period than during the interictal period. Directed violence and self-destructive behavior among epileptics are hallmarks of postictal confusion, according to these authors.

3. *Anxiety, fear, or anger could precipitate a seizure, possibly by inducing hyperventilation.* Aggressive actions or an anxious state could induce hyperventilation. Hyperventilation lowers the seizure threshold and could thereby induce a seizure in an epileptic patient. The confusional state associated with such a seizure or its postictal period might allow continued aggression to occur unhindered by the inhibitions that intact cortical function might bring to bear on the situation. Even if such a seizure were brief, lasting less than half a minute, the postictal period could be much longer (Delgado-Escueta et al., 1981).

4. *Brain damage that predisposes an individual to violence might also cause seizures.* This perspective, forcefully expounded by Stevens and Hermann (1981), and supported by the work of Blake et al. (1995), views epilepsy as an epiphenomenona in relation to violence or any other behavioral deviation. According to this concept, brain damage is a critical etiologic feature in the pathogenesis of psychopathology in epileptics. Brain damage causes violence by disinhibiting violent impulses. Damage to the limbic system or to its connections could make an individual more prone to violence but not because the damage caused epilepsy. Epilepsy, in this view, is an epiphenomenon, an independent manifestation of damage (Woermann et al., 2000).

5. *Violence and epilepsy may be only serendipitously related.* There have been many reports of an association between complex partial seizures and violence. Falconer et al. (1958) reported that 38 percent of patients with temporal lobe epilepsy showed "pathological aggressiveness." Among 666 cases of temporal lobe epilepsy studied by Currie (1971), 7 percent were found to be "aggressive." Glaser (1967) reported "aggressive behavior in 67 of 120 children with limbic epilepsy." Serafetinides (1965) also found "aggressiveness" to be a characteristic of temporal lobe epilepsy. On the other hand, there have also been studies that failed to demonstrate any association between complex partial seizures and violence. In a group of 100 children with a variety of neurological problems including seizures, Ounsted (1969) reported outbursts of rage in 36. But the patients who had only complex partial epilepsy were "uniformly intelligent and conforming children and none of them had rage outbursts at any time." Perhaps the most important of the studies showing no association between complex partial epilepsy and violence was that of Rodin (1973), who evaluated 57 patients with complex partial epilepsy and observed them during their seizures. There were no instances of ictal or postictal aggression. A review of 700 case histories of patients in his epilepsy clinic revealed 34 patients who had committed aggressive acts. The presence or absence of complex partial epilepsy in these 34 patients was not a relevant variable.

The contradictions in these reports may be related to varying definitions of aggression, violence, and complex partial seizures and to the selection of patients. Fighting among children, particularly boys, is certainly not unusual. Physicians who have cared for large numbers of seizure patients would agree that violence and aggressive acts do occur in patients with complex partial seizures, but they would disagree as to whether the incidence of violence in this form of epilepsy is more or less frequent than in the epileptic or general population.

Gunn and Bonn (1971) found no difference in the kind of violent behavior manifested by epileptic and nonepileptic prisoners. In a comparative study of epileptic prisoners and hospitalized epileptic nonprisoners, Gunn (1974) noted great similarities in medical and social factors and psychiatric symptoms; the main difference was more drinking in the group of prisoners. This again raises questions about the hypothesis that violent behavior and seizures per se are related.

Gunn and Fenton (1971) noted a relatively high incidence of epilepsy in prison populations but decided that automatic behavior during actual seizures was a rare explanation for crimes committed by epileptic patients. This study supports Stevens and Herman (1981) and implies that nonictal violence occurs more frequently in brain-damaged prisoners with or without complex partial seizures.

Episodic Dyscontrol

Episodic dyscontrol is a descriptive syndrome manifested by outbursts of rage and violence that seem to be motiveless. It is thought to arise from an epileptic discharge that originates in the brain (often the temporal lobe), and can be controlled with anticonvulsants. The concept of episodic dyscontrol does not provide a comprehensive explanation for more than a few isolated instances of violence (Drake et al., 1992; van Elst et al., 2000). Only one-third of murderers have evidence of temporal lobe abnormality (Blake et al., 1995), and only 5 of 97 incarcerated juvenile delinquents seemed to have an episode of violence that could have been the direct result of a complex partial seizure (Lewis et al., 1982). All five of these youths had other episodes of violence that were clearly not caused by seizures. Any benefit derived from the use of anticonvulsants in treating people with episodic violent behavior may be related to the stabilization of their mood rather than the control of putative epilepsy.

Violent behavior has been reported in patients with lesions of the limbic system secondary to temporolimbic epilepsy (Mark and Ervin; 1970; Ashford et al., 1980; St Hilaire et al., 1980; Devinsky and Bear, 1984) and focal lesions elsewhere, e.g., a patient with a hamartoma of the ventromedial thalamus (Reeves and Plum, 1969). These reports seem to support the concept that violent behavior can arise from cerebral stimulation or destruction. However, there is an alternate explanation: because limbic circuits and limbic impulses are dampened by the frontal lobe, especially the orbitofrontal cortices, the loss of the frontal fibers that reach the limbic system and inhibit it may allow the expression of unacceptable limbic impulses. Lesions in the frontal lobe could do this. Indeed, the case of Phineas Gage has been interpreted this way (Damasio et al., 1994). Patients with orbitofrontal injuries have also been found to display disinhibition, impulsivity, lack of empathy that have justified the appellation "acquired sociopathy" (Tranel, 1994). Lesions in the temporal lobe, by disrupting inhibiting influences that arise in the frontal lobes and travel to the limbic system, could also disinhibit behavior.

CONCLUSION

Acquired damage to the cerebral cortex is often a factor in epilepsy that is clinically relevant. This is true even in epilepsy that is genetically determined. There are forms of epilepsy that are so difficult to differentiate from other causes of abnormal thought and behavior that the EEG can be an indispensable diagnostic tool, even though it is flawed by false negatives and, less often, by false positives. By expanding EEG recording times and using other diagnostic tools, SPECT, PET, fMR, and MRI among them, diagnostic accuracy has been improved. Pseudoseizures of psychogenic origin, usually representing dissociative reactions of formerly physically and sexually abused patients, are especially difficult to distinguish from complex partial seizures without EEG confirmation. Therapy, in the form of anticonvulsant drugs and invasive procedures such as surgical ablation, disconnection, and vagal stimulation has become more effective. Some therapies that have proven effective in controlling epilepsy have either not controlled, exacerbated, or created cognitive and behavioral abnormalities.

There have been several adverse circumstances associated with epilepsy that may be a direct or indirect result of continuing seizures. Seizures may be epileptogenic, leading to a further vulnerability of the patient to seizures. Seizures may cause intellectual deterioration, psychosis, affective disorders, anxiety disorders, personality disorders, disordered sexual behavior, and episodic dyscontrol, a form of violence. This chapter explores the relationship of epilepsy to each of these.

In general, the lesions of the brain that have given rise to epilepsy are probably the major factor in continuing seizures, intellectual deterioration, and psychosis, though epilepsy and its treatment may also play a role in some cases. Much of the schizophrenia-like psychosis encountered among epileptics is probably affective and may be a manifestation of the response of the brain to the presence of an active, discharging epileptic focus. Hyposexuality, encountered in a minority of epileptics, is probably less a manifestation of epilepsy than it is a result of the brain abnormality that also caused epilepsy, though epilepsy and its treatment also may play a role. Violence is rarely a direct manifestation of epilepsy. More commonly, epileptogenic lesions that damage the frontal inhibition of limbic activity cause behavioral vulnerabilities that lead to violence.

Perhaps no other neurological disorder confirms so clearly the role of the brain in psychopathology. Hallucinations, affective changes, panic attacks, sexual disturbances, and other behavioral changes can occur in epileptics. Consequently, the diagnosis of epilepsy must be part of every clinical differential diagnosis in neuropsychiatry, especially if the behavioral disorder runs an episodic course.

REFERENCES

Adamec, R. E., Does kindling model anything clinically relevant? *Biol Psychiatry* 27: 249, 1990.

Adkins, J. C., S. Noble. Tiagabine: A review of its pharmacodynamic and pharmokinetic properties and therapeutic potential in the management of epilepsy. *Drugs* 55:437, 1998.

Aird, R. B., D. M. Woodbury. *The Management of Epilepsy*. C. C. Thomas, Springfield, IL, 1974.

Ajmone-Marsan, C., L. S. Zivin. Factors related to the occurrence of typical paroxysmal abnormalities in the EEG records of epileptic patients. *Epilepsia* 11:361, 1970.

Alemayehu S., G. K. Bergey, E. Barry, et al. Panic attacks as ictal manifestations of parietal lobe seizures. *Epilepsia* 36:824, 1995.

Alper, K., O. Devinsky, K. Perrine, et al. Dissociation in epilepsy and conversion nonepileptic seizures. *Epilepsia* 38:991, 1997.

Altschuler, L., R. Rausch, S. Delrahim, et al. Temporal lobe epilepsy, temporal lobectomy, major depression. *J Neuropsychiary Clin Neurosci* 11:436, 1999.

Alving J. Serum prolactin levels are elevated also after pseudo epileptic seizures. *Seizure* 7:85, 1998.

Andermann, F., B. Zifkin. The benign occipital epilepsies of childhood: an overview of the idiopathic syndromes and of the relationship to migraine. *Epilepsia* 39 Supl 4: S9–23, 1998.

Andermann, L. F., G. Svard, H. J. Meencke, et al. Psychosis after resection of ganglioglioma or DNET: evidence for an association. *Epilepsia* 40:83, 1999.

Andrews, P. I., J. O. McNamara, D. V. Lewis. Clinical and electroencaphelographic correlates in Rasmussen's encephalitis. *Epilepsia* 38:189, 1997.

Andrulonis, P. A., B. C. Glueck, C. F. Stroebel, et al. Borderline personality subcategories. *J Nerv Ment Dis* 170:670, 1982.

Annegers, J. F., W. A. Hauser, L. R. Elveback, et al. Seizure disorders in offspring of parents with a history of seizures—A maternal-paternal difference. *Epilepsia* 17:1, 1976.

Ardinger H. H., J. F. Atkin, R. D. Blackston et al. Verification of the fetal valproate syndrome phenotype. *AM. J. Med. Genet* 29: 171, 1988.

Armon, C. C. Shin, P. Miller, et al. Reversible parkinsonism and cognitive impairment with chronic valproate use. *Neurology* 47:626, 1996.

Arnold, L. M., M. D. Privitera, Psychopathology and trauma in epileptic and psychogenic seizure patients. *Psychosomatics* 37:438, 1996.

Ashford J. W., S. C. Schultz, F. O. Walsh. Violent automatism in a partial complex seizure. *Arch Neurol* 37:120, 1980.

Astradsson, A., E. Olafsson, P. Ludvigsson, et al. Rolandic epilepsy: an incidence study in Iceland. *Epilepsia* 39:884, 1998.

Atre-Vaidya, N., M. Taylor. The sensitization hypothesis and importance Of psychosensory features in mood disorder, *J Neuropsychiatry Clin Neurosci* 9:525, 1997.

Barraclough, B. M. The suicide rate in epilepsy. *Acta Psychiatr Scand* 76:339, 1987.

Bauer, J., C. E. Elger. Anticonvulsive drug therapy. *Nervenarzt* 66:403, 1995.

Bear, D. M., P. Fedio. Quantitative analysis of interictal behavior in temporal lobe epilepsy. *Arch Neurol* 34:454, 1977.

Berg, A., S. Shinnar, A. S. Darefsky, et. al. Predictors of recurrent seizures. *Arch Pediatr Adolesc Med* 151:371, 1997.

Bergen D., S. Daugherty, E. Eckenfels. Reduction of sexual activity in females taking antiepileptic drugs. *Psychopathology* 25:1, 1992.

Berkovic, S. F., A. M. McIntosh, R. M. Kalnins, et al. Preoperative MRI predicts outcome of temporal lobectomy. *Neurology* 45:1358, 1995.

Blake, P. Y., J. H. Pincus, C. Buckner. Neurologic abnormalities in murderers. *Neurology* 45:1641, 1995.

Blumer, D. G. Montouris, B. Herman. Psychiatric morbidity in seizure patients on a neurodiagnostic monitoring unit. *J Neuropsychiatry* 7:445, 1995.

Blumer, D., Antidepressant and double antidepressant treatment for the affective dissorder of epilepsy. *J Clin Psychiatry* 58:3, 1997.

Blumer, D., Wakhlu, K. Davies, et al. Psychiatric outcome of temporal lobectomy for epilepsy: incidence and treatment of psychiatric complications. *Epilepsia* 39:478, 1998.

Boon, P. A., P. D. Williamson, I. Fried, et al. Intracranial, intraaxial space occupying lesions in patients with intractable partial seizures: an anatomoclinical neuropsychological and surgical correlation. *Epilepsia* 32:467, 1991.

Boundy, K. L., C. C. Rowe, A. B. Black, et al. Localization of temporal lobe epileptic foci with iodine-123 iododexetimide cholinergic neuro receptor SPCT. *Neurology* 47: 1014, 1996.

Bourgeois, B. F. Antiepileptic drugs, learning and behavior in childhood epilepsy. *Epilepsia* 39:913, 1998.

Bourgeois, B.F.D., A. C. Prensky, H. S. Palkes, et al. Intelligence in epilepsy: a prospective study in children. *Ann Neurol* 14:438, 1983.

Branford, D., S. Bhaunik, F. Duncan. Epilepsy in adults with learning disorders. *Seizure* 7:473, 1998.

Branford, D., R. A. Collacott. A followup study of adults with learning disabilities and epilepsy. *Seizure* 7:469, 1998.

Bray, P. F., W. C. Wiser. Evidence for a genetic etiology of temporal-central abnormalities in focal epilepsy. *N Engl. J Med.* 27.1:926, 1964.

Bredkjaer, S. R., P. B. Mortensen, J. Parnas. Epilepsy and non-organic, non-affective psychosis. National Epidemiologic Study. *Br J Psychiatry* 712:235, 1998.

Brent, D. A., P. K. Crumrine, R. Varma, et al. Phenobarbital treatment and major depressive disorder in children with epilepsy: a naturalistic follow-up. *Pediatrics* 85: 1086, 1990.

Bridgers, S. L. J. S. Ebersole. The clinical utility of the ambulatory cassette EEG. *Neurology* 35:116, 1985.

Brodal, A. *Neurological Anatomy in Relation to Clinical Medicine*, 3rd ed. Oxford University Press, New York, 1981.

Bruehl C., O. W. Witte. Cellular activity underlying altered brain metabolism during focal epileptic activity. *Ann Neurol* 38:414, 1995.

Bryan, G. E., E. E. Marsh, B. Jabbari, et al. Incidence of seizures in patients receiving tricyclic and tetracyclic antidepressants. *Ann Neurol* 14:153, 1983.

Caplan, R., S. Arbelle, W. Megharious, et al. Psychopathology in pediatric complex partial and primary generalized epilepsy. *Dev Med Child Neurol* 40:805, 1998.

Carrieri, P. B., V. Provitera, B. Iacovetti, et al. Mood disorders in epilepsy. *Acta Neurol (Napoli)* 15:62, 1993.

Chaudry, M. R., D. A. Pond. Mental deterioration in epileptic children. *J Neurol Psychiat* 24:213, 1961.

Cohen, L. M., G. F. Howard. Provocation of pseudoseizures by psychiatric interview during EEG and video monitoring. *Int J Psychiatry Med* 22:131, 1991.

Cohen, R. J., C. Suter. Hysterical seizures: suggestion as a provocative EEG test. *Ann Neurol* 11:391, 1982.

Collins, W. C., O. Lanigan, N. Callaghen. Plasma prolactin concentrations following epileptic and pseudo seizures *J Neurol Neurosurg Psychiatry* 46:505, 1983.

Coons, P. M. The dissociative disorders. *Psychiatric Clin North Am* 21:637, 1998.

Cramer, J., R. H. Mattson, M. L. Prevey, et al. How often is medication taken as prescribed? A novel assessment technique. *JAMA* 261:3273, 1989.

Currie, S., KWG. Heathfield, R. A. Henson, et al. Clinical course and prognosis of temporal lobe epilepsy: a survey of 61 patients. *Brain* 94:173, 1971.

Currier, R. D., S. C. Little, J. F. Suess, O. J. Andy. Sexual seizures. *Arch Neurol* 25:260, 1971.

Damasio, H.,T. Grabowski, R. Frank. The return of Phineas Gage: clues about the brain from the skull of a famous patient. *Science* 264:1102, 1994.

Dantendorfer K., M. Amering, W. Baischer, et al. Is there a pathophysiological and therapeutic link between panic disorder and epilepsy? *Acta Psychiatr Scand* 91:430, 1995

Delgado-Escuta, A.,R. Mattson, L. King, et al. The nature of aggression during epileptic seizures. New Eng. J. Med. 305:711, 1981.

Delgado-Escueta, A. V., D. M. Tremain, G. O. Walsh. The treatable epileptics. *N Engl J Med* 308:1508, 1983.

Demerdash A.,M. Shaalan, A. Midani, et al. Sexual behavior of a sample of females with epilepsy. *Epilepsia* 3282, 1991.

Desai, B. T., R. Porter, J. K. Penry. The psychogenic seizure by video tape analysis: A study of 42 attacks in six patients (Abs.). *Neurology* 29:602, 1979.

Devanand, D. P., A. J. Dwork, E. R. Hutchinson, et al. Does ECT alter brain structure? *Am J Psychiatry* 151:957, 1994.

Devinsky, O., M. S. Duchowny. Seizures after convulsive therapy: a retrospective case survey. *Neurology* 33:921, 1983.

Devinsky O., D. Bear. Varieties of aggressive behavior in temporal lobe epilepsy. *Am J Psychiatry* 141:651, 1984.

Devinsky O., Kelley, R. J. Porter, et al. Clinical and electroencephalographic features of simple partial seizures. *Neurology* 38:1347, 1988.

Devinsky O., H. Abramson, K. Alper, et al. Postictal psychosis: a case control series of 20 patients and 150 controls. *Epilepsy Res* 20:247, 1995.

Devinsky, O., S. Sanchez-Villasenor, B. Vasquez, et al. Clinical profile of patients with epileptic and nonepileptic seizures. *Neurology* 46:1530, 1996.

Diehl, L. W. Schizophrenic syndromes in epilesies. *Psychopathology* 22:65, 1989.

Dodrill, C. B., L. W. Batzel. Interictal behavior fetures of patients with epilepsy. *Epilepsia* 27 (Suppl 2) S64, 1986.

Drake, M. E., A. Pakahis, B. B. Phillips. Neuropsychological and psychiatric correlates of intractable pseudoseizures. *Seizure* 1:11, 1992.

Dulac, O.,A. Kaminska. Use of lamotrigine in Lennox-Gastaut and related epilepsy syndromes. *J Child Neurol* 12 (Suppl 1):23, 1997.

Duncan S.,J. Blacklaw, G. H. Beastall, et al. Sexual function in women with epilepsy. *Epilepsia* 38:1074, 1997.

Ebersole, J. S., R. J. Leroy. An evaluation of ambulatory cassette EEG monitoring. II. Detection of interictal abnormalities. *Neurology* 33:8, 1983a.

Ebersole, J. S., R. J. Leroy. Evaluation of ambulatory cassette EEG monitoring. III. Diagnostic accuracy compared to intensive inpatient EEG monitoring. *Neurology* 33: 853, 1983b.

Eliashev, S. D., S. DeWar, I. Wainwright, et al. Long term follow up after temporal lobe resection for lesions associated with chronic seizures. *Neurology* 48:1383, 1997.

Ellenberg, J. H., K. B. Nelson. Febrile seizures, tested intelligence and learning disorder. *Neurology* 27:342, 1977.

Ellingson, R. J. Incidence of EEG abnormality among patients with mental disorders of apparently nonorganic origin. Critical review. *Am J Phychiatry* 111:263, 1955.

Engel, J. Discussion: epilepsy and behavior. *Epilepsia* 27 (Suppl 2):62, 1986.

Engel, J. PET scanning in partial epilepsy. *Can J Neurol Sci* 18 Suppl 4:588, 1991.

Engel, J. S. Henry, T. R, M. W. Risinger, et al. Presurgical evaluation for partial epilepsy: relative contributions of chronic depth electrode recordings versus FDG-PET and scalp-sphenoidal ictal EEG. *Neurology* 40:1670, 1990.

Engel, J. S. Surgery for seizures, *N Engl J Med* 334:647, 1996.

Falconer, M. Clinical, radiological and EEG correlations with pathological changes in the temporal lobes and their significance in surgical treatment. In: *Temporal Lobe Epilepsy*. M. Baldwin, P. Bailey, eds. C Thomas, Springfield, IL, 1958, p. 306.

Farfel, M. R. Reducing lead exposure in children. *Annu Rev Public Health* 6:333, 1985.

Farwell, J. R., G. Blackner, S. Sulzbacher, et al. First febrile seizures. Characteristics of the child, the seizure, and the illness. *Clin Pediatr* 33:263, 1994.

Farwell, J. R., Y. J. Lee, D. G. Hirtz, et al. Phenobarbital for febrile seizures:effects on intelligence and on seizure recurrence. *N Engl J Med* 322:364, 1990.

Favale, E., V. Rubino, P. Mainardi, et al. Anticonvulsant effect of fluoxetine in humans. *Neurology* 45:1926, 1995.

Fenwick, P., Is dyscontrol epilepsy? In *What is Epilepsy?* Eds. Trimble, M.,E. Reynolds, Churchill Livingstone, 1986, pp. 139–160.

Fenwick, P. B. Antiepileptic drugs and their psychotropic effects. *Epilepsia* 33 (Suppl 6): 33, 1992.

Ferrie, C. D., R. O. Robinson, C. P. Panayiotopoulos. Psychotic and severe behavioral reactions with vigabatrin: a review. *Acta Neurol* Scand 93:1, 1996.

Ferris, G. S. The recognition of non-epileptic seizures. *South Med J* 52:1557, 1972.

Fischer, M., G. Korskjaer, E. Pedersen. Psychotic episodes in Zarondan treatment. Effects and side effects in 105 patients. *Epilepsia* 6:325, 1965.

Flor-Henry, P. Psychosis and temporal lobe epilepsy. *Epilepsia* 10:363, 1969.

Flor-Henry, P. Ictal and interictal psychiatric manifestations in epilepsy: specific or non-specific? *Epilepsia* 13:773, 1972.

Freud, S. *Collected Papers*, Vol. 2. Hogarth, London, 1949.

Fulton, H., Discussion. *Epilepsisa* 2:77, 1953

Gastaut, H., H. Collomb. Étude du comportement sexuel chez les épileptiques psychomoteurs. *Ann Med Psychol* 112:657, 1954.

Gehlert, S. Perceptions of control in adults with epilepsy. *Epilepsia* 35:81, 1994.

Ghaemi, S. N., J. J. Katrow, S. P. Desai, F. K. Goodwin. Gabapentin treatment of mood disorders: a preliminary study. *J Clin Psychiatry*. 59:426, 1998.

Gibbs, F., Ictal and nonictal psychiatric disorders in temporal lobe epilepsy. J Nerv Ment Dis 113:522, 1951.

Gibbs, F. A., E. C. Gibbs. *Atlas of Electroencephalography*, 2nd Ed., Addison-Wesley, Reading, MA, 1952.

Gilman, A., Rall, T., Nies, A., et al. *The Pharmacological Basis of Therapeutics,* 8th ed., Pergoamon Press, NY, pp. 436–462.

Giordani, B., J. C. Sackellares, S. Miller, et al. Improvement in neuropsychological performance in ptients with retractory seizures. *Neurology* 33:489, 1983.

Gissler, J., M. R. Jarvelin, P. Lonhiala, et al. Boys have more health problems in childhood than girls: follow-up of the 1987 Finnish birth cohort. *Acta Paediatr* 88:310, 1999.

Glaser, G. H. The problem of psychosis in psychomotor temporal lobe epileptics. *Epilepsia* 5:271, 1964.

Glaser, G. H. Limbic epilepsy in childhood. *J Nerv Ment Dis* 144:391, 1967.

Glaser, G., J. Pincus Limbic encephalitis. *J Nerv Ment Dis* 144:391, 1969.

Glaser, G. H., R. J. Newman, R. Schafer. Interictal psychosis in complex partial temporal lobe epilepsy: an EEG-psychological study. In: *EEG and Behavior*, G. H. Glaser, ed., Basic Books, New York, 1963, p. 345.

Goddard, G. V., D. C. McIntyre, C. K. Leech. A permanent change in brain functioning resulting from daily electrical stimulation. *Exp Neurol* 25:295, 1969.

Goldensohn, E. S. The relevance of secondary epileptogenesis to the treatment of epilepsy: kindling and the mirror focus. *Eplepsia* 25 Suppl 2:156, 1984.

Good, M. I. The concept of an organic dissociation syndrome: what is the evidence? *Harvard Rev Psychiatry* 1:145, 1993.

Goldman-Rakic, P., L. Selemon, M. Schwartz. Dual pathways connecting the dorsolateral prefrontal cortex with the hippocampal formation and parahippocampal cortex in the rhesus monkey. *Neuroscience* 12:719, 1984.

Gressen, S. P. Mechanisms of cerebral dysgenesis. *Curr Opin Pediatr* 10:556, 1998.

Gunderson, J. G., A. F. Frank, E. F. Ronningstam, et al. Early discontinuance of borderline patients from psychotherapy. *J Nerv Ment Dis* 177:38, 1989.

Gunn J., J. Bonn. Criminality and violence in epileptic prisoners. *Br J Psychiatry* 118: 337, 1971.

Gunn, J., G. Fenton. Epilepsy, automatism and crime. Lancet 1:171, 1971.

Gunn, J., Social factors and epileptics in prison. *Br J Psychiatry* 124:509, 1974.

Gunn, J., Epileptic homicide. *Br J Psychiatry* 132:510, 1978.

Gunn, J., Violence and epilepsy. *New Eng J Med* 306:299, 1982.

Gutnick, M. J., D. A. Prince. Effects of projected cortical epileptiform discharges on neuronal activities in ventrobasal thalamus of the cat; ictal discharge. *Exp Neurol* 46: 418, 1975.

Guze, B. H., M. Gitlin The neuropathologic basis of major affective disorders: neuroanatomic insights. *J Neuropsychiatry Clin Neurosci* 6:114, 1994.

Hancock, E., J. P. Osborn. Vigabatrin in the treatment of infantile spasms in tuberous sclerosis: literature review. *J Child Neurol* 14:71, 1999.

Hart, Y. M., F. Andermann, Y. Robitaille, et al. Double pathology in Rasmussen's Syndrome: a window on the etiology? *Neurology* 50:731, 1998.

Hauser, W. A., J. F. Annegers, L. T. Kurland. Febrile convulsions: Prognosis for subsequent seizures. *Neurology* 27:341, 1977.

Henry, T. R., I. Drury, Non-epileptic seizures in temporal lobectomy candidates with medically refractory seizures. *Neurology* 48:1374, 1997.

Hermann, B. P., P. Riel. Interictal personality and behavioral traits in temporal lobe and generalized epilepsy. *Cortex* 17:125, 1981.

Hermann, B. P., M. Seidenberg, J. Schoenfeld, et al. Neuropsychological characteristics of the syndrome of mesial temporal lobe epilepsy. *Arch Neurol* 54:369, 1997.

Herman-Giddens, M. E., G. Brown, S. Verbiest, et al. Under ascertainment of child abuse mortality in the United States. *JAMA* 282:463, 1999.

Hierons, R., M. Saunders. Impotence in patients with temporal lobe lesions. *Lancet* 2: 761, 1966.

Hill D. The EEG in psychiatry. In: *Electroencephalography*, J.D.N. Hill, G. Parr, eds. Macmilan, Oxford, 1963, p. 368.

Himmelhoch, J., J. Pincus, G. Tucker. Behaviorial features of subacute encephalitis. *Brit J Psychiat* 116:531, 1970.

Holmes, G. L. Benign focal epilepsies of childhood. *Epilepsia* 34 Suppl 3:49, 1993.

Inouye, E. Observations on forty twin index cases with chronic epilepsy and their cotwins. *J Nerv Ment Dis* 130:401, 1960.

Isojarvi, J. I., M. Repo, A. J. Pakarinen Carbamazepine, phenytoin, sex hormones and sexuality. *Epilepsia* 36:366, 1995.

Ito, M. Antiepileptic drug treatment of West syndrome. *Epilepsia* 39 (Suppl 5):38, 1998.

Jay, T., J. Glowinski, A. Thierry. Inhibition of prefrontal cortex excitatory response by the mesocortical DA system. *Neuroreport* 6:1845, 1995.

Jensen, P., S. Jensen, P. Sorensen, et al. Sexual dysfunction in male and emale patients with epilepsy. *Arch Sex Behav* 19:1, 1990.

Johnson, M. V., G. W. Golstein. Selective vulnerability of the develoing brain to lead. *Curr Opin Neurol* 11:689, 1998.

Kalynchuke, L. E., J. P. Pinel, D. Treit, et al. Persistence of the interictal emotionality produced by long-term amygdala kindling in rats. *Neuroscience* 85:1311, 1998.

Kanner, A. M., S. Stagno, P. Kotagai, et al. Postictal psychiatric events during prolonged video-EEG monitoring. *Arch Neurol* 53:258, 1996.

Kanemoto, K., J. Takeuchi, J. Kawasaki, et al. Characteristics of temporal lobe epilepsy with mesial temporal sclerosis, with special reference to psychotic episodes. *Neurology* 47:1199, 1996.

Kanemoto, K., J. Kawasaki, E. Mori. A close relation between violence and epilepsy. Epilepsia 40:107, 1999.

Ketter, T., B. A. Malow, R. Flamini, et al. Anticonvulsant withdrawal-emergent psychopathology. *Neurlogy* 44:55, 1994.

King, D. W., B. B. Gallagher, A. J. Murvin, et al. Pseudoseizures: diagnostic evaluation. *Neurology* 32:18, 1982.

King, M. A., M. R. Newton, G. D. Jackson, et al. Epileptology of the first seizure presentation: a clinical, electroencephalographic and magnetic resonance imaging study of 300 consecutive patients. *Lancet* 352:1007, 1998.

Kluver, H., P. C. Bucy. Preliminary analysis of functions of the temporal lobes in monkeys. *Arch Neurol Psychiatry* 42:979, 1939.

Kolorsky, A., K. Freund, J. Machek, O. Polak. Male sexual deviations. *Arch Gen Psychiatry* 17:735, 1967.

Koo, B. Vigabatrin in the treatment of infantile spasms. *Pediatr Neurol* 20:106, 1999.

Krishnamoorthy, E. S., M. R. Trimble. Forced normalization: clinical and therapeutic relevance. *Epilepsia* 40 (Suppl 10):57, 1999.

Kwan, P., M. J. Brodie. Epilepsy after the first drug fails: substitution or add-on? *Seizure* 9:464, 2000.

Laskowitz, D. T., M. R. Sperling, J. A. French, et al. The syndrome of frontal lobe epilepsy: characteristics and surgical management. *Neurology* 45:780, 1995.

Lennox, W. G. The heredity of epilepsy as told by relatives and twins. *JAMA* 146:529, 1951.

Lennox-Buchtal, M. Febrile convulsions: A reappraisal. *Electroenceph. Clin Neurophysiol* Suppl 32:1, 1973.

Lesser, R. P., H. Leuders, D. D. Dinner. Evidence for epilepsy is rare in patients with psychogenic seizures. *Neurology* 33:502, 1983.

Lewis, D. O., J. H. Pincus, S. S. Shanok, G. H. Glaser. Psychomotor epilepsy and violence in a group of incarcerated adolescent boys. *Am J Psychiatry* 139:882, 1982.

Li, L. M., D. R. Fish, S. M. Sisodiya, et al. High resolution magnetic resonance imaging in adults with partial or secondary generalized epilepsy attending a tertiary referral unit. *J Neurol Neurosurg Psychiatry* 59:384, 1995.

Lilienfeld, A. M., B. Psamanick. Association of maternal and fetal factors with the development of epilepsy. *JAMA* 155:719, 1954.

Lin, Y. Y., M. S., Su, C. H., Yiu. Relationship between mesial temporal seizure focus and elevated prolactin in temporal lobe epilepsy. *Neuorlogy* 49:528, 1997.

Liporace, J., W. Tatum IV, C. L. Morris III, et al. Clinical utility of sleep deprived versus somputer assisted ambulatory 16-channel EEG in epilepsy patients: a multi center study. *Epilepsy Res* 32:357, 1998.

MacLean, P. D., D. W. Ploog. Cerebral representation of penile erection. *J Neurophysiol* 25:29, 1962.

MaClean, P. The limbic system and its hippocampal formation. *J Neurosurg* 11:29, 1954.

Mahaffey, K. R., J. L. Annest, J. Robert. et al. National estimates of blood lead levels: United States 1976–1980: Association with selected demographic and socioeconomic factors. *N. Engl J Med* 307:573, 1982.

Malamud, N. Psychiatric disorder with intracranial tumors of limbic system. *Arch Neurol* 17: 113, 1967.

Malkowicz, D. E., A. Legido, R. A., Jackel, et al. Prolactin secretion after repetitive seizures. *Neuorlogy* 45:448, 1995.

Marcotte, D. Use of topiramat, a new anti-epileptic as a mood stabilizer. *J Affect Disord* 50:245, 1998.

Margerison, J. H., J. Corsellis. Epilepsy and the temporal lobes. *Brain* 89:499, 1966.

Mark, V. H., F. R. Ervin. *Violence and the Brain*. Harper and Row, New York, 1970.

Marshall, A. G., E. O. Hutchinson, J. Honisett. Heredity in common diseases: a retrospective survey of twins in a hospital population. *Br Med J* 1:1, 1962.

Martin, R., R. Kuzniecky, S. Ho, et al. Cognitive effects of topiramate, gabapentin and lamotrigine in healthy young adults. *Neurology* 52:321, 1999.

Mathers, C. Group therapy in the management of epilepsy. *Br J Med Psychol* 65:279, 1992.

Matthews, W., Barabas, G: Suicide and epilepsy. *Psychosomatics* 22:515–524, 1981.

Matsuura, M. Epileptic psychosis and anticonvulsant drug treatment. *J Neurol Neurosurg Psychiatry* 67:231, 1999.

Mattson, R. H., K. L. Pratt, J. R. Calverley. Electroencephalograms of epileptics following sleep deprivation. *Arch Neurol* 13:310, 1965.

Mattson, R. H., J. A. Cramer, J. F. Collins. A comparison of valproate with carbamazapine for the treatment of partial complex seizures and secondarily generalized tonic-clonic seizures in adults. *N Engl J Med* 327:765, 1992.

Maxmen, J.,N. Ward, Psychotropic Drugs Fast Facts, 2nd ed., Norton, NY, 1995.

McConnell, H., P. J. Snyder, J. D. Duffy, et al. Neuropsychiatric side effects related to treatment with felbamate. *J Neuropsychiatry Clin Neurosci* 8:341, 1996.

McConnel, H., Snyder, P. (eds). *Psychiatric Comorbidity in Epilepsy*, American Psychiatric Press, Washington, DC, 1998.

McElligott, R. F. An analysis of the Epilepsy Center at the Veteran's Admiistration Hospital, West Haven, Connecticut, Master's Thesis, Yale University School of Medicine, 1974.

McKenna, P.,J. Kane, K. Parrish, et al. Psychotic syndromes in epilepsy. *Am J Psychiatry* 142:895, 1985.

McNamara, M. E., B. S. Fogel. Anticonvulsant-responsive panic attacks with temporal lobe EEG abnormalities. *J Neuropsychiatry Clin Neurosci* 2: 193, 1990.

Meldrum, B. Physiological changes during prolonged seizures and epileptic brain damage. *Neuropadiatrie* 9:203, 1978.

Mendez, M. F., R. C. Doss, J. L. Taylor. Interictal violence in epilepsy. Relationship to behavioral science variables. *J Nerv Ment Dis* 181:566, 1993.

Mendez, M. F., J. L. Taylor, R. C. Doss, et al. Depression in secondary epilepsy: relation to lesion lateratlity. *J Neurol Neurosurg Psychiatry* 57:232, 1994.

Mesulam, M. *Principles of Behavioral and Cognitive Neurology*, 2nd Ed. Oxford University Press, New York, 2000, p. 55.

Metrakos, K., J. D. Metrakos. Genetics of convulsive disorders: II Genetic and encephalographic studies in centrencephalic epilepsy. *Neurology* 11:474, 1961.

Mignone, R. J., E. F. Donnelly, D. Sadowsky. Psychological and neurological comparisons of psychomotor and nonpsychomotor epileptic patients. *Epilepsia* 11:345, 1970.

Multicenter Study (no author) *Neurology* 45:224, 1995.

Murialdo G., C. A. Galimberti, S. Fonzi, et al. Sex hormones and pituitary function in male epileptics. *Epilepsia* 36:360, 1995.

Nelson, K. B., J. H. Ellenberg. Predictors of epilepsy in children who have experienced febrile seizures. *N Engl J Med* 295:1029, 1976.

Neugebauer, R., M. M. Weissman, R. Ouellette, et al. Comorbidity of panic disorder and seizures. *J Anxiety Disorders* 7:21, 1993.

Ney, G. C., C. Zimerman, N. Schaul, Psychogenic status epilepticus induced by a provocative technique. *Neurology* 46:546, 1996.

Ounstead, C.,J. Lindsay, and R. Norman. *Biologic Factors in Temporal Lobe Epilepsy*. William Heinemann Medical Books, London, 1966.

Ounsted C. Aggression and epilepsy rage in children with temporal lobe epilepsy. *J Psychosom Res* 13:237, 1969.

Pakalnis, A., M. E. Drake, K. John, et al. Forced normalization. *Arch Neurol* 44:289, 1987.

Papez, J. W. A proposed mechanism of emotion. *Arch Neurol Psychiatry* 38:725, 1937.

Perrine, K., B. P. Hermann, K. J. Meador, et al. The relationship of neuropsychological functioning to quality of life in epilepsy. *Arch Neurol* 52:997, 1995.

Petersen, I., O. Erg-Olofsson, U. Selder. Paroxysmal activity in EEG of normal children. In: *Cinical Electroencephalography of Children*, P. Kellaway, I. Petersen eds. Grune & Stratton, New York, 1968, p. 167.

Pirkle, J. L., R. B. Kaufman, D. J. Brody, et al. Exposure of the US population to lead, 1991–1994. *Enviorn Health Perspect* 106:745, 1998.

Polkey, C., Epilepsy surgery. *Acta Neurol Scand* Suppl. 152:183, 1994.

Pond, D. A. Psychiatric aspects of epilepsy. *J Ind Med Prof* 3:1441, 1957.

Popkin, M and G. Tucker, Mental disorders due to a general medical condition and substance induced disorders. Eds widiger, T, A. Frances, h. Pincus et al. In *DSM-IV Sourcebook*, American Psychiatric Press, Washington DC, 1994, p. 243.

Porrino, L. and P. Goldman-Rakic, Brainstem innervation of prefrontal and anterior cingulate cortex in the rhesus monkey revealed by retrograde transport of HRP. *J Comp Neurol* 10:63, 1982.

Post, R. M., T. A. Ketter, P. J. Pazzaglia, et al. Rational polypharmacy in the bipolar affective disorders. *Epilepsy Res Suppl* 11:153, 1996.

Post, R. M., S. R. Weiss, D. M. Chuang. Mechanisms of action of anticonvulsants in affective disorders: comparisons with lithium. *J Clin Psychopharmacol* 12:23S, 1992.

Prichard, P. B., III, B. B. Wannamaker, J. Sagel, et al. Endocrin function following complex partial seizures. *Ann Neurol* 14:27, 1983.

Ramani, V., F. F. Quesney, D. Olson, et al. Diagnosis of hysterical seizures in epileptic patients. *Am J Psychiatry* 137:705, 1980.

Rapin, I. and D. Allen. Syndromes in developmental dysphasia and adult aphasia. *Res Pub Assoc Res Nerv Ment Dis* 66:57, 1988.

Reed, D. M., F. J. Staley. *The Epidemiology of Prematurity*. Urban and Schwarzenberg, Baltimore, 1977.

Regan, K., G. Banks, and R. Beran. Therapeutic recreation programs for children with epilepsy. *Seizure* 2:195, 1993.

Reeves, A. G., F. Plum. Hyperphagia, rage and demential accompanying a ventromedial hypothalamic neoplasm. *Arch Neurol* 20:616, 1969.

Reynolds, E. H. Anticonvulsant drugs, folic acid metabolism, fit frequency and psychiatric illness. *Psychiatr Neurol Neurochirg* 74:167, 1971.

Reynolds, E. H., R. D. Travers. Serum anticonvulsant concentrations in epileptic patients with mental symptoms. *Brit J Psychiat* 124:440, 1974.

Riley, T. L., W. L. Brannon. Recognition of pseudoseizures. *J Fam Pract* 10:213, 1980.

Robertson, M. Mood disorders associated with epilepsy, in McConnel, H., Snyder, P., (eds) *Psychiatric Comorbidity in Epilepsy*, Washington, DC, American Psychiatric Press, 1998, pp. 133–168.

Rodin, E. A. *The Prognosis of Patients with Epilepsy*. C C Thomas, Springfield, IL, 1968.

Rodin, E. A. Psychomotor epilepsy and aggressive behavior. *Arch Gen Psychiatry* 28: 210, 1973.

Rodin, E. A., M. Katz, K. Lennox. Differences between patients with temporal lobe seizures and those with other forms of epileptic attacks. *Epilepsia* 17:313, 1976.

Rossen, R. Electroencephalographic studies in idiopathic epilepsy, idiopathic syncope, and related disorders in a U.S. Naval Hospital. *Am J Psychiatry*. 107:391, 1974.

Roy, A. Hysterical seizures. *Arch Neurol* 36:447, 1979.

Sachdev, P. Schizophrenia-like psychoses and epilepsy: The status of the association. *Am J Psychiatry* 155:325, 1998.

Saint-Hilaire, J. M., M. Gilbert, G. Bouner. Aggression as an epileptic manifestation: two cases with depth electrode study. *Epilepsia* 21:184, 1980.

Schiff, H. B., T. D. Sabin, A. Geller, et al. Lithium in aggressive behavior. *Am J Psychiat* 139:1346, 1982.

Schiottz-Christensen, E., P. Bruhn. Intelligence, behavior and scholastic achievement subsequent to febrile convulsions: An analysis of discordant twin pairs. *Dev Med Child Neurol* 15:565, 1973.

Schmitz, E. B., M. M. Robertson, M. R.Trimble. Depression and schizophrenia in epileps: social and biological risk factors. *Epilepsy Res* 35:59, 1999.

Schorner, W., H. J. Meencke R. Felix. Temporal lobe epilepsy: comparison of CT and MR imaging. *Am J Roent* 149:1231, 1987.

Scolnik, D., I. Nulman, J. Rovet, et al. Neurodevelopment of children exposed in utero to phenytoin and carbamazepine monotherapy. *JAMA* 271:767, 1994.

Septien, L., P. Gras, M. Giroud, et al. Depression and temporal lobe epilepsy. The possible role of laterality of the epileptic foci and gender. *Neurophysiol Clin* 23:327, 1993.

Serafetinides, E. A. Aggressiveness in temporal lobe epileptics and its relation to cerebral dysfunction and environmental factors. Epilepsia 6:33, 1965.

Shamansky, S. L., G. H. Glaser. Socioeconomic characteristics of childhood seizure disorders in the New Haven area: An epidemiologic study. *Epilepsia* 20:457, 1979.

Shaywitz, S. E., B. A. Shaywitz, K. R. Pugh et al. Functional disorganization for reading in the brain in dyslexia. *Proc Natl Acad Sci USA* 95:2636, 1998.

Silveira, D., E. Souza, J. Carvalho, et al. Interictal Hyposexuality inmale patients with epilepsy. *Arq Neuropsiquistr* 59:23, 2001.

Slater, E., A. W. Beard, E. Glithero. The schizophrenia-like psychosis of epilepsy. *Br J Psychiatry* 109:95, 1963.

Small, J. G., V. Milstein, J. R. Stevens. Are complex partial epileptics different: *Arch Neurol* 7:187, 1962.

Smith, J., Episodic rage in *Limbic Epilepsy and the Dyscontrol Syndrome*. M. Grigis and L. Kiloh, eds. Elsevier/North, Holland, Biomedical Press, 1980, p. 255.

Smith, D. B., R. H. Mattson, J. A. Cramer, et al. Results of a nationwide Veteran's Administration Cooperative Study comparing the efficacy and toxicity of carbamazapine, phenobarbitol, phenytoin and primidone. *Epilepsia* 28 (Suppl 3):550, 1987.

Sommerville, E. and J. Bruni. Tonic status epilepticus presenting as confusionsal state. *Ann Neurol* 13:549, 1983.

Southall, D. P., M. C. Plunkett, M. W. Banks, et al. Covert video recordings of life threatening child abuse: lessons for child protection. *Pediatrics* 100:735, 1997.

Spanaki, M. V., I. G. Zubal, J. MacMullen, et al. Periictal SPECT localization verified by simultaneous intracranial EEG. *Epilepsia* 40:267, 1999.

Spencer, S. S. Depth electrode encephalography in selection of refractory epileptics for surgery. *Ann Neurol* 9:207, 1981.

Spencer, S. S., D. D. Spencer, P. D. Williamson, R. H. Mattson. The localizing value of depth electroencephalography in 32 refractory epileptic patients. *Ann Neurol* 12:248, 1982.

Spencer, S. S. Sexual automatisms in complex partial seizures. *Neurology* 33:527, 1983.

Spencer, S. S., D. D. Spencer, G. H. Glaser, et al. More intense focal seizure types after callosal section. The role of inhibition. *Ann Neurol* 16:686, 1984.

Sperling, M. R., M. J. O'Connor, A. J. Saykin, et al. Temporal lobectomy for refractory epilepsy. *JAMA* 276:479, 1996.

Spitz, M. C. Panic disorder in seizure patients: a diagnostic pitfall. *Epilepsia* 32:33, 1991.

Srole, I., et al. *Mental Health in the Metropolis*. McGraw-Hill, New York, 1962.

Staden, U., E. Isaacs, S. G. Boyd, et al. Language disfunction in children with Rolandic Epilepsy. *Neuropediatrics* 29:242, 1998.

Standage, K. F. The etiology of hysterical seizures. *Can Psychiatr Assoc* 20:67, 1975.

Standage, K. G., G. W. Fenton. Psychiatric symptom profiles of patients with epilepsy. *Psychol Med* 5:152, 1975.

Stark-Adamec, C., R. Adamec, J. Graham et al. Complexities in the complex partial seizures personality controversy. Journal of the University of Ottawa 10:231, 1985.

Stevens, J., Psychiatric implications of psychomotor epilepsy. *Arch Gen Psychiat* 14:461, 1966.

Stevens, J., V. Mark, F. Erwin, et al. Deep temporal stimulation in man. *Arch Neurol* 21: 157, 1969.

Stevens J. R., Interictal clinical manifestations of complex partial seizures. *Radiology* 117:113, 1975.

Stevens, J. R, Hermann, B. P. Temporal lobe epilepsy, psychopathology, and violence: the state of the evidence. *Neurology* 31:1127, 1981.

Strauss, E., J. Wada, A. Moll. Depression in male and female subjects with complex partial seizures. *Arch Neurol* 49:391, 1992.

Suter, C. Medical-legal aspects of EEG. Presdntation course at American EEG Society, 34th Annual Meeting, Boston, 1980.

Taylor, D. C. Sexual behavior and temporal lobe epilepsy. *Arch Neurol* 21:510, 1969.

Taylor, D. C. Factors influencing the occurrence of schizophrenia-like psychosis in patients wit htemporal lobe epilepsy. *Psychol Med* 5:249, 1975.

Teicher, M. H., C. A. Glod, J. Surrey. Early childhood abuse and limbic system ratings in adult psychiatric outpatients. *J Neuropsychiatry Clin Neurosci* 5:301, 1993.

Theodore, W. H. R. J. Porter. Removal of sedative-hypnotic antiepileptic drugs from the regimen of patients with intractable epilepsy. *Ann Neurol* 13:320, 1983.

Thomas P. B. Zifkin, O. Migneco, et al. Nonconvulsive status epilepticus of frontal origin. *Neurology* 52:1174, 1999.

Thierry, A., Y. Gioanni, E. Degenetais, et al. Hippocampo-prefrontal cortex pathway. *Hippocampus* 10:411, 2000.

Tranel, D. Acquired sociopathy, the development of sociopathic behavior following focal brain damage. In: *Progress in Experimental Personality and Psychopathology Re-*

search, D.C., Fowles, P. Sutker, S. H. Goodman, eds. New York Springer, 1994.

Trimble, M. Non-monoamine oxidase inhibitor antidepressant and epilepsy: A review. *Epilepsia* 19:241, 1978.

Trimble, MR. Anticonvulsant drugs and cognitive function: a review of the literature. Epilepsia 28 (suppl):S37–S45, 1987.

Trimble, M., Cull, CA. Antiepileptic drugs, cognitive function, and behavior in children. *Clev Clin J Med* 56 Suppl: S140, 1989.

Trimble M. Epilepsy and behavior. *Epilepsy Res* 10: 71, 1991.

Trojaborg, W. Changes in spike foci in children. In: *Clinical Electroencephalography in Children*, P. Kellaway, ed. Grune and Stratton, New York, 1968.

Troupin, A. S., L. M. Ojemann, L. M. Halpern, et al. Carbamazepine (Tegretol): A double blind comparison and phenytoin (Dilantin). *Neurology* 26:342, 1976.

Tucker, G. J. Seizure disorders presenting with psychiatric symptomatology. *Psychiatr Clin North Am* 21:624, 1998.

Tucker, G. J., T. Detre, M. Harrow, G. H. Glaser. Behavior and symptoms of psychiatric patients ands the electroencephalogram. *Arch Gen Psychiat* 12:278, 1965.

Van Elst, L., F. Woerman, L. Lemieux, et al. Affective aggression in patients with temporal lobe epilepsy: a quantiative study of the amygdala. *Brain* 123:234, 2000.

Varney, N. R., M. J. Garvey, B. L. Cook, et al. Identification of treatment-resistant depressives who respond favorably to carbamazepine. *Ann Clin Psychiatry* 5:117, 1993.

Velasco, F., M. Velasco, A. L. Velasco, et al. Electrical stimulation of the centromedian thalamic nuclei in control of seizures: long term studies. *Epilepsia* 36:63, 1995.

Victaroff, J. I., F. Benson, S. T. Grafton, et al. Depression in complex partial seizures. Electroencephalography and cerebral metabolic correlates. *Arch Neurol* 51:155, 1994.

Walden, J., B. Hesslinger, D. VonKalker, et al. Addition of lamotrigine to valproate may enhance efficacy in the treatment of bipolar disorder. *Pharmacopsychiatry* 29:193, 1996.

Watson, C., C. R. Jack, F. Cendes. Volumetric MRI. *Arch Neurol* 54: 521, 1997.

Waxman, S. G., N. Geschwind The interictal behavior syndrome of temporal lobe epilepsy. *Arch Gen Psychiatry* 32:1580, 1975.

Weilberg, J. B., S. Schacter, J. Worth, et al. EEG abnormalities in patients with atypical panic attacks. *J Clin Psychiatry* 56:358, 1995.

Wiebe S., W. T. Blume, J. P. Girvin, et al. A randomized, controlled trial of surgery for temporal lobe epilepsy. *N Engl J Med* 345:311, 2001.

Wilder, G. J., E. R. Ramsey, J. Murphy, et al. Comparison of valproic acid and phenytoin in newly diagnosed tonic-clonic seizures. *Neurology* 12:1474, 1983.

Williams, D. Neural factors related to habitual aggression. *Brain* 92:50, 1969.

Williamson, P. D., S. S. Spencer. Clinical and EEG features of complex partial seizures of extratemporal origin. *Epilepsia* 27 (Suppl 2) :46, 1986.

Williamson, P. D., D. D. Spencer, S. S. Spencer, et al. Complex partial seizures of frontal lobe origin. *Ann Neurol* 18:497, 1985a.

Williamson, P. D., D. Spencer, S. S. Spencer, et al. Complex partial status epilepticus: A depth electrode study. *Ann Neurol* 18:647, 1985b.

Williamson, P. D., V. M. Thadani, T. M. Darcey, et al. Occipital lobe epilepsy: clinical characteristics, seizure spread patterns and results of surgery. *Ann Neurol* 31:3, 1992.

Wilson, S. J., P. Kincade, M. M. Saling, et al. Patient readmission and support utilization following anterior temporal lobectomy. *Seizure* 8:20, 1999.

Wirrell, E. C. Benign epilepsy of childhood with centrotemporal spikes. *Epilepsia* 39 (Suppl 4):S32–41 1998.

Woermann F., L. Van Elst, M. Koepp, et al. Reduction of frontal neocortical grey matter associated with affective aggression in patients with temporal lobe epilepsy: an objective voxel by voxel analysis of automatically segmented MRI. *J Neurol Neurosurg Psychiatry* 68: 162, 2000.

Wyllie, E., J. P. Glazer, S. Benbadis, et al. Psychiatric features of children and adolescents with pseudo seizures. *Arch Pediatr Adolesc Med* 153:244, 1999.

Zivin, L., C. Aimone Marsan. Incidence and prognostic significance of epileptiform activity in the EEG of non-epileptic subjects. *Brain* 91:751, 1968.

Chapter Two

VIOLENCE AND NEUROBIOLOGY

It is impossible to make a one-to-one correlation between violence and specific forms of neurological dysfunction or the brain regions involved. There is no "violence center" in the brain, that, when stimulated or destroyed, always produces violent behavior, though occasional case reports of such a sequence exist (Mark and Ervin, 1970; Ashford et al., 1980; St Hilaire et al., 1980). There is no region of the brain identified on positron emission tomography (PET) or other imaging techniques whose abnormal activity allows doctors to predict that the individual whose brain is abnormal will be violent. If one believes, however, that all thought and behavior derive from the brain, including morality and ethics (Greene et al., 2001), then the brain would be a reasonable starting point for studies of the origins of violence. As we will see below, the neurological status of most violent prisoners is abnormal (Blake et al., 1995); yet the relationship between neurological dysfunction of the brain and the propensity to violence is complex.

BRAIN DAMAGE

To demonstrate brain damage in violent criminals requires a variety of testing procedures. No single test infallibly provides a touchstone to determine the presence or absence of brain damage or brain dysfunction. The history (e.g., learning disorder, epilepsy, brain injury), the physical, neurological examination, neuropsychological tests, the electroencephalogram, and various imaging tests individually may reveal brain dysfunction. (Tranel, 1994; Van Elst et al., 2000). Usually, all these tests are not concordant. Each may fail to identify brain dysfunction, that manifests on another test. In this situation, the abnormal test is definitive. A normal result on one test cannot invalidate or neutralize the diagnostic significance of another abnormal test.

In general, magnetic resonance imaging (MRI) is a very reliable indicator of gross structural disturbances of the brain (tumors, strokes, multiple sclerosis) but seldom provides useful information with regard to primary generalized epilepsy, retardation, dementia, intoxication, learning disorders, clumsiness, and movement disorders. The electroencephalogram (EEG) is better for diagnosing epilepsy than the MRI is. Psychological tests are best for retardation, dementia, and learning disorders. The physical neurological examination is best for clumsiness and movement disorders. A battery of neurological signs provides evidence of diffuse cortical, mainly frontal, dysfunction (Jenkyn et al., 1977, 1985) and the Categories test from the Halstead-Reitan battery, the Wisconsin Card Sorting Test, Trailmaking A and B, and tests of continuous motor performance engage those portions of the brain that subserve executive functions. Each test of brain function can appear normal in patients with moderate to severe brain disorders that have been revealed in another or other tests. In combination, these tests have virtually always revealed evidence of brain dysfunction in violent individuals (Blake et al., 1995; Wong et al., 1997).

Newer imaging techniques that reflect brain metabolism rather than brain structure such as PET scans, single photon emission computed tomography (SPECT) scans, and functional magnetic resonance imaging, (fMR) are only beginning to be used to evaluate cognition in subjects who have been violent (Soderstrom et al., 2000). Position emission tomography scans, performed during frontal lobe activation and compared to controls, have identified dysfunctional regions of the brain in violent individuals (Raine et al., 1994, 1997). Functional MR has revealed abnormalities in the brains of dyslexic children when they were attempting to carry out reading-related tasks (Shaywitz et al., 1998). Though as many as half of prison inmates are dyslexic (Moody et al., 2000), fMR has not yet been applied to violent delinquents.

Many violent individuals have histories of traumatic brain injuries (TBI), and this may be a common source of neurological deficits among them. Repeated mild brain injuries occurring over months or years can result in cumulative neurological and cognitive defects. Mild concussions can have a cumulative effect. In a study of high school football players who were tested before playing and then after apparent recovery from a brain injury sustained in the game, mild concussions caused clinically detectable deficits (McCrea et al., 1997). Athletes who have suffered concussions and who have recovered are more at risk to be detectably and permanently brain damaged by subsequent head injuries than those who have never had a concussion. This is now called the Second Impact Syndrome (MMWR, 1997). This finding has provided the basis for a position statement of the American Academy of Neurology on the management of closed-head injuries among athletes, limiting their return to the sport following concussion to prevent serious brain damage (Kelly and Rosenberg, 1998). Cognitive dysfunction is not only a short-term consequence of concussion but also a predisposing risk factor for brain damage from future concussion (Teasdale and Engberg, 1997). Despite general agreement about the hazards of repeated, mild traumatic brain injuries, it is not possible to determine the exact site of injury in every case nor to define the exact role of each episode in damaging the brain (Kelly and Rosenberg, 1998).

Brain injury, especially the trauma of child abuse, can have devastating effects on children, as the inflicted injuries are usually recurrent. Ewing-Cobbs et al. (1998) reported that single episodes of inflicted TBI, though comparable in severity to noninflicted TBI, were significantly more likely to impair the cognitive function of the victim, even when the TBI did not cause prolonged impairment of consciousness. Mental deficiency was present in 45 percent of the inflicted and 5 percent of the noninflicted TBI groups.

There is no doubt that damage to certain parts of the brain confers a special vulnerability to later violence. Frontal lobe injuries are especially likely to facilitate violent behavior. In a study of Vietnam veterans who sustained penetrating brain injuries, those with frontal lobe damage were significantly more likely to be violent in the succeeding years than the veterans who sustained penetrating injuries elsewhere in the brain. Sustaining frontal lobe injury does not guarantee violence; the majority of the frontally injured veterans had not acted violently at follow-up (Grafman et al., 1996). Reduction of frontal neocortical grey matter may underlie the pathophysiology even of the aggression in some patients with epilepsy of temporal lobe origin (Woermann et al., 2000). The temporal and frontal poles, especially the undersurfaces, are the most likely sites of contusion following traumatic brain injury. Repeated concussions, defined as brain injuries that cause temporary cognitive changes, can cause permanent effects even when each is not severe enough to cause bleeding that is detectable on computed tomography (CT) scans. Presumably this is the result of the shearing effect of injuries upon the axonal nerve processes (Pearl, 1998).

Shaking babies and other abusive acts can produce widespread axonal damage. Beta-amyloid precursor protein has been described by immunohistochemistry in the brain tissue of fatally abused children obtained at autopsy (Shannon et al., 1998). The physical abuse of infants is not rare. In Scotland, for example, the risk of a child suffering nonaccidental head injury by his or her first birthday is 1 in 4065 (Barlow and Minns, 2000). The extent of the changes induced by trauma is comparable to the changes induced by severe hypoxia (Gleckman, 1999).

Brain injuries, including those from conditions that generate epilepsy and mental retardation, can impair executive functioning and lead to the disinhibition of impulses, irritability, and poor judgment. Individuals with violent impulses may express them only when disinhibited.

The temporary encephalopathy of intoxication also provides a neurologic basis for disinhibition. More than half of all homicides are committed by intoxicated individuals (Yarvis, 1994). The extent of encephalopathy caused by intoxicants like alcohol can be assessed with clinical testing and with blood and urine levels at the time of intoxication. All tests of brain structure and function and of body fluids are likely to be normal after the intoxicant has been metabolized. Cocaine and amphetamines are especially likely to result in violence as these drugs induce a sense of invulnerability akin to mania (Post, 1975; McIntyre, 1979). This powerful disinhibiting effect is especially sought out by depressed individuals who are treating themselves with street drugs such as PCP, methamphetamine, and cocaine (Cohen, 1984). Prolonged use of these stimulants induces paranoid delusions and a mental state that is difficult to distinguish from paranoid schizophrenia, except that it ultimately clears after the drug has been fully metabolized (Rosse et al., 1994). Stimulants thus induce a form of neurologically based behavioral disinhibition and paranoia, which we regard as two of the three main vulnerabilites to violence (see below). The prevalence of the use of cocaine correlates with and may predict the rise and fall of violent crime in U.S. cities (Golub and Johnson, 1994; Blumstein et al., 2000)

Despite the association of violence with brain damage and intoxication, it is very clear that most individuals who are damaged, intoxicated, or both are not violent. It is likely that other factors that interact with neurologic brain dysfunction such as mental illness and the experience of abuse in childhood interact with brain damage/intoxication to produce a vulnerability to violent behavior (Loberg, 1983).

ANTISOCIAL PERSONALITY AND THE FRONTAL LOBE

There is a tendency to categorize repeatedly violent behavior as a manifestation of antisocial personality disorder (ASPD). Though there is no doubt that murderers have acted antisocially, this diagnosis does not provide an understanding of their antisocial behavior. It is more a moral label than a medical diagnosis. The list of symptoms that describes ASPD in DSM-IV is very similar to that which might describe patients with frontal lobe damage (e.g., failure to conform to social norms, impulsivity, irritability, recklessness, irresponsibility, lack of remorse, indifference). Thus, ASPD may reflect frontal disease (Damasio et al., 1994).

Quantitative analysis of MRI scans has shown deficient volume of the frontal lobes in people with ASPD as compared with normal controls and drug abusers who did not have antisocial personality disorder (Raine et al., 2000). Raine and colleagues (1994, 1997) have compared PET scans of 41 murderers who pleaded "not guilty by reason of insanity" (NGRI) with 41 controls during a continuous performance test. This visual test activates the frontal region of the brain, as it requires focused attention and mental vigilance for a prolonged period. The premotor frontal cortex in the murderers failed to activate. No deficit was found in the temporal or occipital cortex. Murderers tended to show less activation in the left subcortical regions (amygdala, hippocampus, and thalamus) but higher activation than controls in the homologous regions of the right hemisphere (Raine et al., 1994, 1997). The frontal lobes project to the corpus striatum, the pallidum, the dorsomedial nucleus of the thalamus, the hippocampus, and elsewhere (Chow and Cummings, 1999). Dysfunction in these regions can give rise to disinhibited "frontal" type behavior, even though they are subcortical or not located in the frontal lobes (Mesulum, 2000).

NEUROTRANSMITTERS AND HORMONES

To explain violence, it is not necessary and probably incorrect to reach out to certain commonly invoked factors whose role is uncertain like elevated testosterone levels, low serotonin levels, or genetic influences. Testosterone is not always elevated in violent individuals. It can be elevated in nonviolent individuals and lowering the testosterone levels of violent men does not prevent them from committing future violent crimes (Heim and Hursch, 1979; Raboch et al., 1987; Richer and Crismon, 1993; Hall, 1995; Stalenheim et al., 1998).

For approximately 25 years, biologists have reported a correlation between a low cerebrospinal fluid concentration of serotonin and various behavioral abnormalities, including violent and criminal behavior. The more than 100 studies published so far are not in accord. At first, the behavior that was reported to be associated with low serotonin was depression, later associations were with aggression, then with impulsive, aggression and still later with alcoholism. Not every individual with low serotonin is depressed, aggressive, impulsive or alcoholic nor does every individual with any or all of these behaviors have low serotonin levels. Alper (1995) reviewed this subject and concluded that the relationship of low levels of brain serotonin to behavior was uncertain.

Because discrete behaviors have been associated with specific genetic and chromosomal disorders e.g., OCD (Tourettes), self-destruction (Lesch-Nyhan), and insatiable appetite (Prader-Willi) (Nyhan, 1976; Laurance et al., 1981; Pauls et al., 1986), it might be reasonable to postulate that a genetic propensity to violence may exist. This possibility has been eliminated by extensive studies in Scandanavia by Mednick and his colleagues (1984) who compared the rates of violent crime among the biologic parents and adoptive parents of adopted children. These reports have convincingly shown that violent crime is simply not a genetically transmitted characteristic.

MENTAL ILLNESS

There is strong evidence to support a causal connection between paranoid delusions and violence (Taylor and Gunn, 1984; Taylor, 1985; Soderstrom et al., 2000). The degree of schizophrenic symptoms is a predictor of dangerousness in hospitalized schizophrenics (Yesavage, 1984). Among men convicted of homicide and arson, a high proportion were considered definitely to have been driven by psychotic symptoms to commit offenses (Taylor, 1985). Variability over the course of time in the intensity of paranoia is quite characteristic of depression, mania, schizophrenia, and drug intoxication and may determine the timing of acts of violence. Of 500 British murderers whose psychiatric reports were reviewed, 44 percent had a lifetime history of mental illness, and 14 percent had mental symptoms at the time of the homicide (Shaw et al., 1999). In Sweden, 63 percent of murderers had had prior psychiatric care, 16 percent committed suicide, and 70 percent were intoxicated at the time of the homicide (Lindquist, 1986). Major mental disorder is thus an important factor in violence, especially when comorbid with the encephalopathy of substance abuse (Rasanen et al., 1998; Steadman et al., 1998; Wallace et al., 1998).

There is also a strong link between mood disorder and violent crime. Homicide and depression are closely connected, along with the experience of child abuse (Rosenbaum and Bennett, 1986). Unipolar depression causes irritability and anger (Fava, 1998) and bipolar affective disorder can also cause anger and aggression (Oquendo et al., 2000). Male and female adolescents and adults are more likely to be aggressive when they are clinically depressed (Knox et al., 2000). Intrafamilial violence directed at spouses or children also has been linked to depression (Bourget et al., 2000) and to excessive suspiciousness i.e., paranoia (Rosenbaum and Bennett., 1986). It is not easy to differentiate repetitive and nonrepetitive, paranoid and premeditated violence as opposed to unplanned, impulsive violence. Both share similar underlying vulnerabilities (Wong et al., 1997). Intermittent explosive disorders as defined in DSM-IV probably represent bipolar affective disorder and disinhibition, mainly caused by intoxication (McElroy, 1999).

Paranoia is seen not only in patients with disorders that fall within the scope of psychiatric practice. It exists on a spectrum ranging from mild excessive suspiciousness to delusions of persecution. All degrees of paranoia, even delusions, are nonspecific symptoms. The diseases that can give rise to paranoia vary considerably and include schizophrenia, mania, and depression. Neurological conditions can also cause paranoia. Among these conditions is drug intoxication. In fact, any condition of the brain that can cause cognitive impairment: encephalitis, stroke, epilepsy, thyroid disease, vitamin deficiency, Alzheimer's disease, etc. can lead to paranoid thinking.

Despite a strong correlation of paranoid thinking and depression with violence, how can we explain the fact that most paranoid, depressed, manic, psychotic individuals and most mentally ill individuals are not violent? This question is quite similar to the one that could be asked about neurological damage and the answer is the same. Violent individuals may bring other vulnerabilities to their mental symptoms and neurological damage that, under stress, lead to violence. The most important of these is the experience of child abuse.

ABUSE

The behavioral effects of abuse are noticeable and obvious in primary school years (Feldman et al., 1995). A study of 665 children 9–17 years old revealed a history of abuse in 172. The authors compared the abused with the nonabused children. Associated with the experience of physical abuse were global social impairment, poor social competence, major depression, agoraphobia, generalized anxiety as well as conduct disorder and oppositional defiant disorder (Flisher et al., 1997; Levitan et al., 1998; Ford et al., 1999).

Child abuse can have devastating consequences for children and for the adults they later become. Abuse early in life correlates with depression (DeBellis et al., 1999; Kauffman et al., 2000), aggression, anxiety, suicide (Fergusson et al., 1996), impulsivity, antisocial personality disorder (Luntz and Widom, 1994), borderline personality disorder (Paris et al., 1996a, b; Gudzer et al., 1999), PTSD (Famularo et al., 1996), and conversion disorders (Wyllie et al., 1999).

There is a growing perception that prolonged child abuse can permanently change the structure and function of the brain (Newport and Nemeroff, 2002). Child abuse has thus moved from the purely sociologic and psychological realm of interest into the neurological sphere as well. Abuse can damage the brain by direct trauma. More insidiously and pervasively, it can alter the basic developmental anatomy, physiology, and functioning of the brain.

Though the physical and sexual abuse of infants and children goes beyond emotional neglect in destructive potential, the effects of neglect were described decades ago and confirmed more recently (Spitz and Cobliner, 1966; Provence, 1967; McClellan et al., 1995; Rutter, 1998). The emotional neglect of institutionalized infants in the first years of life can cause long-lasting behavioral–cognitive changes. The early isolation of immature monkeys also induces long-lasting behavioral changes (Harlow et al., 1971). These responses of the immature mammalian brain may be analogous to the imprinting experience of newly hatched goslings (Lorenz, 1970).

What the developing brain registers through its sensory systems about the surrounding environment is increasingly recognized as a critical factor that permanently changes the brain by altering its connections. There is an exuberant development of synaptic connections between nerve cells in the first months and years of life and this connectivity is both pared down and developed by experience. The changes in synaptic function that occur as an individual matures have been correlated with PET measures of cerebral glucose utilization (Chugani, 1998).

Connections that are not used at critical times are lost forever (Huttenlocher and Dabholkar, 1997). The synaptic connections that form in infancy may represent the anatomical substrate for neural plasticity and for early learning as well as the superior capacity of the immature brain to reorganize after injury (Cao et al., 1994). The lack of development of synaptic connections may be the substrate for mental retardation and learning disorders (Huttenlocher, 1991).

Experience is critical for the functional and structural maturation of connections in the mammalian cortex. Through experience, immature circuits are "sculpted." Experience-dependent neural activity endows the brain with an ongoing ability to accommodate to changing inputs during development and throughout life (Katz and Shatz, 1996). Deprived of early experience or presented with an abnormal experience during its early development, the functioning of the cortex is disrupted.

The visual system provides a model of the early sensitivity to the environment shown by the connections of nerve cells in the brain. If an infant is born with a cataract, the cataract must be removed early because if it is not, vision will never develop in the formerly visually deprived eye. This is not true of adults. If dense cataracts are removed from the sightless eye of an adult, blind for years, vision can be restored. Amblyopia ex-anopsia is permanent blindness that develops in a child with strabismus. This form of blindness occurs only in childhood. The development of amblyopia in humans (Grigg et al., 1996; Sengpiel and Blakemore, 1996) illustrates the obliteration of a genetic endowment, present at birth, by abnormal sensory stimulation. Similar permanent changes in the cerebral cortex can occur in other sensory and motor systems when these are manipulated early in life (Singer, 1995). Hearing, somatosensory systems, and motor development all can be permanently affected by early experience (Huntley, 1997), including emotional experience (Joseph, 1998, 1999). Physical abuse can alter the quantitative EEG (Teicher et al., 1997; Ito et al., 1998), the MRI (Bremner and Narayan, 1999), and behavior (George, 1979).

Unbearable early stress from severe physical and sexual abuse might cause neurological changes in a number of different ways. A state of chronic hyperarousal may lead to neurochemical changes in abused children (Kendall-Tackett, 2000). Stress can alter the development of the hypothalamic-pituitary-adrenal axis. In preclinical studies, levels of corticotropin releasing factor (CRF) correlate with brain changes. Corticotropin releasing factor hypersecretion throughout life may result from severe abuse in childhood and this could underlie the psychopathology that follows abuse (Heim et al., 2000). High concentrations of excitatory amino acids have been found in the ventricular cerebrospinal fluid of badly abused children and this could be a source of excitotoxic damage (Ruppel et al., 2001). Nuclear magnetic resonance studies have directly linked abuse, PTSD, and neuronal loss. A low ratio of *N*-acetylaspartate to creatine, implying a loss of neural integrity, was reported in the anterior cingulate of 11 young victims of abuse who had PTSD, compared with age and sex matched controls (De Bellis et al., 2000).

The memory loss of dissociative amnesia in PTSD may result from the toxic action of high, prolonged levels of glucorticosteroids on the hippocampus, which is involved in the storage and retrieval of memories (Joseph, 1999). Quantitative MRI studies of the brain in abused populations reveal decreased brain volumes (Bremner, 1997; Driessen et al., 2000). Positron emission tomography studies of sexually abused women with and without PTSD correlated PTSD with dysfunction of the medial premotor cortex, hippocampus, and visual association cortex (Bremner et al., 1999; Shin et al., 1999). The changes seen clinically and on imaging tests may be the result of developmental and neurochemical factors as indicated above or simple physical injury to the brain.

VIOLENCE AS A COMPLEX PSYCHO-SOCIAL-BIOLOGIC INTERACTION

Raine and his colleagues (1997) classified 4269 male children born and living in Denmark according to two variables. The first was whether there were complications at birth (which loosely correlates with neurological impairment). The second was whether the child had been rejected by the mother (whether the child was unplanned, unwanted, etc.). This correlates, loosely, with neglect. Looking back 18 years later, the authors found that the children who were not rejected and who had no birth complications had roughly the same risk of becoming criminally violent by age 18 years as those with only one of the risk factors, approximately 3 percent. For the children with birth complications who had also been rejected, however, the risk of violence tripled. In fact, the children with both problems accounted for 18 percent of all the violent crimes committed by the 4269 children, even though they made up only 4.5 percent of the group.

It is thus very likely that several factors combine to produce a vulnerability to violent behavior (Cadoret et al., 1995).

A considerable body of data adumbrates a plausible environmental, psychological and neurological interaction that leads to violence. Violent behavior is actually a rare event committed by only a small number of individuals each of whom is not violent all the time. Less than 6 percent of some populations commit up to 70 percent of the violent crimes (Wolfgang, 1975). Considering its rarity, violent crime is abnormal by definition. Certainly one is justified in asking the question, "What is wrong with this (violent) person? Could there be something wrong with his/her brain?" One of us (JHP) has had the opportunity of examining a significant number of murderers and less violent adults and delinquents. This experience has led to a hypothesis of the potential causes of violent behavior (Pincus, 2001). Findings from studies of seriously violent offenders indicate that three factors often crucially influence the likelihood of violence:

1. *Abuse*—The experience of severe, daily, physical and/or sexual abuse in childhood. This abuse has often been sustained for years and is of such a quality that it legitimately makes the child fear for his/her life and corporeal integrity.
2. *Brain damage*—This frequently derives from prenatal, perinatal, and neonatal insults such as maternal alcohol or drug use or other maternal toxic exposures, complicated deliveries, accidental head trauma, sometimes sustained through parental abuse, exposure to toxins, or any of the other myriad causes of brain damage. It is often very difficult to determine which of the many factors that could have caused brain deficits have been the most destructive in an individual patient, and it is often impossible to date and place the damage within the central nervous system.
3. *Paranoia/affective disorder*—This can be the result of mental illness, drug effects, brain damage, or abuse.

All three factors have been found in about two-thirds of violent juveniles (Lewis et al., 1979) and in murderers (Feldman et al., 1986; Lewis et al., 1986; Blake and Pincus, 1995). No violent individual examined by JHP has been free of all three of these factors.

We think it likely that these correlates of violence play an important role in the causation of violence even though most people with only a one of these factors—abuse, brain damage, or paranoid thinking—are not violent. It is also likely that many individuals who have all three factors are not violent or at least not violent all the time. According to our theory, precipitating factors (such as anger or jealousy) that would ordinarily not produce a violent reaction are sufficient only in individuals who carry these vulnerabilities.

The concordance of damage, abuse and paranoid thinking was particularly striking in a group of 14 young men who were awaiting execution for crimes committed before they were 18 years old. The 14 men comprised the entire population of juvenile murderers in four states and represented 38 percent of the entire population of condemned juvenile murderers in the U.S. at that time. All but one had been physically or sexually abused or both. Sixty-four percent had major neurological impairments and only two had full-scale IQ scores over 90. Ten were paranoid, and the rest displayed mood disorders and bizarre behavior. Half had actually been psychotic with psychiatric hospitalizations before committing the capital crime (Lewis et al., 1988).

Of 15 other death row inmates, evaluated only because of the proximity of their execution dates, not because of supposed brain damage, 13 had suffered severe physical abuse, sexual abuse, or both by parents (Feldman et al., 1986). Twelve had neurological deficits and had sustained concussions or worse. Six were chronically psychotic, three had been episodically psychotic; two had bipolar mood disorder. Nine of the 15 subjects suffered psychiatric symptoms during childhood severe enough for consultation. Four had attempted suicide in childhood. Eight expressed paranoid ideas at the time of examination (Lewis et al., 1986).

How do neurological deficits, paranoia, and the experience of abuse relate to the etiology of violence? A follow-up study of 95 delinquent 15-year-old boys 7 years after initial evaluation suggested that paranoid thinking, neurological dysfunction, and abuse were not merely additive, but that *these vulnerabilities interacted* to increase the risk and severity of adult violent criminality. The absence of these variables among incarcerated juvenile delinquents at age 15 predicted future nonviolent behavior over the following 7 years 85 percent of the time (Lewis et al., 1989).

Estimates of the prevalence of previous physical and sexual abuse among incarcerated violent juvenile delinquents have reached up to 80 percent (Lewis et al., 1979). In prisoners held on death row who have been convicted of homicide, both juveniles (Lewis, 1988) and adults (Feldman, 1986; Blake and Pincus, 1995) have prevalence rates of prior sexual and/or physical abuse in their childhoods that has approached 100 percent. Among nondelinquents matched with delinquents for sex, age, race, and socioeconomic level, the prevalence rate of abuse is much lower (13%) (Lewis et al., 1987). The amount of abuse has never been quantified. It seems reasonable to postulate that severity, frequency, duration of episodes, and years of exposure could vary and that the worst abuse would be the most harmful.

Despite the high prevalence of severe abuse among violent criminals, the causal role of abuse in violent behavior must be complex since only a minority of abused children become violent criminals. Follow-up studies of children who have been subjected to abuse have described increased levels of aggressive behavior when compared with controls, but most previously abused children appear to be neither disturbed nor aggressive. In only a minority of families in which abuse was severe enough to lead to outside intervention is there child abuse in the next generation (Widom, 1989). Even if under-reporting of abuse seriously reduced the apparent rate of intergenerational abuse, it is very clear that abuse does not always generate abuse, let alone other violent crimes. Abuse alone is not enough to produce a violent criminal under most circumstances. The capacity of many abused people to lead relatively normal lives is a testament to the resilience of the human spirit (the plasticity of the human brain), yet some formerly abused people do become violent and dangerous to society, and there is a statistical link between the experience of abuse and later violence (Widom, 1989).

SOCIOLOGICAL ASPECTS OF VIOLENCE

The prevalence of violence varies among different groups and it may be worthwhile to utilize the theory of interacting variables to explain this variation. For example, violent crime is much more common among African-Americans. The homicide death rate among all American men aged 15 to 24 rose from 22 per 100,000 in 1987 to 37 per 100,000 in 1994. The homicide death rate for young African-American males in 1993 was 167 per 100,000 (Bureau of Justice Statistics, 1996). This high homicide rate among African-Americans is not likely to be the result of a genetic vulnerability. The theory that an abnormal gene causes human violent criminal behavior has been definitively contradicted by clinical adoption studies (Mednick et al., 1984; Brennan et al., 1996). There is, however, solid evidence that the three factors we believe to underlie violence are disproportionately prevalent in the African-American population.

In 1996 the number of cases of reported child abuse among African-American children was twice their proportion in the general population (Child Maltreatment 1996; Report from the States to the National Child Abuse and Neglect Data System—U.S. Department of Health and Human Services). Conditions that harm the brain besides physical abuse are also more prevalent in the African-American community. These include lead poisoning (Sargent et al., 1995), traumatic brain injuries (Jager et al., 2000), and drug abuse during pregnancy (Wieman et al., 1994). Schizophrenia may also be more prevalent (Strakowski et al., 1996). If the interplay of abuse, neurologic damage, and mental illness causes violent crime, their overrepresentation in the African-American community may explain the demographic facts.

Socioeconomic level is an important factor in violent crimes. Is this a matter of income and housing or rather the unequal prevalence of abuse, brain damage, and mental illness that varies according to socioeconomic level? According to the National Incidence Study (Sedlak and Broadhurst, 1996), the poorest children with family incomes of less than $15,000 per year experienced more than twice the rate of physical abuse as children with annual family incomes of $15,000 to $30,000, and 12 times the rate of those children in families with income of over $30,000. The reason that lower income is associated with increased abuse may reflect a greater tendency among the lowest socioeconomic groups to use illicit drugs (Sedlak and Broadhurst, 1996). Serious mental illness, like schizophrenia, is more common in the lower social classes. Child abuse may generate brain damage. Thus, varying rates of neurological damage, abuse, and mental illness depending on socioeconomic group may explain many of the puzzling demographic features of violent crime.

The thesis that the vulnerability to commit violent crimes is the result of the interaction of severe abuse in childhood (physical and/or sexual) with neurologic disturbances and mental illness can be utilized to explain the gender difference. Although it would be an overstatement to say that women are not violent, it is also true that men commit violent crimes such as homicide more frequently than women by margins of approximately 9 to 1. Men commit 93 to 98 percent of gang-related, drug-related, sex-related, and felony murder. The nearly exclusive focus of whatever violence is commited by women lies within the family relationship. Women commit 37 percent of all homicides of intimates and 39 percent of infanticides. Women, mothers, and stepmothers are responsible primarily for 61 percent of the cases of the physical abuse of children (Bureau of Justice Statistics 1976–99; Child Maltreatment, 1996). If the theory about the interaction of three factors that produces a vulnerability to violence is correct, we must look at the distribution of these factors in groups that are more likely to be violent, in this case males.

Boys and girls are near parity with regard to the prevalence of abuse and mental illness, but neurologic damage is much more common in males. Both the behavioral vulnerability to the effects of abuse and the severity of abuse are worse in males.

In this country, 48 percent of physical abuse victims are girls as are 77 percent of reported sexual abuse victims (Child Maltreatment, 1996). A report from Sweden (Edgardh and Ormstad, 2000) of the prevalence of a history of sexual abuse in a representative sample of almost 2000 teenagers attending secondary school indicated that 2.3 percent of boys and 7.1 percent of girls had been sexually abused. The mean age at the time of first abuse was 9 years for both sexes. 1.2 percent of boys and 3.1 percent of girls reported penetration orally, vaginally, or anally. Suicide attempts or other acts of self-harm were reported by 33 percent of the abused boys (and 5% of the nonabused boys) and by 30 percent of the abused girls (and 9% of the nonabused girls). The sexual penetration of children is always likely to be painful and tissue-destructive, especially given the fact that almost two-thirds of the child victims in the U.S. are prepubertal (less than 11 years old) and 39 percent are less than 7 years old (Child Maltreatment, 1996).

Sexual abuse is more damaging to the psyches of boys than girls. Garnefski and Diekstra (1997) compared 745 high school students (151 boys and 594 girls) who reported a history of sexual abuse with a matched group of students without such a history. A larger proportion of the sexually abused students reported emotional problems, aggressive and criminal behaviors, addiction-risk behaviors and suicidality. Sexually abused boys had considerably more problems in each of these areas than sexually abused girls did. The differences could not be attributed to the finding that the sexually abused boys were also more likely to have been physically abused than were the sexually abused girls. This study indicated that the aftermath of sexual abuse for boys is even worse than it is for girls.

Boys are also more likely to be seriously physically injured by physical abuse (nonsexual) as evidenced by the fact that 56 percent of the children killed by abuse are boys (Child Maltreatment, 1996; Mahoney et al., 2000). This is a meaningful gender difference but cannot explain the order of magnitude difference between the sexes in the numbers of homicides committed by men and the almost exclusive focus of serious violence by women within a family relationship.

The distribution of mental illness does not explain the greater male propensity to violence. Males do not have higher rates of mental illness. The prevalence of serious mental illnesses that can cause paranoid delusions, like schizophrenia and bipolar affective disorder, is about equal by gender (Bijl et al., 1998). Schizophrenia starts a bit earlier in men and is generally somewhat more severe, probably because of a preexistent neurologic vulnerability (Leung and Chue, 2000). Males with schizophrenia consistently show poorer cognitive functioning than women before becoming schizophrenic. Males also demonstrate more "negative" symptoms such as withdrawal, apathy, and inability to relate to others. These negative symptoms do not respond well to antipsychotic drug treatment. Male schizophrenics have more cognitive deficits, structural brain abnormalities, and neurophysiologic abnormalities. These findings suggest that there is more neurologic disablity among male schizophrenics (Hendrick et al., 2000).

Mania has about the same prevalence in both sexes (Hendrick et al., 2000). Unipolar depression is actually 1.5 to 3 times more prevalent among women (Ustun, 2000), but the overall morbidity of mental illness is approximately the same for both genders in large-population studies (Bijl et al., 1998).

On the other hand, neurological dysfunction is much more common among boys. Attention-deficit hyperactivity disorder (Arnold, 1996), childhood autism (Smalley et al., 1988), pervasive developmental disorders (Volkman et al., 1993), dyslexia (Flannery et al., 2000), developmental dysphasia (Rapin and Allen, 1998), and certain forms of mental retardation are more prevalent among males by margins of up to 4 or 5 to 1. These abnormalities may be inherited as X-linked traits, like the Fragile X syndrome, a chromosomal abnormality that causes more cases of mental retardation than Trisomy 21 (mongolism) and affects only males (Boue et al., 1997). Even normal boys demonstrate patterns of behavior that seem to reflect delayed brain development much more frequently than girls do. The behavior of little girls in primary school is, in general, better modulated and mature.

"Immaturity" and "as yet undeveloped" are related concepts given that immaturity has a physiologic and anatomic basis. There is some preliminary evidence that the development of the circuitry of the brain is slower in males than in females (Benes et al., 1994; Overman et al., 1996; DeBellis et al., 2001). This supports the old hypothesis that testosterone, the male hormone, impedes aspects of brain development and makes the male brain more vulnerable to a variety of learning and behavioral disorders (Rapin and Allen, 1988) and to the kinds of unmodulated, careless motor activity that can result in traumatic brain injury, which is also much more common in boys (Consensus Conference, 1999; Jager et al., 2000).

The unequal distribution of neurologic dysfunction between the sexes may account for much of the greater vulnerability of males to violence. The abnormal behavioral patterns imposed by neurologic deficits and delayed development can elicit severe parental responses, especially in abusive homes. In this way neurologic deficits can contribute to abuse and to the alienation of victims who, as a result of abuse, may tend to mistrust others (paranoia).

Supporting the link between abuse and neurologic damage is the fact that in developmentally disabled children, reported abuse is more common than in nondisabled children. In a population-based epidemiologic study (Sullivan and Knutson, 2000), a link between neurologic, educationally relevant disablility and abuse was discovered. Fully 31 percent of disabled children were abused, a rate 3.4 times greater than their nondisabled peers.

Not only are males more likely to be neurologically disabled, and not only does disability impose a greater risk of abuse, but males with disability are more likely than females with disability to be abused. In a study of 1834 abused children, disabled boys represented a significantly larger proportion of physically abused, sexually abused, and neglected children than would be expected from the respective proportion of abused and neglected children without disabilities; though half of abused children without disabilities were boys, 65 percent of abused children with disabilities were boys (Sobsey et al., 1997).

The combination of neurologic defects with abuse and mental illness is severalfold more common in boys because neurologic defects are severalfold more common in boys, The abuse of damaged boys is more common than that of damaged girls and is more harmful to the boys. These links between neurologic deficit and abuse adequately explain the increased prevalence of violence among males and these considerations also support the theory of the origins of violence that we have presented.

Abuse is humiliating, degrading, and is likely to impose a sense of worthlessness, helplessness, anxiety, hopelessness, social incompetence, and guilt on children from which they can escape temporarily by exerting the greatest effort to control themselves throughout the remainder of their lives or by employing force in order to victimize others. It takes a good brain to keep violent urges in check. Damaged by neurological illness or mental illness, the brain may not provide effective social inhibitions to control violence.

To deal with the horrid feelings that abuse imposes, abused women more often than men have a tendency to become sexually active at an early age (Edgardh and Ormstad, 2000), to become promiscuous and/or prostitutes (Widom and Kuhns, 1996), to bear children at an early age (Dietz et al., 1999), and to abuse their children. None of these behaviors is obligatory for abused women, but there is evidence that such behavior is more likely in abused females.

It seems probable that mothers would have greater access than fathers to the children with respect to the opportunity to abuse them (Rudin et al., 1995), hence the violence of women is focused in the home. The options available to women for temporarily lifting their morale (attracting the opposite sex repeatedly in a short time, becoming pregnant, and abusing their children) are not as available to men. Consequently, for men, the use of their physical size in conflicts with outsiders is a more likely outcome of the same destructive combination of factors that is the root of violence for both men and women: the interaction of abuse, mental illness, and neurological damage.

CONCLUSION

Neurologic damage, mental illness, and the experience of unremitting physical and/or sexual abuse in childhood interact to create a vulnerability to violent behavior. To explain variations in the rate of violence in different social groups one must start with the estimation of the prevalence of these three factors in the groups being studied. Variations in the distributions and prevalence of the three factors by gender, race, and socioeconomic level explain variations in the prevalance of violence in different groups. Violence in any group can probably be understood by focusing on these factors.

REFERENCES

Alper, J. S. Biological influences on criminal behavior: how good is the evidence? *BMJ* 310: 272, 1995.

Arnold, L. E. Sex differences in ADHD: conference summary. *J Abnorm Child Psychol* 24:555, 1996.

Ashford, J. W., S. C. Schultz, F. O. Walsh. Violent automatism in a partial complex seizure. *Arch Neurol* 37:120, 1980.

Barlow, K. M. R. A. Minns. Annual incidence of shaken impact syndrome in young children. *Lancet* 356:1571–1572, 2000.

Benes F. M., M. Turtle, Y. Khan, et al. Myelination of a key relay zone in the hippocampal formation occurs in the human brain during childhood, adolescence, and adulthood. *Arch Gen Psychiatry* 51:477, 1994.

Bijl R. V., A. Ravelli, G. van Zessen. Prevalence of psychiatric disorder in the general population: results of The Netherlands Mental Health Survey and Incidence Study (NEMESIS). *Soc Psychiatry Psychiatr Epidemiol* 33:587, 1998.

Blake P. Y., J. H. Pincus, G. Buckner. Neurologic abnormalities in murderers. *Neurology* 45: 1641, 1995.

Blumstein A., F. P. Rivera, R. Rosenfeld the rise and decline of homicide and why. *Ann Rev Public Health* 21:505, 2000.

Boue J., B. Simon-Bouy. Genetics of fragile X syndrome and its prevention. *J Gynecol Obstet Biol Reprod (Paris)* 26:273, 1997.

Bourget D., P., Gagne J. Moami. Spousal homicide and suicide in Quebec. *J Am Acad Law* 28:179, 2000.

Bremner, J. D., M. Narayan L. H. Staib, et al. Neural correlates of memories of childhood sexual abuse in women with and without posttraumatic stress disorder. *Am J Psychiatry* 156:1787, 1999.

Bremner, J. D., P. Randall, E. Vermetten, et al. Magnetic resonance imaging-based measurement of hippocampal volume in post-traumatic stress disorder related to childhood physical and sexual abuse. *Biol Psychiatry* 41:23, 1997.

Brennan, P. A., S. A. Mednick, B. Jacobsen. Assessing the role of genetics in crime using adoption cohorts. *Ciba Found Symp* 194:115, 1996.

Bureau of Justice Statistics Homicide Trends in the United States 1976–1999. Department of Justice. http://www.ojp.usdoj.gov:80/bjs/homicide/gender.htm.

Cadoret, R. J., W. R. Yates, E. Troughton. Genetic-environmental interaction in the genesis of aggressivity and conduct disorders. *Arch Gen Psychiatry* 52:916, 1995.

Cao, Y., E. M. Vikingstad, P. R. Huttenlocher, et al. Functional magnetic resonance studies of the reorganization of the sensorimotor area after unilateral brain injury in the perinatal period. *Proc Natl Acad Sci* 91:9612, 1994.

Child Maltreatment 1996: Reports from the states to the National Child Abuse and Neglect Data System U.S. Department of Health and Human Services pp. 2–14.

Chow, T. W., J. L. Cummings. Frontal-subcortical circuits. In: *The Human Frontal Lobes—Functions and Disorders*, B. L. Miller, J. L. Cummings, eds. Guilford Press, New York, 1999, p. 3.

Chugani, H. T. A critical period of brain development: Studies of cerebral glucose utilization with PET. *Prev Med* 27:184, 1998.

Cohen, S. Recent developments in the use of cocaine. *Bull Narc* 36:3, 1984.

Consensus Conference: Rehabilitation of persons with traumatic brain injury. NIH Consensus development panel on rehabilitation of persons with traumatic brain injury. *JAMA* 282: 974, 1999.

Damasio, H. T. Grabowski, R. Frank. The return of Phineas Gage: clues about the brain from the skull of a famous patient. *Science* 264:1102, 1994.

DeBillis, M., M. Keshavan, S. Spencer et al. N-Acetylaspartate concentration in the anterior cingulate of maltreated children and adolescents with PTSD. *Amer J Psychiatry* 157:1175, 2000.

De Bellis, M. D., M. S. Keshavan, S. R. Beers, J. Hall, K. Frustaci, A. Masalehdan, J. Noll. Sex differences in brain maturation during childhood and adolescence. *Cereb Cortex* 11:552–557, 2001.

De Bellis, M. D., M. S. Keshaven, et al. Developmental traumatology. Part II Brain development. *Biol Psychiatry* 45:1271, 1999.

Dietz, P. M., A. M. Spitz, R. F. Anda, et al. Unintended pregnancy among adult women exposed to abuse or household dysfunction during their childhood. *JAMA* 282: 1359, 1999.

Driessen, M., J. Herrmann, K. Stahl, et al. Magnetic resonance imaging volumes of the hippocampus and the amygdala in women with borderline personality disorder and early traumatization. *Arch Gen Psychiatry* 57:1115, 2000.

Edgardh, K., K. Ormstad. Prevalence and characteristics of sexual abuse in a national sample of Swedish seventeen-year-old boys and girls. *Acta Paediatr* 89:310, 2000.

Ewing-Cobbs, L., L. Kramer, M. Prasad, et al. Neuroimaging, physical, and developmental findings after inflicted and non-inflicted traumatic brain injury in young children. *Pediatrics* 102: 300, 1998.

Famularo, R., T. Fenton, R. Kinscherff, et al. Psychiatric comorbidity in childhood post traumatic stress disorder. *Child Abuse Negl* 20:953, 1996.

Fava, M. Depression with anger attacks. *J. Clin. Psychiatry* 59 (Suppl 18):18, 1998.

Feldman M., K. Malhoun, D. O. Lewis. Filicidal abuse in the histories of fifteen condemned murderers. *Bull Am Acad Psychiatry Law* 14:345, 1986.

Feldman, R. S., S. Salzinger, M. Zrosario, et al. Parent, teacher, and peer ratings of physically abused and nonmaltreated children's behavior. *J Abnorm Child Psychol* 23:317, 1995.

Fergusson, D. M., L. J., Horwood, M. T. Lynskey. Childhood sexual abuse and psychiatric disorder in young adulthood: II. Psychiatric outcomes of childhood sexual abuse. *J Am Acad Child Adolesc Psychiatry* 35:1365, 1996.

Flannery, K. A., J. Liederman, L. Daly, et al. Male prevalence for reading disability is found in a large sample of black and white children free from ascertainment bias. *J Int Neuropsychol Soc* 6:433, 2000.

Flisher, A. J., R. A. Kramer, C. W. Hoven, et al. Psychosocial characteristics of physically abused children and adolescents. *J Am Acad Child Adolesc Psychiatry* 36:123–231, 1997.

Ford, J. D., R. Racusin, W. B. Daviss, et al. Trauma exposure among children with oppositional defiant disorder and attention deficit-hyperactivity disorder. *J Consult Clin Psychol* 67:786, 1999.

Garnefski, N., R. F. Diekstra. Child sexual abuse and emotional and behavioral problems in adolescence: gender differences. *J Am Acad Child Adolesc Psychiatry* 36:323, 1997.

George, C. Social interactions of young abused children: approach, avoidance, and aggression. *Child Dev* 50:306,1979.

Gleckman, A. Diffuse axonal injury in infants with nonaccidental craniocerebral trauma: enhanced detection by beta-amyloid precursor protein immunohistochemical staining. *Arch Pathol Lab Med* 123:146, 1999.

Golub, A., B. D. Johnson. A recent decline in cocaine use among youthful arrestees in Manhattan 1987 through 1993. *Am J Public Health* 84:1250, 1994.

Grafman, J, et al. Frontal lobe injuries, violence, and aggression: a report of the Vietnam Head Injury Study. *Neurology* 46:1231, 1996.

Greene, J. D., R. B. Sommerville, L. E. Nystrom, et al. An fMRI investigation of emotional engagement in moral judgment. *Science* 293:2105, 2001.

Grigg, J., R. Thomas, F. Billson. Neuronal basis of amblyopia: a review. *Indian J Ophthalmol* 44:69, 1996.

Gudzer, J., J. Paris, P. Zelkowitz, et al. Psychological risk factors for borderline pathology in school aged children. *J Am Acad Child Adolesc Psychiatry* 38:206, 1999.

Hall, G. C. Sexual offender recidivism revisited: a meta analysis of recent treatment studies. *Consult Clin Psychology* 63:802, 1995.

Harlow, H. F., M. K. Harlow, S. J. Suomi. From thought to therapy: lessons from a primate laboratory. How investigation of the learning capability of rhesus monkeys has led to the study of their behavioral abnormalities and rehabilitation *Am. Sci* 59:538, 1971.

Heim, C., D. J. Newport, S. Heit, et al. Pituitary-adrenal and autonomic responses to stress in women after sexual and physical abuse in childhood. *JAMA* 284:592, 2000.

Heim, N., C. J. Hursch. Castration for sex offenders: treatment or punishment? Review and critique of European literature. *Arch Sex Behav* 8:281, 1979.

Hendrick, V., L. L. Altshuler, M. J. Gitlin, et al. Gender and bipolar illness. *J Clin Psychiatry* 61:393, 2000.

Huntley, G. W. Differential effects of abnormal tactile experience on shaping representation patterns in developing and adult motor cortex. *J Neurosci* 17:9220, 1997.

Huttenlocher, P. R. Dendritic and synaptic pathology in mental retardation. *Pediatri Neurol* 7:79, 1991.

Huttenlocher, P. R., A. S. Dabholkar. Regional differences in synaptogenesis in human cerebral cortex. *J Comp Neurol* 387:167, 1997.

Ito, Y., M. H. Teicher, C. A. Glod, et al. Preliminary evidence for aberrant cortical development in abused children: a quantitative EEG study. *J Neuropsychiatry* 10:298, 1998.

Jager, T. E., H. B. Weiss, J. H. Cohen, et al. Traumatic brain injuries evaluated in U.S. emergency departments 1992–1994. *Acad Emerg Med* 7:134, 2000.

Jenkyn, L. R., D. B. Walsh, C. M. Culver, A. G. Reeves. Clinical signs in diffuse cerebral dysfunction. *J Neurol Neurosurg Psychiatry* 40:956, 1977.

Jenkyn, L. R., A. G. Reeves, T. Warren. Neurologic signs in senescence. *Arch Neurol* 42: 1154, 1985.

Joseph, R. Traumatic amnesia, repression, and hippocampus injury due to emotional stress, corticosteroids, and enkephalins. *Child Psychiatry Hum Dev* 29:169, 1998.

Joseph, R. The neurology of traumatic "dissociative" amnesia: commentary and literature review. *Child Abuse Negl* 23:715, 1999.

Katz, L. C., A. Shatz. Synaptic activity and the construction of cortical circuits. *Science* 4:1133, 1996.

Kaufman, J., P. M. Plotsky, C. B. Nemeroff, et al. Effects of early adverse experiences on brain structure and function. Clinical implications. *Biol Psychiatry* 48:778, 2000.

Kelly, J. P., J. H. Rosenberg. The development of guidelines for the management of concussion in sports. *JH Trauma Rehabil* 13:53, 1998.

Kendall-Tacket, K. A. Physiological correlates of childhood abuse: chronic hyperarousal in PTSD, depression, and irritable bowel syndrome. *Child Abuse Negl* 24:799, 2000.

Knox, M, C. King, G. L. Hanna, et al. Aggressive behavior in clinically depressed adolescents. *J Am Acad Child Adolesc Psychiatry* 39:611, 2000.

Laurance, B. M., A. Brito, J. Wilkinson. Prader-Willi syndrome after age 15 years. *Arch Dis Child* 56:181, 1981.

Leung, A., P. Chue. Sex differences in schizophrenia, a review of the literature. *Acta Psychiatr Scand* (Suppl) 401:3, 2000.

Levitan, R. D., S. V. Parikh, A. D. Lesage, et al. Major depression in individuals with a history of childhood physical or sexual abuse: relationship to neurovegetative features, mania, and gender. *Am J Psychiatry* 155:1746, 1998.

Lewis, D., S. Shanock, J. Pincus, et al. Violent juvenile delinquents. *J Amer Acad Child Adolesc Psychiat.* 18:307, 1979.

Lewis, D. O., J. H. Pincus, B. Bard, et al. Neuro-psychiatric, psychoeducational and family characteristics of fourteen juveniles condemned to death in the United States. *Am J Psychiatry* 145:584, 1988.

Lewis, D. O., J. H. Pincus, M. Feldman, et al. Psychiatric, neurological, and psychoeducational characteristics of 15 death row inmates in the United States. *Am J Psychiatry* 143:838, 1986.

Lewis, D., R. Lovely, C. Yeager, et al. Toward a theory of violence. *J Amer Acad Child Adolesc Psychiat.* 29:150, 1989.

Lewis, D. O., J. H. Pincus, R. Lovely, et al. Biosocial characteristics of matched samples of delinquents and non-delinquents. *J Am Acad Child Adolsc Psychiatry* 26:744, 1987.

Lindquist, P. Criminal homicide in northern Sweden 1970–1981:alcohol intoxication, alcohol abuse, and mental disease. *Int J Psychiatry* 8:19, 1986.

Loberg, T. Belligerence in alcohol dependence. *Scand J Psychol* 24:285, 1983.

Lorenz, K. *Studies in Animal and Human Behavior*, Vol. 1. Translated by Robert Martin Methuen and Co. Ltd., London, 1970.

Luntz, B. K., C. S. Widom. Antisocial personality disorder in abused and neglected children grown up. *Am J Psychiatry*.151:670, 1994.

Mahoney, A., W. O. Donnelly, T. Lewis, et al. Mother and father self-reports of corporal punishment and severe physical aggression toward clinic-referred youth. *J Clin Child Psychology* 29:266, 2000.

Mark, V. H., F. Ervin. *Violence and the Brain*. Harper and Row, New York, 1970.

McClellan, J., J. Adams, D. Douglas, et al. Clinical characteristics related to severity of sexual abuse: a study of seriously mentally ill youth. *Child Abuse Negl* 10:1245, 1995.

McCrea, M., J. P. Kelly, J. Kluge, et al. Standardized assessment of concussion in football players. *Neurology* 48:586, 1997.

McElroy, S. Recognition and treatment of DSM IV intermittent explosive disorder. *J Clin Psychiatry*, 60(Suppl 15):12, 1999.

McIntyre, J. S. Mania: the common symptom of several illnesses. *Postgrad Med* 66:145, 1979.

Mednick, S. A. W. F. Gabrielli, Jr., B. Hutchings. Genetic influences in criminal convictions: Evidence from an adoption cohort. *Science* 224:891, 1984.

Mesulum, M. *Principles of Behavioral and Cognitive Neurology*, 2nd Ed. Oxford University Press, New York, 2000, p. 55.

MMWR. Sports related recurrent brain injuries—United States, *MMWR* 46:224,1997.

Moody, K. C., C. E. Holzer 3rd, M. J. Roman, et al. Prevalence of dyslexia among Texas prison inmates. *Tex Med* 96:69, 2000.

Newport, J., C. Nemeroff. Childhood trauma: psychiatric and neurobiologic consequences. of aggressivity and conduct disorders. *Arch Gen Psychiary*, 52:916, 1995.

Newport, J. and Nemeroff, C. Childhood Trauma, Semin Clin Neuropsychiatry (2), 2002.

Nyhan, W. L. Behavior in the Lesch-Nyhan Syndrome. *J Autism Child Schizophr* 6:235, 1976.

Oquendo, M. A., C. Waternaux, B. Brodsky, et al. Suicidal behavior in bipolar mood disorder: clinical characteristics of attempters and nonattempters. *J Affect Disord* 59: 107, 2000.

Overman, W. H., J. Bachevalier, E. Schuhmann, et al. Cognitive gender differences in very young children parallel biologically based cognitive gender differences in monkeys. *Behav Neurosci* 110:673–684, 1996.

Paris, J., H. Zweig-Frank, J. Gudzer. Risk factors for borderline personality in male outpatients. *J Nerv Ment Dis* 182:375, 1994a.

Paris Psychological risk factors for borderline personality disorder in female patients. *Compr Psychiatry* 35:301, 1994b.

Pauls, D. L., J. F. Leckman. The inheritance of Gilles de la Tourette syndrome and associated behaviors. Evidence for autosomal dominant transmission. *N Engl J Med* 315:993, 1986.

Pearl, G. S. Traumatic neuropathology. *Clin Lab Med* 18:39, 1998.

Pincus, J. H. Base Instincts: What Makes Killers Kill. Norton, New York, 2001.

Post, R. M. Cocaine psychoses: a continuum model. *Am J Psychiatry* 132:225, 1975.

Provence, S. *Infants in Institutions: A Comparison of their Development Through the First Year of Life With Family Reared Children.* International Universities Press, New York, 1967.

Raboch, J., H. Cerna, P. Zemek. Sexual aggressivity and androgens. *Br J Psychiatry* 151: 398, 1987.

Raine, A., P. Brennan, S. A. Mednick Interaction between birth complications and early maternal rejection in predisposing individuals to adult violence: specificity to serious early-onset violence. *Am J Psychiatry* 154:1265, 1997.

Raine, A., M. S. Buchsbaum, D. LaCasse. Brain abnormalities in murderers indicated by positron emission tomography. *Biol Psychiatry* 42:495, 1997.

Raine, A., M. S. Buchsbaum, J. Stanley, et al. Selective reductions in prefrontal glucose metabolism in murderers. *Biol Psychiatry*, 36:365, 1994.

Raine, A., T. Lencz, S. Bihrle, et al. Reduced frontal prefrontal gray matter volume and reduced automatic activity in antisocial personality disorder *Arch Gen Psychiatry* 57: 119, 2000.

Rapin, I., D. A. Allen Syndromes in developmental dysphasia and adult aphasia. Assoc for Res in Nerv Ment Dis 66:57, 1988.

Rasanen, P., J. Tiihonen, M. Isohanni, et al. Schizophrenia, alcohol abuse, and violent behavior: a 26-year follow-up study of an unselected birth cohort. *Schizophr Bull* 24: 437, 1998.

Richer, M., M. L. Crismon. Pharmacotherapy for sexual offenders. *Am J Psychiatry* 143: 367, 1986.

Rosnebaum, M., B. Bennett. Homicide and depression. *Amer J Psychiatry* 143:367, 1986.

Rosse, R. B., J. P. Collins, M. Fay-McCarthy, et al. Phenomenologic comparison of the idiopathic psychosis of schizophrenia and drug induced psychoses: a retrospective study. *Clin Neuropharmacol* 17: 359, 1994.

Rudin, M. M., C. Zalewski, J. Bodmer-Turner. Characteristics of child sexual abuse victims according to perpetrator gender. *Child Abuse Negl* 19:963, 1995.

Ruppell, R. A., P. M. Kochanek, P. D. Adelson, et al. Excitatory amino acid concentrations in ventricular cerebrospinal fluid after severe traumatic brain injury in infants and children: the role of child abuse *J Pediatr* 138:18, 2001.

Rutter, M. Developmental catch-up and deficit following adoption after severe global, early privation. English and Romanian Adoptees (ERA) Study Team. *J Child Psychol Psychiatry*, 39:405, 1998.

Saint-Hilaire, J. M., M. Gilbert, G. Bouner. Aggression as an epileptic manifestation: two cases with depth electrode study. *Epilepsia* 21:184, 1980.

Sargent, J. D., M. J. Brown, J. L. Freeman, et al. Childhood lead poisoning in Massachusetts communities: its association with socioeconomic and housing characteristics. *Am J Public Health* 85:528, 1995.

Sedlak, A. J., D. D. Broadhurst. U.S. Department of Health and Human Services, *National Incidence Study*, September 3, 1996.

Sengpiel, F., C. Blakemore. The neural basis of suppression and amblyopia in strabismus. *Eye* 10:250, 1996.

Shannon, P., C. R. Smith, J. Deck, et al. Axonal injury and the neuropathology of shaken baby syndrome. *Acta Neuropathol* 95:625, 1998.

Shaw, J. L., T. Appleby, G. Amos, et al. Mental disorder and clinical care in people convicted of homicide: national clinical survey. *BMJ* 318:1240, 1999.

Shaywitz, S. E., B. A. Shaywitz, K. R. Pugh, et al. Functional disorganization for reading in the brain in dyslexia. *Proc Nat Acad Sci USA* 95:2636, 1998.

Shin, L. M., R. J. McNally, S. M. Kosslyn, et al. Regional cerebral blood flow during script-driven imagery in childhood sexual abuse-related PTSD: a PET investigation. *Am J Psychiatry* 156:575, 1999.

Singer, W. Development and plasticity of cortical processing architectures. *Science* 270: 758, 1995.

Smalley, S. L., R. F. Asarnow, M. A. Spence. Autism and genetics. *Arch Gen Psychiatry* 45:953, 1988.

Sobsey, D., W. Randall, R. K. Parilla. Gender differences in abused children with and without disabilities. *Child Abuse Negl* 21:707, 1997.

Soderstrom, H., M. Tullberg, C. Wikkelso, et al. Reduced regional blood flow in non-psychotic violent offenders. *Psychiatry Res* 98:29, 2000.

Spitz, R., G. Cobliner. *First Year of Life: A Psychoanalytic Study of Normal and Deviant Development of Objective Relations.* International Universities Press, Madison, CT, 1966.

Stalenheim, E. G. Testosterone as a biologic marker in psychopaths *Psychiatry Res* 77: 79, 1998.

Steadman, H. J., E. P. Mulvey, J. Monahan, et al. Violence by people discharged from acute psychiatric inpatient facilities and by others in the same neighborhoods. *Arch Gen Psychiatry* 55:393, 1998.

Strakowski, S. M., M. Flaum, X. Amandor, et al. Racial differences in the diagnosis of psychosis. *Schizophr Res* 21:117, 1996.

Sullivan, P. M., J. F. Knutson. Maltreatment and disabilities: a population-based epidemiological study. *Child Abuse Negl* 24:1257, 2000.

Taylor, P. J. Motives for offending among violent psychotic men. *Br J Psychiatry* 147: 491, 1985.

Taylor, P. J., J. Gunn. Violence and psychosis. I. Risk of violence among psychotic men. *BMJ* 30;288, 1984.

Teasdale, T. W., A. Engberg. Duration of cognitive dysfunction after concussion and cognitive dysfunction as a risk factor: a population study of young men. *BMJ* 315: 569, 1997.

Teicher, M. H., et al. Preliminary evidence for abnormal cortical development in physically and sexually abused children using EEG coherence and MRI. *Ann NY Acad Sci* 821: 160, 1997.

Tranel, D. Acquired sociopathy, the development of sociopathic behavior following focal brain damage. *Prog Exp Pers Psychopathol Res* 17:285, 1994.

Ustun, T. B. Cross-national epidemiology of depression and gender. *J Gend Spec Med* 3:54, 2000.

Van Elst, L., F. Woerman, L. Lemieux, et al. Affective aggression in patients with temporal lobe epilepsy: a quantitative study of the amygdala. *Brain* 123:234, 2000.

Volkman, F. R., P. Szatmari, S. S. Sparrow. Sex differences in pervasive developmental disorders *J Autism Dev Disord* 23: 579, 1993.

Wallace, C., P. Muller, P. Burgess, et al. Serious criminal offending and mental disorder case linkage study. *Br J Psychiatry* 172:477, 1998.

Widom, C. S. The cycle of violence. *Science* 244:160,1989.

Widom, C. S., Kuhns, J. B. Childhood victimization and subsequent risk for promiscuity, prostitution, and teenage pregnancy: a prospective study. *Am J Public Health* 86: 1607, 1996.

Wiemann, C. M., A. B. Berenson, V. V. San Miguel. Tobacco, alcohol, and illicit drug use among pregnant women. Age and racial/ethnic differences *J Reprod Med* 39:769, 1994.

Woermann, F., L. van Elst, M. Koepp, et al. Reduction of frontal neocortical grey matter associated with affective aggression in patients with temporal lobe epilepsy: an objective voxel by voxel analysis of automatically segmented MRI. *J Neurol Neurosurg Psychiatry* 68:162, 2000.

Wolfgang, M. Delinquency and violence from the viewpoint of criminality. In: *Neural Bases of Violence and Aggression*, W. S. Fields, W. H. Sweet, eds. Warren Green, St. Louis, 1975, p. 456.

Wong, M., P. Fenwick, G. Fenton, et al. Repetitive and non-repetitive violent offending behavior in male patients in a maximum security mental hospital-clinical and neuroimaging findings. *Med Sci Law* 37:150, 1997.

Wyllie, E., J. P. Glazer, S. Benbadis, et al. Psychiatric features of children and adolescents with pseudoseizures. *Arch Pediatr Adolesc Med* 153:244, 1999.

Yarvis, R. M., Patterns of substance abuse and intoxication among murderers. *Bull Am Acad Psychiatry Law* 22:133, 1994.

Yesavage, J. A., Correlates of dangerous behavior by schizophrenics in a hospital. *J Psychiatr Res* 18:225, 1984.

Chapter Three

SCHIZOPHRENIA

Since the first edition of this book was published in 1974, there has been little change in our ability to diagnose schizophrenia. We now have greater consensus on the diagnostic criteria (DSM-III, DSM-IIIR, and DSM-IV) and we have standardized interviews to reliably apply these criteria. Even with this increased precision, however, the diagnosis is still solely based on history and observation; we do not yet have a laboratory test that can confirm the diagnosis of schizophrenia.

In the early 1970s schizophrenia was the common label for any psychosis. In the U.S., DSM-II (1968) embodied diagnostic criteria that were much broader than European criteria (Hordern et al., 1968; Kendell, 1975). Consequently, schizophrenia was the most common diagnosis for acutely psychotic patients being treated on the newly emerging general hospital psychiatric units. It later became apparent that many of these psychotic patients were not schizophrenic. Many other causes of psychosis emerged: affective disorder, drug reactions, head trauma, seizure disorders, encephalitis, and metabolic disturbances can all mimic schizophrenia. The recent DSM editions have narrowed the definition of schizophrenia and currently we apply the schizophrenic label to a much smaller group of patients, but there is still great variability in probable etiology within this group.

Quite dissimilar patients can meet the current diagnostic criteria for schizophrenia. Is it valid to compare a patient whose onset of symptoms occurred at the age of 15 with one whose onset was at age 35; one who has always had positive symptoms with one who has always had negative symptoms; a patient who shows great disorganization and confusion to a patient with a fixed delusion who is otherwise well organized; someone who has never needed or been given any psychopharmacologic agent with someone who has been treated with many different antipsychotic drugs; a patient with birth complications with a patient who had no birth complications; a patient whose cerebral ventricles are enlarged with a patient whose cerebral ventricles are normal? When one considers the variability of the clinical features of patients who can fit under the rubric of "schizophrenia," it is no wonder that the research findings vary. This leaves many studies to conclude that "these findings are valid for a subgroup of schizophrenic patients." American psychiatry's recent attempts at diagnostic rigor are a vast improvement and have brought us into closer agreement with our colleagues in other countries. Our diagnostic criteria are still basically descriptive, however, and real diagnostic vigor will come only with either biologic or etiologic criteria.

Despite these diagnostic problems, there was an enormous amount of research on schizophrenia during the 1990s, often with conflicting results. There was renewed interest in the gross and microscopic anatomy of the brains of schizophrenic patients. Although no definitive anatomic area of dysfunction has been identified, abnormalities in the frontal lobes and the hippocampus have been described (Bogerts and Falki, 1995). Molecular neurobiologists have made major advances in defining the neurotransmitter systems of the brain but no specific neurotransmitter defect has been definitively linked to the disease, though the roles of dopamine and glutamate in the disease are becoming clearer (Olney and Farber, 1995, Carlsson, 1988). Similarly, there have been many sophisticated genetic studies of schizophrenic families, but no specific gene for schizophrenia has yet been isolated.

In published work over the past decade, there has been less emphasis on psychopathological description. Now the clinician only needs to look for the symptoms required by DSM-IV to make a diagnosis of schizophrenia. There has also been less emphasis on the classical subtypes of schizophrenia (hebephrenic, paranoid, etc.), in favor of dividing schizophrenics into those with positive and negative symptoms (Table 3–1). Although several new antipsychotic drugs have been developed, treatment remains symptom oriented rather than curative.

Schizophrenia is a very complex illness and the answers will not be simple. We do have a better understanding of how the antipsychotic medications work. We also have an intriguing emerging glutamatergic hypothesis that possibly explains some of the clinical phenomenology of schizophrenia. And at last we seem to have research methods that match the complexity of the illness.

Table 3–1 Symptomatic Diagnostic Criteria

Kraepelin (1896)[a]

Disturbances of attention and comprehension
Hallucinations, especially auditory
Audible thoughts
Influenced thoughts
Loosening of Associations
Impaired cognitive function and judgment
Affective flattening
Morbid Behavior (reduced drive, stereotypy, negativism, etc.)
  Course
    Psychic Invalidity

Bleuler (1911)[a]

Fundamental Symptoms (Only fundamental necessary)
  Loose associations
  Impaired affect
  Ambivalence
  Autism

Intact Functions
  Sensation and perception
  Orientation
  Memory
  Consciousness
  Motility

Accessory or secondary symptoms
  Hallucinations and delusions
  Catatonia
  Depressive symptoms

Schnieder's First Rank Symptoms (1939)[a] (any one confirms the diagnosis)

Auditory Hallucinations
  Audible thoughts (voices speaking patient's thoughts aloud)
  Voices arguing (two or more voices arguing usually about patient, refer to patient in third person)
  Voices commenting on patient's actions

Delusional Experiences
  Bodily sensations imposed on patient by some external source
  Thoughts being taken from his mind
  Thoughts ascribed to others
  Diffusion of thoughts (patient's thoughts experienced as all around him)
  Feelings, impulses, volitional acts imposed on him or under control of external sources

(continued)

Table 3–1 Symptomatic Diagnostic Criteria (*continued*)

Delusional Perception (private meaning of a consensually validated perception)

Negative Symptoms of Schizophrenia (1982)[b]

Affective flattening
Alogia (poverty of speech, content of speech, blocking)
Avolition
Apathy
Anhedonia
Asociality
Inattentiveness

Positive Symptoms of Schizophrenia (1982)[b]

Hallucinations
Delusions
Bizarre behavior
Thought disorder
Tangentiality, illogicality, affective lability

DSM-IV (1994)[c]

A. Characteristic Symptoms
Two (or more)[d] of the following, each present for a significant portion of time during a 1-month period (or less if successfully treated):
- Delusions
- Hallucinations
- Disorganized speech (e.g., frequent derailment or incoherence)
- Grossly disorganized or catatonic behavior
- Negative symptoms, i.e., affective flattening, alogia, avolition

B. Social/Occupational Dysfunction
Continuous signs of the disturbance persist for at least 6 months.
(Must include 1 month of symptoms that meet the criteria in A and may include prodromal or residual symptoms.)
Excludes schizoaffective and mood disorders, substance abuse, and general medical conditions

[a] Berner et al. (1983).

[b] Andreasen (1982).

[c] mAPA (1994).

[d] Note: Only one criterion symptom is required if delusions are bizarre or hallucinations consist of a voice keeping up a running commentary on the person's behavior or thoughts, or two or more voices conversing with each other.

CLINICAL FEATURES

Schizophrenia occurs in approximately 1 percent of the population worldwide. The first symptoms usually develop in late adolescence. The primary symptoms are disorganized thinking, delusions, hallucinations, and deteriorating social function. These symptoms usually persist leading to a chronic course (Table 3–2).

In most classifications of schizophrenia, thought disturbance is considered a fundamental symptom. Though all patients may not manifest a specific type of thought disorder to warrant the diagnosis, some defect in cognition must be present during the course of the illness. Certainly one could consider hallucinations and delusions as disturbances of thinking; however, to classify them as such fails to make the distinction between a disturbance of the formal aspects of language structure and a perception or thought that is not consensually validated. A patient with paranoid delusions can appear both coherent and logical but yet be quite delusional. Hallucinations and delusions refer more to perceptions or thoughts that lack consensual validation. It is not usually difficult to recognize delusions and hallucinations, but other types of conceptual disorganization in schizophrenics are often more difficult to grasp (Andreasen, 1979; Taylor and Abrams, 1984).

Bleuler (1950) defined the thought disorder of schizophrenia as *loose associations*. Loose associations were essential for establishing a diagnosis of schizophrenia. Loosening of associations means an absence of normal connections between expressed thoughts. Bleuler gave an extreme example of this symptom. "My last teacher in that subject was Professor A. He was a man with black eyes. I also like black eyes. There are also blue and gray eyes and other sorts too. I have heard it said that snakes have green eyes. All people have eyes" (Bleuler, 1950). In a milder form, the patient's thought pattern may not immediately appear to be abnormal, but after 10 or 15 minutes of conversation, one may not be quite sure what the patient is talking about or how he arrived at a particular point. If the examiner then pays attention to the associative pattern, he or she will find that the patient is constantly switching from one topic to another, often introducing new ideas that are unrelated to what has gone before.

In DSM-IV *derailment* means the same thing as loose associations. *Incoherence,* another manifestation of thought disorder, means that the person's speech is incomprehensible, almost a word salad, with little meaning. At times the speech of schizophrenics is so disorganized that it has an almost aphasic quality, with many word finding difficulties, and neologisms (Critchley, 1964). Faber et al. (1983) explored this by comparing the verbal behavior of schizophrenics with that of aphasics. Although observers were able to distinguish the two groups, there was some overlap. Paraphasic (word finding) errors were equally present in both groups, but the schizophrenics showed more illogicality, loose

Table 3–2 Follow-up Studies of Schizophrenic Patients

AUTHOR	DATES OF STUDY	NUMBER OF SUBJECTS	RESULTS	DURATION OF FOLLOW-UP
Bleuler (1950)	1898–1905	515	After 1st episode 60% able to support selves (mild deterioration) 22% deteriorate (severe) 18% medium deterioration (medium)	
Freyham (1955)	1920–1955	100	54% (sudden onset) out of hospital 24% (gradual onset) out of hospital	35 years
	1940–1955	100	71% (sudden onset) out of hospital 49% (gradual onset) out of hospital	15 years
Israel (1956)	1913–1952	4,254	64.1% discharged 24% permanent hospitalization 60% of all discharged never readmitted	40 years
Mandelbrote (1970)	1963–1963[a]	63	46% discharged in 12 months 64% 1st admissions out for 2 years 26% 1st admissions out and discharged but readmitted	3 years
Roder (1970)	1951–1955	310	28% of admissions under 5 months' stay	3 years
	1956–1960		58% of admissions under 5 months' stay	
	1951–1952		20.8% not readmitted	
	1959–1960		44.4% not readmitted	
Huber (1980)	1945–1973	502	22% complete remission 43% residual but no psychosis	22.4 years
Ciompi (1980)	1963	289	27% recovery 20% mild	37 years
Harding (1987)	1965–1988	269	34% fully recovered 34% considerably recovered 32% no recovery	32 years

[a]Phenothiazines introduced in 1954.

associations, and complex word usage. By giving tests for aphasia to chronic schizophrenics, Goren et al. (1996) were also able to show some similarities between the two disorders.

Another abnormal pattern of thought that has been characterized as fundamental to schizophrenia is overinclusion. This refers to the patient's apparent failure to exclude from his consciousness competing, contradictory, or merely irrelevant thoughts so that his thinking is encumbered with ideas that are insufficiently connected to his main train of thought (Cameron, 1963). Overinclusion, in our view, can be placed under the rubric of loose association.

Another defect in the thought patterns of schizophrenics lies in what has been called the abstract-concrete dimension. The Russian psychologist Vygotsky felt that schizophrenic thought disorder essentially represented a loss of the ability to think abstractly and a tendency toward concreteness (Vygotsky, 1962). Concreteness has been defined as an attitude that is determined by and cannot proceed beyond some immediate experience, object, or stimulus (Mayer-Gross et al., 1969). From his work on patients with brain injuries, Kurt Goldstein developed a similar concept of the "concrete attitude," which be applied to the problem of schizophrenic thinking. Goldstein believed that many of the peculiarities in the behavior of schizophrenics became understandable when they were considered an expression of abnormal concreteness (Goldstein, 1944). He was quick to point out, however, that the level and type of concreteness is not identical with that seen in neurological cases, primarily because of the intrusion of idiosyncratic and personalized ideas in schizophrenic thinking (Goldstein, 1958). Not all schizophrenics seem to be concrete or literal, and some patients, especially those with markedly paranoid features, have even been described as overly abstract.

Among the most striking of the abnormalities of thought and speech in schizophrenics is the idiosyncratic, personalized, and often bizarre character of their verbal expressions (Harrow et al., 1972; Tucker and Rosenberg, 1975). When it is bizarre, this quality is easy to notice, but it may be subtle and become apparent only during a formal mental status examination. The part of the examination that is especially useful for this purpose is proverb interpretation and discernment of similarities and differences. For example, when asked the meaning of "People in glass houses should not throw stones," one of our patients replied, "Because people would see me in my house and throw stones at me." Another, when asked the similarity between an apple and an orange, said, "An apple is round and symbolizes perfection but none of us can be perfect." In these responses one can see aspects of many of the disturbances of thinking mentioned above. During the mental status examination, one may be able to determine not only personalized, bizarre, and idiosyncratic concept formation in schizophrenics but also abnormal concreteness, loose associations, and overinclusive thought. Obviously, there is much overlap in these descriptions of schizophrenic thought patterns. When examining for schizophrenia it is important to use several proverbs and similarities, since abnormal responses may occur only after several adequate answers. Disjointedness, idiosyncrasy, and bizarreness seem to be more characteristic of schizophrenia than of any other psychiatric or neurological condition. If this type of thinking is present, one must suspect schizophrenia.

The other "fundamental" symptoms described by Bleuler are not only still observed, but also pertinent to understanding the clinical phenomenology. He felt that disturbances of affect, ambivalence, and autism were also characteristic of schizophrenic patients, but we now realize are also common to many psychotic and brain damaged patients. *Affect* in schizophrenics is classically described as *flattened*: emotional expression is absent or its range is limited. This is found to be true more frequently in chronic patients; in acute schizophrenic breaks, it is uncommon. The affect may also be *inappropriate* in that a patient can tell a happy story and appear sad or vice versa.

Ambivalence is the capacity of schizophrenic patients to feel intense contradictory emotions at the same time, for instance, to express both hate and love for a person in almost the same breath: "I hate that Dr. X and want to strangle him, that wonderful man who saved my life." Neither ambivalence nor flattened affect is consistently present in schizophrenia; therefore, we do not feel that either is necessary for diagnosis.

Bleuler defined *autism* as a break with external reality, in which the patient becomes preoccupied with his inner life. External events may become so blended with subjective feelings or fantasy that the patient sees them as relating specifically to him; at this point such symptoms could be called delusional or hallucinatory, an example is the patient thinks that the people in the television show, that all the patients in the day room are watching, are commenting on his behavior and specifically telling him what to do. Autism in schizophrenics appears to be a behavioral result of thought disorder.

AGE AT ONSET AND GENDER

Schizophrenia is primarily a disease of young people. Kraeplin noted that most patients were under the age of 35 at the time of diagnosis, a finding that has been confirmed in many studies. The first clear-cut symptoms appear before the age of 25 in 50 percent of the cases; onset after the age of 40 is unusual (Kraeplin, 1925). Although Jeste and colleagues (Jeste et al., 1995, 1998) have described a group of patients (most frequently women), with a history of good social functioning, who had their first episode of schizophrenia after the age of 45. This late-onset schizophrenia seems unrelated to any dementing process or cerebral insult. These patients meet all the diagnostic criteria for schizophrenia.

Symptoms of schizophrenia rarely begin in the first decade, but when they do, they virtually always occur in the latter half, seldom before the age of 5. Childhood schizophrenia has often been confused with infantile autism; a condition that usually begins in the first year of life and that always appears before age 5 (see p. 162).

Recent studies of schizophrenia have also delineated interesting gender differences. Szymanski et al. (1995) reported that the onset of schizophrenic symptoms tends to occur between the ages of 15 and 25 in men and between the ages of 25 and 35 in women. They also presented evidence that the course of the illness is milder in women. Men seem to have poorer outcomes, higher relapse rates, and more hospitalizations. These gender differences are interesting findings in light of recent studies that have shown consistent neural differences by gender. Shaywitz et al. (1995) have shown that women have more diffuse neural networks for language. Harasty et al., (1997) demonstrated that women's temporal lobes have larger volumes than men's do. There is also a whole range of well-known neuroendocrine differences.

CHANGING DIAGNOSTIC CRITERIA AND SYMPTOMATIC CLASSIFICATIONS

In 1980, the publication of the American Psychiatric Association's Diagnostic and Statistical Manual III (DSM-III) made the diagnostic criteria very specific, but the symptoms used were not new. From Table 3–1 it is clear that the symptoms used to establish the DSM-III diagnostic criteria were a mixture of the diagnostic symptoms used by Krapelin, Bleuler, and Schneider. In 1987, DSM-IIIR changed the diagnostic criteria again, reducing the requirement that acute schizophrenic symptoms be present from 1 month to a single week. DSM-IIIR also did away with the criterion that the onset of illness had to occur before the age of 45 years. In 1994, DSM-IV returned to the 1-month acute phase criterion and added negative symptoms to the positive ones. These rapid changes in diagnostic criteria not only highlight the descriptive and arbitrary nature of the diagnostic process but also make it hard to compare research using diagnostic criteria developed at different times.

The historical diagnostic subtypes of schizophrenia (hebephrenic, catatonic, undifferentiated, etc.) have proven to be of little clinical utility. A symptomatic distinction that does seem to have some clinical value has been the categorization by positive and negative symptoms (Table 3–1). Negative symptoms are characterized by an absence of affect and few verbal productions. Patients with positive symptoms have hallucinations, delusions, and the more vivid florid symptoms (Andreasen, 1982; Andreasen and Olsen, 1982; Andreasen et al., 1995; Buchanan and Carpenter, 1997). This distinction is similar to the older and well-studied concept of *process* and *reactive* schizophrenia, with the process schizophrenic having a preponderance of negative symptoms and a poor prognosis and the reactive having the more florid positive symptoms with a better prognosis (Phillips, 1953; Kantor and Herron, 1966). Both of these symptomatic distinctions recognize the difficulty in treating the patient's negative symptoms. The positive symptoms have always seemed more amenable to antipsychotic treatment than the negative symptoms. Recently, however, investigators have observed that the new atypical antipsychotic medications are wholly or partially effective for the treatment of negative symptoms (Buchanan et al., 1996; Rosenheck et al., 1997). (The term *atypical* is used for the recently developed antipsychotics such as clozapine, olanzapine, risperidone, quetiapine, sertindole, and ziprasidone, whose mechanisms of action seem somewhat different from the older neuroleptics. These new atypical drugs have fewer extrapyramidal side effects, and are weak D2 antagonists.) However the positive and negative distinction may be artificial. It is not clear if positive (reactive) or negative (process) symptoms represent something about schizophrenia, psychosis in general, or brain damage. At some point in their illness, the same schizophrenic patient can manifest either predominantly positive or negative symptoms; and many schizophrenic patients will have both types of symptoms during the same episode of illness (Carpenter, 1992). Negative symptoms have also been observed in patients with Alzheimer's disease who are not psychotic (Reichman et al., 1996). A recent study by Ratakonda et al. (1998) of a large sample of schizophrenic and nonschizophrenic psychotic patients ($n = 412$) has shown great overlap in both positive and negative symptoms in both groups. Consequently the effectiveness of the new atypicals for negative symptoms may simply represent another nonspecific effect of these drugs in the treatment of psychosis.

SCHIZOAFFECTIVE DISORDER

The term *schizoaffective* is used to indicate the presence of both schizophrenic and affective symptoms that meet the DSM-IV criteria for schizophrenia and affective disorder (DSM-IV 1994). How this disorder relates to either schizophrenia or bipolar affective disorder is still in question. There are indications that it is primarily an affective disorder (Pope et al., 1980; Winokur, 1989). From a study of 39 schizoaffective patients, their family histories, and first-degree relatives, Clayton et al. (1968) found more affective disease in the families and concluded that schizoaffective disorder is a genetic variant of affective illness. This conclusion was supported by data from a review of 420 twin pairs selected from military veterans in which one or both twins were psychotic (Cohen et al., 1972). The concordance rate for schizoaffective disorder in this group was the same as that for manic-depressive illness (50%) and more than twice as high as that for schizophrenia.

Clayton (1982) noted that the manic schizoaffective cases seemed more of a variant of bipolar disorder (perhaps a more severe form). The depressed cases seemed more heterogeneous, consisting of both depressed schizophrenics and patients with primary affective disorders. Schizoaffective patients are less successfully treated than typical bipolar patients (Strakowski et al., 1999) and the psychosis in a group of schizoaffective patients persists despite treatment compared to the psychosis of typical bipolar patients. The difficulty in successfully treating schizoaffective symptoms places the condition closer to schizophrenia.

PERSONALITY DISORDERS AND SCHIZOPHRENIA

Paranoid, borderline, avoidant (social inhibition), schizoid (a pattern of poor social contacts and little emotional expression), and schizotypal (poor social contacts plus cognitive or perceptual distortions and eccentricities) personality disorders have been associated with schizophrenia. In a case-controlled study of 534 schizophrenics and 2043 of their relatives, Kendler et al. (1993) clarified this relationship. Schizotypal personality disorders have a strong familial link to schizophrenia. Paranoid, schizoid, and avoidant personality disorders are modestly but significantly associated with schizophrenia. Borderline personality disorder is not related to schizophrenia.

Some have classified these personality disorders (schizoid, schizotypal, paranoid disorders) as schizophrenia spectrum disorders. Thaker et al. (1993) found a much higher rate of schizophrenia and schizophrenia spectrum personality disorders in the relatives of schizophrenia spectrum personality disorders than in controls. These findings indicate that the schizophrenia spectrum disorders are probably genetic variants of schizophrenia and, like schizophrenia, are genetically transmitted.

COURSE AND NATURAL HISTORY

Kraepelin's original clinical delineation of schizophrenia as a disease entity was made primarily on the basis of its poor prognosis; he postulated that schizophrenic patients manifested a consistently progressive deteriorating course over time without full recovery. Psychotic patients who recovered were not schizophrenic by definition. In recent years, this has been questioned. Manfred Bleuler, for instance, described several patterns of evolution of the disease. One pattern, which varies in severity, is characterized by gradual deterioration over time, and another pattern is episodic. In the episodic course, complete or partial remissions are punctuated by acute exacerbation (Bleuler, 1968). Bleuler also noted that the milder chronic conditions have increased in frequency and that the severe chronic conditions have diminished. This trend has been observed by others, who also noted shorter psychotic episodes and less bizarre, generally more moderate symptoms (Grinker, 1972; Remar and Hagopian, 1972; Harding et al., 1987). Some of the investigators believe this change in the phenomenology may be related to the increased use of psychopharmacological agents. Others feel that it represents less repression and greater tolerance of deviance in our contemporary society and take this as evidence that schizophrenia is a culturally determined disorder.

However, the actual symptoms seem to have changed very little. In a study of the charts of schizophrenic patients hospitalized in 1850 and 1950, only minor differences were noted in the symptoms and course (Klaf and Hamilton, 1961). The most marked differences between the two groups were in the kind of delusions the patients had. Patients in 1850 tended to be preoccupied with religion, whereas patients in 1950 were more preoccupied with sex. The average age, the proportion of married to single patients, and the incidence of mental illness in the patients' families were the same. Though hospital stays were twice as long in the nineteenth as in the twentieth century, the percentages of cure in both centuries were the same. The remarkable similarity of the symptoms, family history, age of patients, and clinical course lends credence to the concept that schizophrenia is a disease of the brain rather than an individual response to environmental stimuli.

It is notable that Kraepelin studied his patients over a long period of time. Though many of these patients made short-term recoveries, they all ultimately deteriorated. Current data suggest that his prognostic view was unnecessarily gloomy (Huber et al., 1975; Ciompi, 1980; Harding et al., 1987). Harding et al. (1987) in a 30-year follow-up of schizophrenic patients, using DSM-III criteria for diagnosis and standardized rating scales, found that one-half to two-thirds had achieved improvement or had recovered. An interesting and unexplained empirical finding in the natural history of schizophrenia is an inordinately high death rate. Ciompi (1980) noted that the average mortality in his study group of schizophrenics was almost twice as high as is expected in a normal population of the same age. This high rate of death in schizophrenics has been noted by others (Niswander et al., 1963; Tsuang et al., 1979; Schwab et al., 1988; Winokur and Tsuang, 1996).

One of the main obstacles to long-term prospective studies in this country is the strong tradition of divorcing hospital treatment from outpatient treatment. The hospital psychiatrist seldom follows his patient through into outpatient treatment. After discharge, the patients return to their homes, group homes or other community facilities, or to the streets in the metropolitan areas where attempts to establish outpatient treatment are made. Often all contacts with the patient are lost. This not only complicates patient care but makes good follow-up studies much more difficult. Table 3–2 is a summary of some of the follow-up studies done over the years.

Various forms of psychoeducational treatment (a form of patient and family education about the illness rather than a strict psychotherapeutic approach) have been reported to yield better outcomes for schizophrenic patients, preventing relapse and improving quality of life (Davis et al., 1993; Penn and Mueser, 1996). When 151 schizophrenics, who had been ill 6–10 years, were treated with a form of individual psychoeducational therapy and medication, only 29 percent had recurrent psychotic episodes resulting in hospitalization during the 3-year study period (Hogarty et al., 1997).

DIFFERENTIAL DIAGNOSIS

Differentiating from Other Psychiatric Disorders

It is often difficult on the basis of the clinical presentation alone, to accurately diagnose a patient during an acute psychotic state, particularly if this is the patient's first psychotic episode. If one took a 5-minute video tape of a patient with schizophrenia, mania, psychotic depression, or an other patient who has delusions and hallucinations it would be almost impossible to make the diagnosis from the video tape alone. The phenomenology of all acutely psychotic patients is very similar. The key factors in differentiating schizophrenia from other psychiatric disorders are the history of the illness, the demographics of each condition, and the family history. For example with the manic patient there is usually a history of mood swings and alternating depressive and manic episodes, with periods of normality between; the psychotic depressive is usually older and shows clear symptoms of affective disorder with mood congruent delusions. The young patient who is experiencing his first psychotic break poses the most difficult diagnostic problem. Often we must treat the psychosis symptomatically and follow the patient over a period of time before making a definitive diagnosis. In a young patient with acute psychosis bipolar disorder, intoxication, drug withdrawal, metabolic encephalopathy, infection, seizures, thyroid disease, organ failure, and hypoglycemia are important considerations.

Brief psychotic disorders (DSM-IV) have the symptoms of schizophrenia for at least a day but for no longer than a month. Many Europeans call such episodes hysterical or psychogenic psychosis. Hirsch and Hollender (1969) described hysterical psychosis as a "state marked by a sudden and dramatic onset, temporarily related to a profoundly upsetting event." Patients may have hallucinations and delusions, and they may engage in unusual behavior; thought disorder is transient and circumscribed, and affect is volatile rather than flat. The acute episode typically lasts 1 to 3 weeks and leaves no residual symptoms. Most clinicians have seen dramatic cases of this type, which are more common in some subcultures than in others, but the question arises as to the relation of these episodes to the psychotic disorders they resemble, especially schizophrenia. European psychiatrists make a clear distinction between schizophrenia and psychogenic psychosis. Stromgren (1974) describes psychogenic psychosis as follows: *(1)* the psychosis would not have arisen without some distinct mental trauma, which often makes it easy to understand the etiology. *(2)* There tends to be a psychological predisposition, of a neurotic or psychopathic nature, to the reactions that represent hysterical psychosis, but no genetic relationship with schizophrenia exists. *(3)* There must be a close temporal relation between the onset of trauma and of psychosis, and the psychosis often ends shortly after the trauma does. There are no residual symptoms. Hysterical psychosis takes three common forms: *(1)* emotional reactions that are usually depressive, *(2)* alterations of consciousness or clouded states (see Chapter 6, pp. 97–98), and *(3)* paranoid states and delusions. These conditions can be distinguished from schizophrenia by applying the diagnostic criteria for the latter.

Neurological Diseases

Any disease of the central nervous system or disruption of its function (e.g., by drugs, sleep deprivation, etc.) may cause behavioral manifestations that mimic schizophrenia. The differential diagnosis rests heavily on the type of symptoms present, the mode of onset, the family history of mental illness, the medical history, and the clinical course (Yudofsky and Hales, 1997; Tucker, 1997, 1998).

Schizophrenia is not the only condition that can cause disturbances of thinking, though schizophrenia, affective disorder, and drug-induced psychoses are by far the most common causes of such symptoms in young adults. Because of its high incidence, there is a strong temptation to make the diagnosis of schizophrenia whenever a young person develops a serious cognitive disturbance. Schizophrenia-like episodes, however, have been described in association with other psychiatric disorders and with other neurological conditions such as cerebral trauma, tumor, encephalitis, presenile degeneration and other degenerative diseases of the gray and white matter, narcolepsy, vascular disorders, and a host of metabolic or toxic disorders, such as endocrinopathies, cerebral anoxia, and hypercapnia (Davison and Bagley, 1969). Though psychoses are commonly seen in these conditions, they rarely mimic the symptoms of schizophrenia exactly; the disorientation, memory deficit, confusion, and fluctuating states of consciousness that are characteristic of some neurological diseases are seldom encountered in schizophrenia. The difficulty in differentiating schizophrenia from neurological conditions arises mainly in the initial onset of neurological disease.

Most neurological diseases will either progress to overt neurological symptoms or else clear up completely. So our comments deal mostly with diagnostic problems of acute onset. The mistake often made by inexperienced clinicians is to label as schizophrenic any bizarre, delusional, or mute behavior that cannot be easily explained by a familiar medical condition. Clinicians faced with delusions and hallucinations, often overlook such overt signs of disorientation, dysmnesia, tremor, myoclonic jerks, Babinski reflexes, and asterixis or other clear evidence that the disorder is neurological.

In addition to disorientation and dysmnesia, there are a few simple guidelines for the differentiation of acute neurological disease from classical schizophrenia. In the former there are usually: *(1)* A good premorbid social history. The patient does not have problems at work and his family is generally warm and supportive rather than disturbed, as is so often the case in schizophrenia (Wynne, 1968). Sociability is characteristically preserved in most neurological disorders until a very late stage of deterioration, long after disorientation and dysmnesia have appeared. In schizophrenia, early loss of sociabiliy is common. *(2)* An abrupt change in personality, mood, and ability to function at work and at home of less than 6 months' duration. The abruptness of the onset of such symptoms supports a neurological cause. *(3)* Rapid fluctuations in mental status. The patient has a clouded sensorium and is disoriented one day, then completely oriented the next. Though fluctuations can also be seen in some schizophrenics, they are generally not so rapid. Even when the schizophrenic's mental status seems to clear suddenly, he will still show some signs of bizarre behavior or delusional thinking. Marked fluctuations in mental status are, in general, more characteristic of acute neurological disease than schizophrenia, but this is not necessarily true of chronic neurological disease. The fluctuations in mental status of neurological patients may also be accompanied by fluctuating motor behavior. The patient may display aggressive impulses and engage in assaultive behavior at one moment but at the next apologize profusely and try to befriend the people be has just abused. The mode of behavior during this period frequently has a driven quality to it, as has been described in brain-injured patients by Goldstein and Scheerer (1941) and Kahn (1934). *(4)* A patient with an acute neurological problem is usually unresponsive to psychiatric intervention, whether psychotherapeutic or pharmacological. Rather than controlling behavior, psychopharmacological agents may precipitate a stuporous or comatose state depending on the underlying condition.

Many patients who present with bizarre behavior and mute states are shunted immediately to the psychiatrist. Even major neurological signs can be overlooked or interpreted as part of the patient's "functional" disturbance. It goes without saying that marked behavioral aberrations should not blind clinicians to neurological symptoms.

Drug Reactions

Symptoms suggesting schizophrenia are commonly seen in patients who have taken amphetamines, cocaine, LSD, mescaline, ketamine, and belladonna alkaloids. Hallucinations and psychosis may also accompany alcohol and barbiturate withdrawal. These states of intoxication and withdrawal may cause a psychosis without major disorientation (though this is rare) as well as any of the physical changes seen in the neurological impaired. The presence of visual hallucinations, however, should always suggest the possibility of a drug reaction or a toxic or metabolic encephalopathy. Formed visual hallucinations are unusual in schizophrenia and in diseases that affect the macroscopic structure of the brain (e.g., brain tumors). Auditory hallucinations, however, are common in schizophrenia and unusual in drug reactions.

Sleep Disorders

Prolonged inability to sleep may produce disorganized thought patterns and even such major distortions of reality as illusions, delusions, and hallucinations. It is possible that this happens only in individuals with a schizophrenic predisposition. Resumption of a normal sleep pattern in such individuals will resolve their symptoms quickly. Residual thought disorder persists in most schizophrenics even after normal sleep has been restored (Berger and Oswald, 1962).

BIOLOGIC BASIS OF SCHIZOPHRENIA

Early editions of this book properly emphasized the genetic and neurological findings in schizophrenic patients to make the case that schizophrenia was a disorder of the brain. At that time the identification of schizophrenia with the brain was controversial; many conceptualized schizophrenia as primarily a "psychological" reaction to an abnormal environment, a view that is no longer respectable. We now look at the genetic and neurological findings in schizophrenia as clues to the etiology of this disorder and no longer argue about whether such findings exist.

Genetics

The incidence of schizophrenia in the general population is approximately 1 percent. The data obtained in epidemiological surveys of schizophrenia in different countries and cultures are similar, and all investigators agree that the incidence is increased in families of schizophrenics and is highest in their first-degree relatives. The rate is roughly 10 to 15 percent in the parents, siblings, and children of schizophrenics. This consistency is remarkable considering the differences and imprecision of the various diagnostic criteria applied.

There have been many twin studies of schizophrenia in the U.S., the U.K., Japan, Germany, and Scandinavia. In all but one (Tienari, 1963), the incidence of schizophrenia is much higher in monozygote than dizygotic twins of schizophrenics (Gottesman and Sheilds, 1982; McGuffin et al., 1995). The overall incidence of schizophrenia in the monozygotic twins of schizophrenics is 61 percent. In the dizygotic twins studied, there was a 12 percent concordance rate. These figures do not change in twin studies that use more modern diagnostic criteria (DSM-III and IIIR) for schizophrenia (Farmer et al., 1987; Onstad et al., 1991).

Another approach to testing the environmental hypothesis was taken in a study of the psychosocial adjustment of 47 adults born to schizophrenic mothers and permanently separated from their mothers in the first few days of life (Heston, 1966). They were compared to 50 control adults with nonschizophrenic mothers who had also been permanently separated from their natural mothers in the first few days of life. The comparison was based on a review of school, police, army, and hospital records, plus a personal interview and personality testing using the Minnesota Multiphasic Personality Inventory (MMPI). Social-class determinations and IQ testing were also done, and three psychiatrists independently rated the subjects. In this study, schizophrenia was significantly more prevalent in the individuals born to schizophrenic mothers. Of 47 persons with schizophrenic mothers, 5 were schizophrenic. No cases of schizophrenia were found in the 50 control subjects. The age-corrected rate for schizophrenia in the experimental group was 16.6 percent, a finding consistent with that of all the family studies that had been done on children raised by schizophrenic biological parents. In addition, serious psychosocial disability, that is, psychiatric diagnosis other than schizophrenia was found in approximately half of the persons born to schizophrenic mothers. An increased incidence of schizophrenia-related personality disorders has also been noted in the families of schizophrenic patients (Kendler et al., 1985). Many had been discharged from the armed forces for behavioral reasons; others had police records or a history of alcoholism. The diagnosis of sociopathic personality was more than 4 times as common in the experimental group, in which 5 times as many persons spent more than 1 year in a penal or psychiatric institution.

These findings were substantiated by an independent study (Kety, 1976). In this study, 364 first-degree relatives of 33 schizophrenic adoptees and controls (nonschizophrenic adoptees) living in Copenhagen, Denmark, were interviewed by a man who did not know the relationship of the person he was interviewing to the adoptee. In almost all cases, the relative being interviewed did not know of the relationship or the adoptee's diagnosis. From summaries of these interviews, three independent raters made a psychiatric diagnosis. After a consensus was reached among these three psychiatrists, the subjects were divided into four groups: biological or adoptive relatives of schizophrenic index adoptees (two groups) and biological or adoptive relatives of control adoptees (two groups). The prevalence of schizophrenic illness (chronic schizophrenia, latent schizophrenia, and uncertain schizophrenia) in subjects genetically related to the schizophrenic index cases was 13.9 percent. The prevalence of schizophrenic illness among the adoptive relatives of schizophrenics was 2.7 percent, and it was 3.8 percent in all subjects not genetically related to a schizophrenic index case. The difference between the group genetically related to the schizophrenic index cases and the group not so related is highly significant. These relatives did not differ from the rest, however, with regard to mental illness other than schizophrenia. This study was replicated in the entire population of Denmark in 1994 with similar results (Kety et al., 1994; Ingraham and Kety, 2000) and in Finland (Tienari et al., 2000).

Although molecular genetic techniques hold much promise for unraveling the genetic basis of schizophrenia, the results to date of molecular approaches have not been conclusive. Neither association studies nor linkage studies have identified a specific genetic locus for schizophrenia. Suggestive sites that have been implicated but only variably replicated include the short arms of chromosomes 6 and 8, the long arm of chromosomes 2, 11, 22 as well as the X and Y chromosomes; and the HLA region of 6p. Attempts to locate specific defects in the chromosomal areas of genes that control neurotransmitter systems such as dopamine have also been inconclusive (Kendler, 1999).

Molecular genetics demands a precise identification of the disorder to be studied. Perhaps we do not yet have this precision in the study of complex behavioral disorders. In Huntington's disease, an autosomal dominant disorder for which the exact genetic defect has been identified, several different psychiatric syndromes can occur during the illness, ranging from affective to schizophrenia-like symptoms. Jason et al. (1997) have shown that although the severity of the cognitive decline and early onset of Huntington's disease is related to the number of trinucleotide repeats (CAG) on the Huntington's gene, the number of repeats was not associated with the varied psychiatric manifestations seen in Huntington's that is, the patients with more repeats were not more or less likely to be psychotic as their dementia progressed (Zappacosta et al., 1996). Similarly, the newly described Velo-cardio-facial syndrome has been associated with schizophrenia, bipolar disorder, and attention-deficit hyperactivity dsiorder (ADHD) and is clearly related to a deletion on chromosome 22q11 (Lachman et al., 1996). The deletion of this chromosome leads to a lack of catechol-o-methyltransferase, one of the enzymes that catabolizes dopamine. Varied psychiatric manifestations have also been noted in the fragile X syndrome (Levitas, 1996). It is possible that what is genetically transmitted is a general predisposition to psychosis or behavioral disorder that could be modified by the individual's environment (Kendler et al., 1985, 1997; Cloninger, 1994; Crow, 1994) or other genes that modify behavior. Erlenmeyer-Kimling et al. (1995, 1997) studied the offspring of patients with schizophrenia and found many unspecified psychotic conditions and affective psychoses in them.

A recent postmortem study examined the brains of 15 patients with schizophrenia, 15 with bipolar disorder (11 psychotic), 15 with nonpsychotic unipolar depression, and 15 controls. Compared to the controls and the nonpsychotic bipolar and unipolar depressed patients, the psychotic patients, both those with schizophrenia and bipolar disorders, had 50 percent reduction in the messenger RNA for reelin and glutamate decarboxylase in the prefrontal cortex. Reelin is a large intracellular lipoprotein that is involved in the develoment of architectonic patterns in hippocampus and in cortex and seems to be involved in learning and the early growth and development of neuronal architecture (Guidotti et al., 2000). Reduction in reelin and glutamate decarboxylase may represent genetically transmitted nonspecific factors that lead to a vulnerability to psychosis; this vulnerability, interacting with other genetic disorders, may produce a variety of diseases, such as schizophrenia, bipolar disorder, Huntington's disease, etc.

In summary, there is a clear genetic component in schizophrenia. The risk increases with the number of relatives already affected. McGuffin et al. (1995) noted that the risk of becoming schizophrenic increases from 9 percent to 16 percent when both a parent and sibling have the disorder. The risk is slightly higher than 10 percent if the mother alone is schizophrenic and developed the condition early in her adolescence. The risk is even higher (46%) when both parents have the disorder. Still, 60 percent of schizophrenics do not have first- or second-degree relatives with the disease. (Bleuler, 1978). The most credible contemporary hypothesis at this stage is that what is transmitted is a predisposition or vulnerability to develop schizophrenia; also required are the presence of other genes and environmental factors to produce the illness (Kendell, 1991; Maier et al., 1993; McGuffin et al., 1995).

Biochemical Findings

Molecular biology has greatly expanded our capacity to identify and to localize neurotransmitter receptors in the brain in specific anatomic areas, and it has considerably amplified our view of the complexity the central nervous system. Instead of one dopamine receptor, for example, at least five have been identified, conveniently titled D1–D5; as many as 15 serotonin receptor subtypes have also been identified (Cooper et. al., 1996). The fact that most of the agents that are effective in treating schizophrenia block dopamine has led to the hypothesis that schizophrenia is related to an excess of dopamine (Breier, 1996).

The anatomic localization of the dopamine receptors is consistent with the functional imaging and neuropathologic abnormalities described in schizophrenia. The five postsynaptic dopamine receptors are distributed differently in the brain. In the brain the D1 receptors are found chiefly in the cortex; D2 receptors are prominent in the striatum (presumably the source of drug induced Parkinsonism and other extrapyramidal symptoms caused by dopamine receptor blocking drugs); the D3 and D4 receptors are found mainly in the limbic system; and D5 receptors are mainly in the hippocampus and to some extent in the thalamus. Actually, all five dopamine receptors have some representation in the thalamus and hippocampus. There are three major pathways taken by the dopaminergic axons whose terminals lead to dopaminergic receptors. All three dopamine pathways originate from cell bodies in the substantia nigra in the midbrain's ventral tegmentum. The first set projects to the caudate and putamen (nigrostriatal); The second set to the medial prefrontal, cingulate, and entorhinal cortex (mesocortical); and the third projects to the septum, nucleus accumbens, amygdala, olfactory tubercle, and piriform cortex (mesolimbic). There are also localized sites of dopaminergic neurons in the olfactory bulbs, the pituitary, and the hypothalamus.

Evidence that schizophrenia derives from excessive sensitivity to dopamine is inferential. Most antipsychotic drugs block D2 receptors. Direct evidence for dopamine hyperactivity in schizophrenia has been minimal. An increased quantity of D2 receptors has been reported in the postmortem brains of schizophrenic patients. This has been presumed to be the basis for excessive dopaminergic function in schizophrenia (Cooper et al., 1996). The increase, however, in D2 receptor density may well be the result of neuroleptic use in the patients rather than the primary cause of the illness. The fact that clozapine, an effective antipsychotic drug, has its primary action on the D4 receptors and almost none on the D2 receptors raises a question about the role of the D2 receptors in mediating psychosis.

Actually, clozapine has at least some blocking action at all five of the dopamine receptors, as well as four of the serotonin receptors. Serotonin excess has been proposed as an alternative cause of schizophrenia. The major serotonin receptors fall into three classes: those that use protein G transduction as a second messenger, those that use phosphoinositol transduction, and those that use ion-gated channel transduction. Serotonergic neurons send their axons over two major pathways in the brain originating from the raphe nuclei, where their cell bodies are located. One projects from the dorsal raphe to the cortex and striatal regions, and the other from the median raphe to the limbic regions (Kapur et al., 1996). Serotonin neurons tend to inhibit dopamine neurons. Blocking serotonin might improve a postulated dopamine hypofunction in the prefrontal areas by disinhibiting the dopamine neurons. The beneficial effect of the atypical antipsychotic drugs on the negative symptoms of schizophrenia has been thought to result from the frontal lobe stimulation that serotonin blockade produces. This concept questions the hypothesis of schizophrenia being related to a hyperdopaminergic state. The fact that clozapine is also a potent antagonist of adrenergic, muscarinic, and histaminic systems also potentially implicates these neurotransmitters in the drug's therapeutic actions and in systems that may be altered in schizophrenia.

Although some studies have shown increased norepinephrine levels in schizophrenic patients, it has been difficult to separate these levels from the possibility of a secondary stress-induced reaction (Litman and Pickar, 1996). There is some evidence that an experimental alpha-2 adrenergic blocking agent may improve treatment response (Litman and Pickar, 1996). Some have also postulated that the muscarinic cholinergic system may be important in establishing a balance with dopamine to ameliorate the positive symptoms of schizophrenia and that increased muscarinic activity in itself may intensify the negative symptoms of schizophrenia (Tandon and Greden, 1991). To complicate the picture even further, Sharma et al. (1997) presented rather convincing data indicating that low neurotensin levels in schizophrenia become elevated with antipsychotic drug treatment. It is clear that there are many systems that interact with dopamine; and it also clear that blocking dopamine receptors ameliorates many of the symptoms but does not cure schizophrenia. It is also likely that dopamine plays some role in the complex and dynamic biochemical processes that underlie schizophrenia.

Using similarities in the biochemical and clinical effects of pharmacologic agents, some have postulated a role for glutamate in schizophrenia. Glutamate neurons are located in the pyramidal cells of the cerebral cortex, the granule cells of the hippocampus, and the pathways from the thalamus to the cortex. All are areas in which abnormalities have been found in the neuroimaging and neuropathologic studies of schizophrenic brains. Drugs that inhibit the activity of glutamate neurons can reproduce many of the clinical symptoms of schizophrenia and one of the most interesting of these is phencyclidine (PCP), a major antagonist of the glutamate NMDA receptor. Clinically, this produces a psychosis that is similar to schizophrenia, manifested by delusions and hallucinations and disorganization of thoughts and speech. When injected repeatedly into rat brains for 3 to 4 days, PCP and other NMDA antagonists, cause subtle, permanent neurodegenerative changes in the corticolimbic region. These changes and their distribution are very similar to those that have been described in postmortem studies of schizophrenic brains (Benes et al., 1991). The changes are age-dependent in that rats do not become susceptible to them until they are approximately 10 months of age. This has a human parallel, as children seem not to be as susceptible to the psychotogenic effects of PCP as are adults.

On the basis of these observations, it has been proposed that schizophrenia could result from a genetic deficit of NMDA receptors. The clinical, behavioral, and cognitive disorganization and gating defects noted in schizophrenic patients are also evident in PCP-induced psychosis. Hypofunction of the excitatory glutamate NMDA receptors on inhibitory gamma-aminobutyric acid (GABA) neurons would have a net excitatory effect. When GABA neurons are not stimulated, there is less inhibition and hence more excitation. This might cause the cortical areas in which these neurons are located to lose their ability to filter incoming information. This might be the cellular explanation for the clinical experience of the schizophrenic patient who describes being flooded with unmodulated information. Dopamine inhibits glutamate release and could also lead to disinhibition. Dopamine blocking drugs, by correcting this, could reverse psychosis (Olney and Farber, 1995; Coyle, 1996). The consideration of glutamate's role in schizophrenia has added another dimension to the complex biochemical state that schizophrenia seems to represent.

Neurological Abnormalities in Schizophrenic Patients

Minor physical and neurological abnormalities are commonly found in schizophrenia (Heinrichs and Buchanan, 1988). Although the effects of medication, malnutrition, and multiple electrical shock treatment may have something to do with these abnormalities they have been most often related to environmental influences such as perinatal trauma, prenatal infection, autoimmune disorders, and prenatal malnutrition (Susser, 1999). Abnormalities include minor motor and sensory (soft) neurological signs on physical examination, electroencephalographic abnormalities, changes in information processing, and organic patterns on psychological tests. All of these minor neurological findings no longer seem inexplicable or incidental in light of the recent histological and structural changes observed in the brains of schizophrenics. The question has now turned to the implications of these findings, e.g., do these findings imply that schizophrenia is a neurodegenerative process, such as Alzheimer's, or is it more related to a prenatal maldevelopment process (Woods, 1998).

Minor, nonlocalizing neurological abnormalities. Soft signs have been noted in many studies of acute schizophrenic adult patients (Kennard, 1960; Larsen, 1964; Pollin and Stabenau, 1968; Rochford et al., 1970, Heinrichs and Buchanan, 1988; Flashman et al., 1996; Arango et al., 1999; Karp et al., 2001) and adolescent schizophrenics (Hertzig and Birch, 1966, 1968). Rochford and colleagues (1970) examined 65 hospitalized, untreated psychiatric patients for the presence of the following minor signs: *(1)* motor impersistence; *(2)* astereognosis; *(3)* agraphesthesia; *(4)* extinction during bilateral simultaneous stimulation; *(5)* excessive bilateral hyperreflexia; *(6)* coordination defects; *(7)* disturbance of balance and gait; *(8)* cortical sensory abnormalities; *(9)* mild movement disorders; *(10)* speech defects; *(11)* abnormal motor activity; *(12)* defective auditory-visual integration; *(13)* choreiform movements and adventitious motor overflow (tremor); *(14)* cranial nerve abnormalities, such as slight anisocoria, esotropia, auditory deficit, and visual field and retinal defects; and *(15)* unequivocally abnormal EEGs. He found neurological abnormalities in 36.8 percent of the psychiatric patients (all diagnostic groups). This was significantly different from an age-matched normal control population (5%). Neurological soft signs were found in 65.5 percent of the schizophrenic patients. By way of comparison, there were no soft signs in patients with primary affective disorders.

In 72.5 percent of schizophrenics, Pollin and Stabenau (1968) found at least one neurological sign. The most common neurological abnormalities in Pollin's schizophrenic patients were defects in stereognosis; graphesthesia; difficulty in coordination, balance, and gait; and tremor. There was also some difficulty in the integration of auditory-visual stimuli.

In several studies, not only has an increased incidence of soft signs in schizophrenic patients been observed, but also a high correlation between these signs and thought disorder, especially overinclusive thinking. The relation of neurological impairment to thought disorder is stronger than its relations to the diagnostic category of schizophrenia (Tucker et al., 1974; Tucker and Silberfarb, 1975). The main tests for these neurological impairments were specific sensorimotor portions of the Halstead-Reitan battery (e.g., finger agnosia, fingertip writing, tactile form recognition, and the tactile performance test). Davies et al. (1975) found a high correlation of neurological soft signs and behavioral symptoms in schizophrenics, especially those with paroxysmally abnormal EEGs. Quitkin et al. (1976) found more neurological soft signs in schizophrenics with premorbid asocial behavior as well as in individuals with emotionally unstable character disorders—two conditions that are generally chronic. Rosenbaum (1971) noted defects in schizophrenic patients with regard to weight discrimination and proprioception. He postulated that these defects are related to "insufficiently articulated proprioceptive signals . . . in schizophrenic persons." The abnormalities he found can be considered soft signs, similar to those observed in the studies cited above.

Abnormalities in the frontal lobes and prefrontal cortex of schizophrenic patients and their nonschizophrenic relatives have been increasingly identified neuropsychological studies (Weinberger et al., 1986; Liddle and Morris, 1991; Goldman-Rakic, 1995; Park et al., 1995). An extensive review of motor and sensory abnormalities in schizophrenic patients by Heinrichs and Buchanan (1988) confirms their prevalence in 50%–65% of schizophrenic patients. They noted that the majority of these minor neurologic abnormalities are in the areas of integrative sensory function, motor coordination, and the sequencing of complex motor acts, i.e., executive functions usually associated with frontal lobe dysfunction. Flashman et al. (1996) observed a similar array of impairments in schizophrenic disorders unrelated to the cognitive disorders that characterize posterior brain functions (parietal, occipital, temporal). Hoff et al. (1999) has shown that these neuropsychological impairments are stable over the first 4–5 years of illness.

Chatterjee et al. (1995) reported a 17 percent incidence of extrapyramidal signs in first-episode schizophrenic patients prior to any treatment with neuroleptics. The signs included akinesia, rigidity, cogwheeling, and even a case of dyskinesia; the patients with these signs were more likely to develop parkinsonian side effects with antipsychotics medications and seemed to have a poorer short-term prognosis with relation to the control of their psychosis. Choreoathetoid movements, indistinguishable from tardive dyskinesia, occur in 20 percent of schizophrenic patients before treatment (Buckley et al., 1996, 1998; Fenn et al., 1996).

Fish (1975) has described neurointegrative defects in infancy that she considers signs of dysregulation of maturation in neurological systems that represent a biological continuum with schizophrenic disorders in later life. The prospective study of persons at high risk for schizophrenia, particularly the offspring of schizophrenic parents, is an important area of research, not only for the evaluation of the role of the central nervous system but also for an understanding of the spectrum concept of schizophrenia (Campion and Tucker, 1973). Rieder et al. (1975) compared the offspring of schizophrenics with a matched control group to find a surprising increase in the incidence of fetal and neonatal deaths among the children of schizophrenics. This was confirmed by Walker and Emory (1983) but found not to be true in a British perinatal mortality survey for schizophrenic offspring; but they did note a higher mortality in the offspring from mothers with affective psychosis (Done et al., 1991).

The growing awareness of neurological abnormalities and reproductive problems in schizophrenia logically has led to consideration of the role of obstetrical complications in the abnormal neurodevelopment observed in schizophrenia. With few exceptions (Sacker et al., 1995), studies bearing on this issue show a high prevalence of obstetrical complications in schizophrenics ranging from 21 to 40 percent (Dalman et al., 1999). Schizophrenic patients also have a high prevalence of general physical anomalies that imply congenital maldevelopement of the brain such as low set ears, and a high arched palate (Buckley et al., 1998). There is a clear relationship between maternal influenza, obstetrical complications, and the development of schizophrenia in the offspring, at an early age (Wright et al., 1995; Verdoux et al., 1997).

The increased frequency of events known to produce brain injury, like obstetric complications, and the high prevalence of neurological abnormalities among schizophrenics suggests that brain damage can play a role in the etiology of schizophrenia. Some investigators argue that the birth complications and neurological abnormalities are caused by an already compromised fetus (Weinberger, 1995). Brain damage may also contribute to the severity of schizophrenia and may determine which carrier of the genotype becomes symptomatic. There is considerable data that the early onset group of schizophrenics has smaller cerebral volumes and lower IQs (Alaghband-Rad et al., 1997; Russell et al.,

1997). Emphasizing the role of brain damage in the expression of genetic psychosis, Kinney et al. (1998) and Zornberg et al. (2000) have also noted that the birth histories of bipolar patients reveal many obstetrical complications.

The upshot of these studies is that we need to reexamine the idea that there are no localizing neurological findings in schizophrenia. When schizophrenic patients are tested, it is not uncommon to find deficits in motor and sensory function, in visual and auditory perception, in verbal and nonverbal memory, or in executive functions. All of these deficits indicate that there is some dysfunction of the frontal lobes in schizophrenia (Blanchard and Neele, 1994). Another indication of brain dysfunction, particularly in frontal lobe dysfunction, are the reports by Holzman et al. (1973) that abnormal smooth pursuit eye movements during pendulum tracking characterize schizophrenic patients and their families. Shagass et al. (1974) observed the same characteristic jerky eye movements but found they related more to psychosis in general than to schizophrenia specifically. More recent studies found saccadic (jerky) eye movements during what should have been smooth pursuit in schizophrenics and their relatives (Thaker et al., 1996; Keefe et al., 1997; Lencer et al., 2000). Visual tracking defects have become one of the most widely investigated phenomena in schizophrenic patients. These smooth pursuit defects may serve as an important biologic marker for schizophrenics as they occur in 50%–80% of schizophrenic patients and in 40 percent of their relatives. But they may not be as specific as once was thought given that similar defects have been also reported in affective disorders, obsessive-compulsive disorder (OCD), and in Parkinson's and Alzheimer's diseases. In each of these disorders there is abundant independent evidence of frontal lobe dysfunction (Hutton et al., 1998; Hutton and Kennard, 1998).

Aberrant vestibular function has been widely observed in schizophrenic patients. The vestibular system integrates sensation with motor functions and behavior. Studies made by 11 different groups over the past 50 years have all shown reduced nystagmus in schizophrenic patients in response to caloric and rotational stimulation of the vestibular system (Ornitz, 1970; Myers et al., 1973). Whereas the reduced nystagmus response is directly related to duration of illness in many studies, the relation of vestibular alterations to schizophrenia remains unclear. In some studies auditory and visual hallucinations have followed pharmacological suppression of vestibular sensibility, but the possibility of direct toxic effects of the drugs occurring elsewhere in the brain was not ruled out (Tice, 1968). Prolonged use of psychotropic drugs may induce vestibular changes in chronic patients, which may obscure the association between vestibular defects and schizophrenia in recent studies. In the older studies, however, these psychotropic drugs were not used because they were not yet available. The existence of these minor neurological abnormalities has led to theories that the behavior of schizophrenics reflects a disturbance of the sensory integrative functions of the brain (Andreasen, 1999).

Two experimental approaches have lent more credence to the idea of sensory dysfunction in schizophrenia. Braff et al. (1992, 1995) have used the startle reflex as a way of exploring sensory gating. In an experimental setting they gave schizophrenic patients a prestimulus acoustic noise followed by a loud acoustic or forceful tactile stimulus to create a startle response. This response is measured by eye blinks and changes in skin conductance. The prestimulus reduces or *gates* the amplitude of the startle response in normal individuals but not in schizophrenics, thus implying that the schizophrenics have deficits in adjusting, modulating, or controlling stimuli from the environment. This inability to modulate external stimuli could lead to cognitive disorganization and withdrawal under the bombardment of unfiltered stimuli from the environment. There is increasing evidence that schizophrenics have trouble in habituating to the effects of the startle, indicating that this is a persistent problem of sensory integration. The inability to integrate sensory stimuli (e.g., prioritizing and sorting external stimuli) is the type of defect that again implicates a disturbance in frontal lobe functions. Using evoked auditory potentials in a similar stimulus/prestimulus paradigm, Freedman et al. (1994, 1996) have shown that schizophrenics do not suppress the response to the second stimuli over time, indicating a defect in sensory gating or inhibition. Freedman has found similar gating defects in non-schizophrenic family members of schizophrenics, which means that this impairment may serve as a marker for genetic studies of schizophrenic patients (Young et al., 1996; Freedman et al., 1997). Interestingly, this particular gating phenomenon is partially mediated by cholinergic nicotinic receptors in the hippocampus, an anatomic area that has been identified as abnormal in histologic, neuropathologic, and imaging studies of schizophrenics (Bogerts and Falkai, 1995; Leonard et al., 1996; Bunney and Bunney, 1999).

Braff et al. (1992, 1995) developed a rat model that shows great similarity to the sensory gating defect and the effects of doapamine seen in schizophrenic patients. With lesions in the premotor cortex and the hippocampus, the rats responded normally to startle stimuli, but when treated with a dopaminergic agonist, the lesioned animals manifested a gating defect. If the rats were lesioned in the neonatal period, the gating defect was not evident until the rat reached the postpubertal period (Lipska et al., 1995; Swerdlow et al., 1995). This may be relevant to schizophrenia as the vulnerability to it is genetic and presumably present from birth but the disease only becomes symptomatic in late adolescence.

The relation of the individual to the environment is obviously very important to cognitive function. Gross disruptions of perceptual and sensory integrative functions produced by drugs and sensory deprivation regularly lead to psychotic-like states the symptoms of which can resemble those of schizophrenia. It has long been known that people in such isolated situations as Arctic camps and solitary prison confinement, patients in iron lungs, and survivors at sea experience a variety of disturbing subjective alterations. In fact, any environment that is unvarying and that offers only a limited range of sensory stimuli can give rise to *(1)* difficulty in focusing and organizing thoughts, *(2)* illusions and delusions, *(3)* a sharp sense of the need for variation in extrinsic stimuli, *(4)* a distortion of the sense of time passing, and *(5)* the hallucinatory experiences that occur during prolonged deprivation. These alterations are not limited to the period of deprivation but persist briefly after it has ended. Objects continue to appear to swirl, and shapes and lines seem distorted (Solomon et al., 1957).

Electroencephalographic data. Most of the available data relating electroencephalographic (EEG) abnormalities to abnormal mental states are discussed in chapter 1. The EEG changes described in schizophrenia do not have a specific diagnostic or therapeutic significance. Reports of electroencephalographic abnormality in schizophrenic patients referred at random range from 5 to 80 percent, with an average of approximately 25 percent (Abenson, 1970); but the vagaries of EEG interpretation and the variability in diagnosing schizophrenia obscure the meaning of these data. Patients diagnosed as catatonic schizophrenics seem to show consistently higher rates of EEG abnormality, usually manifested as nonspecific slowing. Given that catatonic states are often acute and have a relatively good prognosis, one wonders if all cases so labeled are really catatonic schizophrenia. We have seen patients with seizures, toxic/metabolic encephalopathy, encephalitis, occult hydrocephalus, and left middle cerebral artery occlusion presenting with speechlessness, waxy flexibility, and other psychotic behavioral abnormalities; they were mistakenly thought to have catatonic schizophrenia. The result, a higher rate of EEG abnormality in catatonic schizophrenics, raises some question about the diagnosis (Liberson et al., 1958; Tucker et al., 1965). Still the increased prevalence of EEG abnormalities among schizophrenics in general seems well documented (Small et al., 1964; Treffert, 1964; Tucker et al., 1965). Studies using quantitative EEG's (QEEG) have been surprisingly few, however, a recent study demonstrated QEEG differences between schizophrenics with positive and negative symptoms (Harris et al., 1999). Older studies using QEEG have shown decreased variability and high mean energy content (Goldstein et al., 1963). In several studies, this stability or hyperregulation in the EEGs of schizophrenics correlated with a poor prognosis, whereas dysrhythmic records correlated with a better prognosis (Yamada, 1960; Igert and Lairy, 1962).

Many of the EEG studies of schizophrenics are complicated by the treatment given the patients. Fukuda and Matsuda (1969) found high voltage slow-wave changes after five electroconvulsant treatments (ECTs) in 40 to 70 percent of patients, and in 80 to 87 percent after 10 ECTs. Though they reported that almost all EEGs returned to normal in 3 days, Muscovitch and Katzelenbogen (1948) claimed that such abnormalities could last for up to 10 months. Phenothiazines and other psychotropic drugs complicate EEG studies even more; they typically cause slowing of alpha rhythms and an increase in amplitude, with superimposed sharp fast activity (Steiner and Pollack, 1965). These changes may persist for up to 3 months after medications are stopped (Fink and Kahn, 1956; Swain and Litteral, 1960). To make interpretation more difficult, predrug EEGs have not usually been recorded. In a study of schizophrenic patients on phenothiazines, Steiner found patterns characteristic of sleep activity in 65 percent and significant amounts of diffuse delta and theta activity in 43 percent. Since all the atypical antipsychotics, particularly clozapine, have been associated with seizures in nonepileptic patients they would also be likely to produce EEG changes (Alldredge, 1999).

In summary, electroencephalographic abnormalities are seen in schizophrenics, especially catatonic schizophrenics, more often than in the general population. This statement seems valid even when allowances are made for an occasional misdiagnosis of schizophrenia or an EEG abnormality caused by drugs or shock therapy. It is not known whether the schizophrenic process or an underlying biochemical defect causes these electroencephalographic abnormalities. It seems likely that neurologic features that cause brain damage, so often associated with schizophrenia, may be variably reflected in the EEG.

Neuroimaging. Over the past 25 years examinations of schizophrenics using static types of imaging e.g., computerized tomography (CT) and magnetic resonance imaging (MRI) have found structural changes in sub groups of patients. There have been inconsistent reports of ventricular enlargement, decreased size of the frontal lobes, and cerebellar atrophy in schizophrenic patients with CT scans (Johnstone et al., 1976; Golden et al., 1980; Weinberger et al., 1980; Andreasen, 1999). These investigators have correlated these changes with neuropsychological impairment, poor response to treatment, and poor premorbid adjustment. The ventricular enlargements that these authors have demonstrated would often not be called abnormal by radiologists but rather are subtle variations within the normal range. The authors also clearly stated that these changes were not present in all the schizophrenics they studied. Other investigations have not confirmed their findings of ventricular enlargement (Andreasen et al., 1982; Jerinigan et al., 1982).

There has been some question about temporal lobe abnormalities revealed by MRI. Kulynych et al. (1996) found no significant difference in the volume of the superior temporal gyrus of schizophrenics. Petty et al. (1995) and Barta et al. (1997) showed that the gray matter was smaller bilaterally in the planum temporale in right-handed schizophrenics. Usually, lateralized abnormalities in schizophrenics implicate the left hemisphere. Marsh et al. (1997) also showed that a group of early onset schizophrenic patients had smaller gray matter volumes in the temporal lobes but not the hippocampus. However, Jacobsen et al.

(1996, 1997a, b) were not able to show any temporal lobe volume changes in childhood schizophrenics. Almost all the studies in this area, whatever their results, suffer from serious methodologic problems, such as: *(1)* The study populations have been disparate, ranging from old to young, chronic to acute, rigidly diagnosed to less rigidly diagnosed. *(2)* The techniques of measuring ventricular size in each study were not standardized and vary from actual manual measurements to computerized measurements; consequently, there is great variation from study to study in the incidence of abnormal findings, as well as in their comparability. *(3)* The control populations have varied from none to reported norms in the literature, to normal populations, to neurologic patients who are referred for evaluation for headaches, and so on. Very few of these studies have compared other chronic psychiatric patients to the schizophrenic patients, and none have utilized a "blind" technique for reading CAT scans. When this comparison has been made, significant differences often disappear in the schizophrenic group (Weinberger et al., 1980).

The functional imaging studies using positron emission tomography (PET), functional magnetic resonance (FMR) tomography, magnetic resonance spectroscopy (MRS), and single photon emission tomography (SPECT) make possible the study of cerebral function in the living patient. These studies have done much to expand our knowledge, particularly in terms of complimenting some of the recent neuroanatomical findings in schizophrenia. Positron emission tomography, SPECT, and FMR are dynamic techniques that access the metabolic activity of the brain. These techniques depend on blood flow. In general, the more metabolically active the region, the greater its blood flow. Dramatic changes in PET and FMR can be produced by moving a limb, reading, solving mathematical problems, etc. These tests are used to best advantage when there is a reliable way to activate a specific part of the cortex. For example, Shaywitz et al. (1998) compared normal and dyslexic children at rest and while reading. At rest, the FMRs in both groups were comparable, as were the MRIs. When attempting to read, the left parietal lobe was activated in normal children; the dyslexics activated their frontal lobes. Apparently the frontal lobes do not carry out reading functions as well as the left parietal lobe but the brain recruits the frontal lobe if the left parietal lobe is not functioning.

These functional imaging techniques have begun to show consistent abnormalities in the temporal lobes, the basal ganglia, and the frontal lobes in schizophrenic patients. In 1990, Buchsbaum reviewed 20 PET studies of schizophrenia that showed lowered activity in all or one of these three areas (Buchsbaum, 1990). More recent studies have added the thalamus to this group (Flaum et al., 1995; Vita et al., 1995; Buchsbaum et al., 1996). Single photon emission computed tomography and FMR, as well as PET have demonstrated lower activity in the frontal lobes, temporal lobes, basal ganglia, and thalamus of drug naïve patients and first episode schizophrenic patients (Nopoulos et al., 1995; Vita et al., 1995; Buchsbaum et al., 1996; Bertolino et al., 1998). Some studies have shown a diminished size of the cerebellum but others have not confirmed this finding (Jacobson et al., 1997a,b). Some studies have shown greater differences in men but many other studies have found the changes to be unrelated to gender (Flaum et al., 1995; Lauriello et al., 1997).

The dynamic imaging techniques have also been useful in illuminating neurotransmitter pathways. Using PET, Nordstrom et al. (1995) showed that clozapine in vivo occupied D1 and 5-HT receptors and had low D2 occupancy. Holcomb et al. (1996) used PET to study glucose metabolism and found that it was the same 5 days after withdrawal of haloperidol as when the patient was receiving haloperidol. But when the same patients were studied 30 days after haloperidol cessation, there was a decrease in glucose metabolism in the caudate, putamen, and anterior thalamus, whereas glucose metabolism increased in the frontal cortex and anterior cingulate gyrus. Because haloperidol blocks D2 receptors, these findings implied that the D2 pathways in the brain control parts of the basal ganglia and thalamus and that these regions are involved in schizophrenia. As improved radioligands are developed such studies should become even more precise in mapping neurotransmitter sites and their actions (Ito et al., 1998).

Using nuclear magnetic resonance (NMR), Stanley and associates (1995) demonstrated a breakdown of membrane phospholipid products in the prefrontal areas in drug naïve and chronic schizophrenic patients as compared to controls, which confirmed an earlier study by Pettegrew et al. (1991). This study again implicates a defect in the frontal lobes that occurs early in the schizophrenic process and persists in chronicity. Single photon emission computed tomography studies have also begun to show some potential for clinical use in predicting drug response. Klemm and collegues (1996) used a raclopride derivative with high affinity for D2 receptors to quantitate D2 receptor blockade in patients taking neuroleptics. He suggested this may be a way of monitoring neuroleptic treatment. In a SPECT study, Rodriguez (1996) showed that patients who had lower prefrontal perfusion responded more poorly to clozapine than those who had high rates of perfusion.

Dynamic imaging has also been useful in exploring specific aspects of psychopathology. Woodruff et al. (1997) used FMR to investigate auditory hallucinations in schizophrenic patients and found that when the patient was having auditory hallucinations, there was reduced blood flow in the temporal cortical regions associated with registering external speech. They postulated that this might represent competition for a common neurophysiological resource for language. Carter et al. (1997) hypothesized that schizophrenic patients taking the Stroop test (used to evaluate selective attention when there are competing stimuli) would not activate the anterior cingulate gyrus as normals do when they take this test; he confirmed this hypothesis in a PET study. This study demonstrates that it is now possible to use functional imaging in humans to test hypotheses derived from studies on animals, and to study regions of a living patient's brain that have been identified as abnormal in other studies, including postmortem studies, of the brains of schizophrenics.

These dynamic imaging techniques also have the potential to play a role in the diagnosis and clinical management of schizophrenia. But some caution is in order. Schizophrenic patients who have been treated with antipsychotic drugs cannot be compared with normal individuals if the purpose is to discover a deficit that is unique to schizophrenia. In several studies, schizophrenic patients have been compared to other nonschizophrenic psychiatric patients, particularly those with mood disorders. Many changes noted in schizophrenic patients compared to normal controls are also present in the nonschizophrenic, psychiatric controls (Elkis et al., 1995; Pearlson et al., 1995; Cannon et al., 1997). Thus, the changes noted may not be specific to schizophrenia. This has been the historical fate of many findings in schizophrenic patients. When the schizophrenic is compared to normal patients there are differences, but when the schizophrenic is compared to other psychiatric patients, particularly patients with nonschizophrenic psychoses, the differences disappear. The findings then seem to be a common property of psychoses or of some factor-like treatment that has no etiological relationship to schizophrenia.

Neuropathological findings. Reports of neuropathologic findings whether gross or microscopic in the brains of schizophrenic patients have been scarce. Older studies observed nonspecific abnormalities. As more precise neuropathological techniques have become available, more consistent findings are emerging. This effort has been facilitated by the development of *brain banks* that have collected tissue from carefully diagnosed schizophrenics. Even some of the older findings that were considered random and inconclusive now correlate with many of the functional imaging studies (Bogerts and Falkai, 1995). In the limbic region, reduced cell volumes have been reported in the hippocampus as well as disturbed cellular architecture that often extends to the cingulate gyrus and the entorhinal cortex.

Neuropathological studies of schizophrenics indicate that the total number of neurons in the frontal area appears intact but there is an increase in cell density in the premotor cortex; in addition there are decreases in the density of dendritic spines of pyramidal neurons in cortical layer III and decreased signs of synaptic activity (Lewis and Anderson, 1995). Neurophysiological studies of the frontal premotor area, in nonhuman primates, implicate this area in working memory (Goldman-Rakic, 1987) and control in the temporal integration of information (Fuster, 1993). Because portions of the frontal lobes (cortical and subcortical) appear to be dysfunctional in schizophrenics, the animal studies may help explain the difficulties in sensory integration that have been observed in schizophrenics. The frontal lobes permit subjects to keep events in their working memory and to sequence temporal events. The dysfunctions of the frontal areas that have been described in schizophrenics could explain both their conceptual and language disturbances.

Increases in basal ganglia volumes have also been observed in schizophrenics, but most researchers attribute these changes to the use of antipsychotic medications. Kung et al. (1998), however, found an increase in the density of synapses in the caudate nucleus and striatum but not the putamen in schizophrenic patients. These changes were not evident in normal controls or in other psychiatric patients. Neuroleptics act on the caudate and the putamen, the location of many dopamine receptors. The fact that the changes were found in the caudate but not in the putamen would suggest that perhaps the increases in the caudate are not caused by neuroleptic use alone but reflect some abnormality specific to schizophrenia.

The nature of some of the neuropathological findings also provides support for the theory that schizophrenia may be congenital in origin, a disorder of early pre- or postnatal brain development. The changes found in the brains of schizophrenics are usually of the following types: alterations of cytoarchitecture; a persistence of a cavity in the septum pellucidum (which should disappear with normal development); and an absence of normal cerebral structural asymmetries (Bogerts and Falki, 1995). This type of pathology is usually associated with prenatal or perinatal developmental problems. Few of the neuropathological studies have found any gliosis, which is usually a hallmark of aquired damage and neuronal degeneration.

The onset of schizophrenia in late adolescence or early adulthood, once was thought to imply an acquired as opposed to a genetic condition. Actually, in humans and primates, as postnatal development proceeds, there is a progressive reduction of excitatory synapses, particularly in the premotor frontal lobes (Bourgeois et al., 1994). This pruning continues during adolescence. The symptoms of schizophrenia develop as the cortex develops during young adulthood. Myelinization and synapse development advance during the first two decades, bringing the premotor frontal cortex and anterior temporal regions fully into the functional brain circuitry. The effects of genetically abnormal frontal lobes or hippocampus may not become apparent until the frontal lobes and hippocampus are fully attached to the brain's electrical grid. In the schizophrenic, in other words, development may permit the symptoms of schizophrenia to develop as the brain matures (Arnold, 1999; Keshavan and Hogarty, 1999).

PSYCHOLOGICAL TESTING FOR SCHIZOPHRENIA

The early psychological testing of schizophrenia using projective techniques and personality inventories was aimed at validating various theories about the psychodynamic etiology of schizophrenia. Currently, the major use for psychological tests in schizophrenia is to assess cognitive function. The major tools have been standardized tests such as the Halstead Neuropsychological Test Battery and the Continuous Performance Test (Hoff, 1995; Calev, 1999). Personality inventories usually deal with long-standing personality traits. Though helpful in raising a suspicion of chronic schizophrenia or schizoid personality, they also fail to discriminate acute schizophrenia from acute neurological syndromes.

The tests developed to assess brain damage also cannot distinguish the chronic schizophrenic from the brain-damaged patient. This has been demonstrated quite clearly by two detailed studies in which the Halstead Neuropsychological Test Battery was used (Watson et al., 1968); in these studies, the organics could not be distinguished from the chronic schizophrenics. Vega and Parsons (1967) and Lacks et al. (1970) repeated these findings.

For the past three decades, the thrust of neuropsychological research into schizophrenia shifted to testing specific cognitive functions such as memory, frontal lobe function, attention, and psychomotor performance. In most cases there is little to differentiate schizophrenic patients from patients with neurological lesions that affect these performance parameters (Calev, 1999). Abnormalities identified on neuropsychological tests in schizophrenia may not be specific as tests results can be affected by medication, age, education, gender, and even handedness (Conuit et al., 1994). In a carefully done study of schizophrenics and matched controls, schizophrenics displayed impairments of motor, sensory, and perceptual functioning, verbal and nonverbal memory, and frontal lobe functioning. This study did not identify any lateralized cognitive impairments in schizophrenics (Blanchard and Neale, 1994).

The extent of the cognitive impairment in schizophrenia was further highlighted by studies that compared the disorder with Alzheimer's disease. Davidson and colleagues (1996) using the Mini-Mental Status Examination found that schizophrenic patients performed worse on the tests of naming and constructional praxis than Alzheimer's disease patients, whereas the Alzheimer's disease patients were more impaired on global recall. Grouping the patients by the severity of illness the scores showed no differences; both were impaired. Hutton et al. (1998) shed some light on executive function in schizophrenic patients. They studied first-episode schizophrenics and found in addition to performing poorly on memory tasks, the schizophrenics had significant deficits in executive functions, particularly in planning and strategy tasks, whereas more chronic patients also had trouble in tasks that required shifting attention. By studying acute and chronic patients and showing that the cognitive deficits become more severe with chronicity, the authors suggest that schizophrenia is a progressive disease that affects the frontal lobes and its connections.

AROUSAL

Many studies have identified the schizophrenic as *hyperaroused*, a term that refers to an abnormally heightened state of neurophysiological activity (Grossberg, 2000; Pryor, 2000). Some feel that this state may actually cause thought disorders. The term *arousal* is not clearly defined, but, in general, it refers to a state of alertness with increased physiological measurements of the kind often associated with high levels of anxiety. These include increased galvanic skin resistance, increased muscle tension as measured by electromyography, desynchronization of the EEG with alpha suppression, and increased pulse rate. This evidence of hyperarousal has been speculatively linked with statements by acute schizophrenics indicating that they are "flooded" with stimuli, that is, "When I try to read something, each bit I read starts me thinking in ten different directions at once." It has been suggested that the hyperarousal leads to a "low threshold for disorganization under increasing stress" (Epstein and Coleman, 1970). It may also refelect the defects in sensory gating noted earlier (p. 110, Braff et al. 1992, 1995) The psychophysiological disorganization caused by stimulus overload is hypothesized as the primary causal factor in the thought disturbance typical of schizophrenic patients. When the physiological parameters of arousal are studied in samples of schizophrenic and nonschizophrenic patients, the symptoms related to feeling flooded by stimuli correlate highly with measures of anxiety (Tucker et al., 1969). Consequently, hyperarousal, though frequently present in schizophrenics, may simply be a manifestation of heightened anxiety, rather than something specific to schizophrenia.

TREATMENT

The use of antipsychotic drugs is essential to the treatment of schizophrenia (Tucker et al., 1984; Brier, 1996). Not only are these drugs more effective than placebos for schizophrenics (Brier, 1996), but they are also more effective than any type of psychotherapy alone (Grinspoon et al., 1968; May et al., 1981). Psychological forms of therapy can be useful adjuncts to drugs, but no one can claim that they offer an alternative to drugs.

The antipsychotics have now been in use for close to 50 years, and although they have brought major changes in the places where the schizophrenic is treated (now the majority of schizophrenic patients are treated in the community rather than large remote state hospitals), it is not clear that they have altered the long-term outcome. They are neither curative of schizophrenia nor do they always control the symptoms in all cases (Davis, 1993). It is still true that approximately one-third of the schizophrenics get better, approximately one-third have major residual symptoms, and approximately one-third deteriorate (see Table 3–2). Approximately 15 percent of schizophrenic patients show no effect from antipsychotic medications, another 15 percent will experience almost complete symptom control, and the remainder will have a mixture of residual symptoms of varying severity.

The new atypical antipsychotics have been very welcome. Clozapine provides clinical improvement for 40%–60% of the chronic patients who have failed to respond to other antipsychotics, while it and the other atypicals seem to have fewer extrapyramidal side effects (Brier and Buchanan, 1996). Clozapine, introduced in 1989, was the first radically different drug introduced since the early 1950s. Recently a whole new generation of clozapine-like drugs have been released: risperidone, olanzapine, quetiapine, sertindole, and ziprasidone. All of these drugs differ from the older antipsychotics with regard to their neuronal receptor sites of action. The traditional or typical antipsychotics primarily interact with the D2 receptor. The atypical drugs affect a whole range of receptor sites: low D1, D2 binding, high affinity for 5HT2, alpha-adrenergic 1 and 2, histaminic 1, and muscarinic receptors in varying degrees. Each of the atypical drugs has minor variations in this pattern but most are similar to each other. These new drugs seem to create less extrapyramidal effects because they occupy the D2 receptor site only transiently or at a lower occupancy rate than the traditional neuroleptics (Kapur et al., 2000). However, all the atypicals make Parkinson's symptoms worse in patients with Parkinson's disease. Only clozapine and quetiapine can be used without risk of worsening Parkinson's symptoms (Goetz et al., 2000). Risperidone produces dose-related extrapyramidal symptoms; but causes only transient rises in serum prolactin levels (the D2 receptor blockers all cause variable increases in serum prolactin related to their D2 receptor occupancy). Other major side effects of the atypicals are sedation, weight gain, hypotension, and salivation. Even though clozapine has caused seizures, the epileptogenic potential of the other drugs seems to be less. Since the atypical antipsychotics produce fewer extrapyramidal symptoms and less tardive dyskinesia (TD) they may lead to better patient compliance. With the older antipsychotics, patients often experienced uncomfortable bodily sensations, probably related to subtle extrapyramidal effects. These feelings often led them to discontinue the antipsychotic medication. Among patients taking typical antipsychotic medication, approximately 4%–5%/year will develop tardive dyskinesia. Fortunately 60 percent of the cases of TD ultimately remit spontaneously (see Chapter 5). But for those that do not remit, it is a socially disabling side effect of antipsychotic therapy. The lower rate of TD with the new antipsychotics is a major step forward.

CONCLUSION

It is obvious that schizophrenia is a complex disorder. But it is a disorder that has been clearly described for over a hundred years. Although the etiology and curative treatments are not yet known, we have made significant progress in delineating many of the central nervous system abnormalities associated with schizophrenia. For the first time investigators using different methodologies are identifying the same anatomical sites in the brain as being dysfunctional in schizophrenia. There are consistent reports from neuroanatomists, molecular biologists, neuropsychologists, and those doing functional imaging that there seem to be dysfunctions in the frontal lobes, the hippocampus, and the entorhinal cortex of schizophrenics. And although no specific gene has yet been identified, the course of the illness with onset in late adolescence and the common clinical and laboratory neurological findings indicate that schizophrenia is a disease of neurodevelopment. As these biologic findings accumulate, we may soon have biologic markers with which to diagnose and define schizophrenia. Once we can define the disorder biologically, we will be better able to determine the etiology and treatment.

REFERENCES

Abenson, M. H. EEG's in chronic schizophrenia. *Br J Psychiatry* 116:421, 1970.

Alaghband-Rad, J., S. D. Hamburger, J. N. Giedd, et al. Childhood-onset schizophrenia: biological markers in relation to clinical characteristics. *Am J Psychiatry* 154:64, 1997.

Alldredge, B. K. Seizure risk associated with psychotropic drugs. *Neurology* 53 (Suppl 2):68, 1999.

American Psychiatric Association. *Diagnostic and Statistical Manual of Mental Disorders*, 2nd ed. American Psychiatric Association, Washington, DC, 1968.

American Psychiatric Association. *Diagnostic and Statistical Manual of Mental Disorders*, 4th ed. American Psychiatric Association, Washington, DC, 1994.

Andreasen, N. C. Thought, language and communication disorders. *Arch. Gen Psychiatry* 36:1315, 1979.

Andreasen, N. C. Negative symptoms in schizophrenia. *Arch Gen Psychiatry* 39:784, 1982.

Andreasen, N. C., S. Olsen. Negative versus positive schizophrenia. *Arch Gen Psychiatry* 39:789, 1982.

Andreasen, N. C., M. R. Smith, C. Jacoby, J. Dennert, S. Olsen. Ventricular enlargement in schizophrenia. *Am J Psychiatry* 139:292, 1982.

Andreasen, N. C., S. Arndt, R. Alliger, et al. Symptoms of schizophrenia. methods, meanings, and mechanisms. *Arch Gen Psychiatry* 52:341, 1995.

Andreasen, N. C., A unitary model for schizophrenia. *Arch Gen Psychiatry* 56:781, 1999.

Arango, C., J. Bartko, J. Gold, Prediction of neuropsychological performance by neurological signs in schizophrenia. *Am J Psychiatry* 156:1349, 1999.

Arnold, S. E., Neurodevelopmental abnormalities in schizophrenia. *Dev Psychopathol* 11: 439, 1999.

Barta, P. E., G. D. Pearlson, L. B. Brill, et al. Planum temporale asymmetry reversal in schizophrenia: replication and relationship to gray matter abnormalities. *Am J Psychiatry* 154:661, 1997.

Benes, F. M., J. McSparren, E. D. Bird, et al. Deficits in small interneurons in prefrontal and cingulate cortices of schizophrenic and schizoaffective patients. *Arch Gen Psychiatry* 48:996, 1991.

Berger, R. J., I. Oswald. Effects of sleep deprivation, subsequent sleep and dreaming. *Br J. Psychiatry* 108:457,1962.

Berner, P., E. Gabriel, H. Katschnig, et al. *Diagnostic Criteria for Schizophrenia and Affective Psychosis*. World Psychiatric Association, American Psychiatric Press, Washington, DC, 1983.

Bertolino, A., J. H. Callicott, I. Elman, et al. Regionally specific neuronal pathology in untreated patients with schizophrenia: a proton magnetic resonance spectroscopic imaging study. *Biol Psychiatry* 43:641, 1998.

Blanchard, J. J., J. M. Neale. The neuropsychological signature of schizophrenia: generalized or differential deficit? *Am J Psychiatry* 151:40, 1994.

Bleuler, E. *Dementia Praecox or the Group of Schizophrenias*. Zinkin, trans. International Universities Press, New York, 1950.

Bleuler, M. A 23-year longitudinal study of 208 schizophrenics. In: *Transmission of Schizophrenia*, D. Rosenthal, S. Kety, eds. Pergamon, London, 1968, p. 3–14.

Bleuler, M. *The Schizophrenic Disorders*. Yale University Press, New Haven, CT, 1978.

Bogerts, B., P. Falkai, Postmortem Brain Abnormalities in Schizophrenia. In: *Contmporary Issues in the Treatment of Schizophrenia*, American Psichiatric Press, Washington DC, 1995, p. 43

Bourgeois, J. P., P. S. Goldman-Rakic, P. Rakic, Synaptogenesis in the prefrontal cortex of rhesus monkeys. *Cerebral Cortex* 4:78, 1994.

Braff, D. L., C. Grillon, M. A. Geyer. Gating and habituation of the startle reflex in schizophrenic patients. *Arch Gen Psychiatry* 49:206, 1992.

Braff, D. L., N. R. Swerdlow, M. A. Geyer. Gating and habituation deficits in the schizophrenia disorders. *Clin Neurosi* 3:131, 1995.

Breier, A. *The New Pharmacotherapy of Schizophrenia*. American Psychiatric Press, Washington, DC, 1996.

Breir, A., R. W. Buchanan. Clozapine. In: *The New Pharmacotherapy of Schizophrenia*, A. Breir, ed. American Psychiatric Press, Washington, DC, 1996, p. 1.

Buchanan, R. W., M. Brandes, A. Brier. Treating negative symptoms. In: *The New Pharmacotherapy of Schizophrenia*, A. Breier, ed. American Psychiatric Press, Washington DC, 1996, p. 179

Buchanan, R. W., W. T. Carpenter, Jr. The Neuroanatomies of schizophrenia. *Schizophr Bull*, 23:367, 1997.

Buchsbaum, M. The frontal lobes, basal ganglia, and temporal lobes as sites for schizophrenia. *Schizophr Bul* 16:377, 1990.

Buchsbaum, M., S. Toshiyuki, C. Ying Teng, et al. PET and MRI of the Thalamus in never-medicated patients with schizophrenia. *Am J Psychiatry* 153:191, 1996.

Buckley, P., R. W. Buchanan, S. C. Schulz, C. A. Tamminga. Catching up on schizophrenia. The Fifth International Congress on Schizophrenia Research, Warm Springs, VA, April 8–12, 1995. *Arch Gen Psychiatry* 53:456, 1996.

Buckley, P. The clinical stigmata of aberrant neurodevelopment in schizophrenia. *J Nerv Ment Dis* 186:79,1998.

Bunney, W. E., B. G. Bunney. Neurodevelopmental hypothesis of scizophrenia. In: *Neurobiology of Mental Illness*, D. Charney, E. Nestler, B. Bunney, eds. Oxford University Press, New York, 1999, pp. 225–235.

Calev, A. *Assessment of Neuropsychological Functions in Psychiatric Disorders.* American Psychiatric Press, Washington, DC, 1999, pp. 33–66.

Cameron, N. *Personality Development and Psychopathology.* Houghton Mifflin, Boston, 1963.

Campion, E. W., G. J. Tucker. A note on twin studies, schizophrenia and neurological impairment. *Arch Gen Psychiatry* 35:60, 1973.

Cannon, M, P. Jones, C. Gilvarry, et al. Premorbid social functioning in schizophrenia and bipolar disorder: similarities and differences. *Am J Psychiatry* 154:1544, 1997.

Carlsson, A. The current status of the dopamine hypothesis of schizophrenia. *Neuropsychoparmacology* 1:179, 1988.

Carpenter, W. T., Jr. The negative symptom challenge. *Arch Gen Psychiatry* 49:236–237, 1992.

Carter, C. S., M. Mintun, T. Nichols, J. D. Cohen. Anterior cingulate gyrus dysfunction and selective attention deficits in schizophrenia: [^{15}O] H_2O PET Study during single-trial Stroop task performance. *Am J Psychiatry* 154:1670, 1997.

Chatterjee, A., M. Chakos, A. Koreen, et al. Prevalence and clinical correlates of extrapyramidal signs and spontaneous dyskinesia in never-medicated schizophrenia patients. *Am J Psychiatry* 152:1724, 1995.

Ciompi, L. Catamnestic long-term study on the course of life and aging of schizophrenics. *Schizophr Bull.* 6:606, 1980.

Clayton, P. J., L. Rodin, G. Winokur. Family history studies III: Schizoaffective disorder. *Comp Psychiatry* 9:31, 1968.

Clayton, P. J. Schizoaffective Disorders. J Nerv Ment Disease 170:646, 1982.

Cloninger, R. Tests of alternative models of the relationship of schizophrenic and affective psychoses. In: *Genetic Approaches to Mental Disorders*, E. Gershon, R. Cloninger, American Psychiatric Press, Washington, DC, 1994, pp. 149–162.

Cohen, S. M., M. G. Allen, W. Pollin, Z. Hrubec. Relationship of schizoaffective psychoses to manic depressive psychosis and schizophrenia. *Arch Gen Psychiatry* 26: 539, 1972.

Convit, A., J. Volavka, P. Czobor, et al. Effect of subtle neurological dysfunction on response to Haloperidol treatment in schizophrenia. *Am J Psychiatry* 151:49, 1994.

Cooper, J. F., Bloom, R. Roth. *The Biochemical Basis of Neuropharmacology*, 7th Ed., Oxford University Press, New York, 1996.

Coyle, J. T. The glutamatergic dysfunction hypothesis for schizophrenia. *Harvard Rev Psychiatry* 3:241, 1996.

Critchley, M. The neurology of psychotic speech. *Br J Psychiatry* 110: 353, 1964.

Crow, T. J., The failure of the kraepelinian binary concept and the search for the psychosis gene. In: *Concepts of Mental Disorders*, A. Kerr. H. McClelland, eds. Gaskell, London, 1991, pp. 31–4.

Crow, T. J. The demise of the Kraeplinian binary system as a prelude to genetic advance. in *Genetic Approaches to Mental Disorders*, E. Gershon, R. Cloninger, American Psychiatric Press, Washington, DC, 1994, pp. 163–92.

Dalman, C., P. Allebeck, J. Culberg, et al. Obstetric complications and the risk of schizophrenia. *Arch Gen Psychiatry* 56:234, 1999.

Davidson, M., P. Harvey, K. A. Welsh, et al. Cognitive functioning in late-life schizophrenia: a comparison of elderly schizophrenic patients and patients with Alzheimer's disease. *Am J Psychiatry* 153:1274, 1996.

Davies, R., J. Neil, J. Himmelhoch. Cerebral dysthymias in schizophrenics receiving phenothiazines. *Clin Electroencephalogr* 6:103, 1975.

Davis J. M., J. M Kane, S. R. Marder, et al. Dose response of prophylactic antipsychotics. *J Clin Psychiatry* 54(3 Suppl):24, 1993.

Davison, K., C. R. Bagley. Schizophrenia-like psychoses associated with organic disorders of the central nervous system: A review of the literature. In: *Current Problems in Neuropsychiatry*, R. N. Herrington, ed. Headley Bros., Ashford, Kent, 1969.

Done, D. J., E. C. Johnstone, C. D. Firth, et al. Complications of pregnancy and delivery in relation to psychosis of adult life. *BMJ* 302:1576, 1991.

Elkis, H. L. Friedman, A. Wise, H. Y. Meltzer. Meta-analyses of studies of ventricular enlargement and cortical sulcal prominence in mood disorders. Comparisons with controls or patients with schizophrenia. *Arch Gen Psychiatry* 52:735, 1995.

Epstein, S., M. Coleman. Drive theories of schizophrenia. *Psychosom Med* 32:113, 1970.

Erlenmeyer-Kimling, L., U. H. Adamo, D. Rock, et al. The New York High-Risk Project: prevalence and Comorbidity of Axis I Disorders in Offspring of Schizophrenic Parents at 25-Year Follow-up. *Arch Gen Psychiatry* 54:1096, 1997.

Erlenmeyer-Kimling, L. E. Squires-Wheeler, U. H. Adamo, et al. The New York High-Risk Project: Psychoses and Cluster A personality disorders in offspring of schizophrenic parents at 23 years of follow-up. *Arch Gen Psychiatry* 52:857, 1995.

Faber, R., R. Abrams, M. Taylor, et al. Comparison of schizophrenic patients with formal thought disorder and neurologically impaired patients with aphasia. *Am J Psychiatry* 140:348, 1983

Farmer, A. P. McGuffin, I. Gottesman. Twin concordance and DSM III schizophrenia. *Arch Gen Psychiatry* 44:634, 1987.

Fenn, D. S., D. Moussaoui, W. F. Hoffman, et al. Movements in never-medicated schizophrenics: a preliminary study. *Psychopharmacology* 123:206, 1996.

Fink, M., R. C. Kahn. Relation of EEG delta activity to behavioral response in electroshock. *Arch Neurol Psychiatry* 78:516, 1956.

Fish, B. Biologic antecedents of psychosis in children. In: *Biology of* Major *Psychosis*, D. X. Freedman, ed. Raven Press, New York, 1975.

Flashman, L. A., M. Flaum, S. Gupta, N. C. Andreasen. Soft signs and neuropsychological performance in schizophrenia. *Am J Psychiatry* 153:526, 1996.

Flaum, M., V. W. Swayze, D. S. O'Leary, et al. Effects of diagnosis, laterality, and gender on brain morphology in schizophrenia. *Am J Psychiatry* 152:704, 1995.

Frazier, J. A., J. N. Giedd, D. Kaysen, et al. Childhood-onset schizophrenia: brain MRI rescan after 2 years of Clozapine maintenance treatment. *Am J Psychiatry* 153:564, 1996.

Freedman, R., L. E. Adler, P. Bickford, et al. Schizophrenia and nicotinic receptors. *Harv Rev Psychiatry* 2:179, 1994.

Freedman, R., L. E. Adler, M. Myles-Worsley, et al. Inhibitory gating of an evoked response to repeated auditory stimuli in schizophrenic and normal subjects. Human recordings, computer simulation, and an animal model. *Arch Gen Psychiatry* 53:1114, 1996.

Freedman, R., H. Coon, M. Myles-Worsley, et al. Linkage of a neurophysiological deficit in schizophrenia to a chromosome 15 locus. *Proc Natl Acad Sci USA* 94:587, 1997.

Fukuda, T., Y. Matsuda. Comparative characteristics of slow wave EEG, autonomic function and clinical picture in typical and atypical schizophrenia during and following electroconvulsive treatment. *Int Pharmacopsychiatry* 3:13, 1969.

Fuster, J. M. Frontal lobes. *Curr Opin Neurobiol* 3:160, 1993.

Goetz, C., L. Blasucci, S. Leurgans, et al. Olanzapine and clozapine. *Neurology* 55:789, 2000

Golden, C. J., J. A. Moses, R. Zelogowski, et al. Cerebral ventricular size and neuropsychological impairment in young chronic schizophrenics. *Arch Gen Psychiatry* 37: 619, 1980.

Goldman-Rakic, P. S. Circuitry of primate prefrontal cortex and regulation of behavior by representational memory. In *Handbook of Physiology. The Nervous System, Vol. 5,* F. Plum, V. Mountcastle, ed. American Physiological Society, Bethesda, MD, 1987, p. 373.

Goldman-Rakic, P. More clues on "latent" schizophrenia point to a developmental origin. *Am J Psychiatry* 152:1701, 1995.

Goldstein, K. Methodological approach to the study of schizophrenia thought disorder. In: *Language and Thoughts in Schizophrenia*, J. S. Kasanin, ed. W. W. Norton, New York, 1944.

Goldstein, K., M. Scheerer. Abstract and concrete behavior, an experimental study with special tests. *Psychol Med Monogr Suppl*, 53(2): 239, 1941.

Goldstein, K. Concerning the concreteness in schizophrenia. *J Abnorm Soc Psychol* 57: 146, 1958.

Goldstein, L., H. B. Murphree, A. A. Sugarman, et al. Quantitative electroencephalographic analysis of naturally occurring (schizophrenic) and drug-induced psychotic states in human males. *Clin Pharmacol Ther* 4:1O, 1963.

Goren, A., G. Tucker, G. Ginsberg. Language of dysfunction in schizophrenia. *Eur J Disord Commun* 31:153, 1996.

Grinker, R. R. Changing Styles in Psychiatric Syndromes: Psychoses and Borderline States. Presented at 12th Annual Meeting, American Psychiatric Association, Dallas, Texas, May 1972.

Grinspoon, L., J. R. Ewalt, R. Sbader. Psychotherapy and pharmacotherapy in chronic schizophrenia. *Am J Psychiatry* 124:1645, 1968.

Grossberg, S. The imbalanced brain. *Biol Psychiatry* 15:81, 2000.

Guidotti, A., J. Auta, V. Gervevini, et al. Decrease in reelin and glutamic acid decarboxylase 67 expression in schizophrenia and bipolar disorder. *Arch Gen Psychiatry* 57: 1061, 2000.

Harasty, J, et al. Language associated corticol regions are proportionally larger in the female brain. *Arch Neurol* 54:171, 1997.

Harding, C., G. Brooks, T. Ashikaga, et al. The Vermont longitudinal study of persons with severe mental illness. *Am J Psychiatry* 144:718, 1987.

Harris, A., L. Williams, G. Bahramali, et al. Different psychopathological models and quantified EEG in schizophrenia. *Psychol Med* 29:1175, 1999.

Harrison, G., P. Mason, C. Glazebrook, et al. Residence of incident cohort of psychotic patients after 13 years of follow-up, *BMJ* 308:813, 1994.

Harvey, P., E. Howanitz, M. Parrella, et al. Symptoms, cognitive functioning and adaptive skills in geriatric patients with life long schizophrenia *Am J Psychiatry* 155: 1080, 1998.

Harrow, M., G. J. Tucker, P. Shield. II. Stimulus overinclusion in schizophrenic disorders. *Arch Gen Psychiatry* 27:40, 1972.

Heinrichs, D. W., Buchanan R. W. Significance and meaning of neurological signs in schizophrenia. *Am J Psychiatry* 145:11, 1988.

Hermann, B. P., M. Seidenberg, J. Schoenfeld, K. Davies. Neuropsychological characteristics of the syndrome of mesial temporal lobe epilepsy. *Arch Neurol* 54:369–376, 1997.

Hertzig, M. A., H. G. Birch. Neurologic organization in psychiatrically disturbed adolescent girls. *Arch Gen Psychiatry* 15:590, 1966.

Hertzig, M. A. and H. G. Birch. Neurologic organization in psychiatrically disturbed adolescents. *Arch Gen Psychiatry* 19:528, 1968.

Heston, L. L. Psychiatric disorders in foster home reared children of schizophrenic mothers. *Br J Psychiatry* 112:819, 1966.

Hirsch, S., M. Hollender. Hysterical psychosis. *Am J Psychiatry* 125: 909, 1969.

Hoff, A. L. Neuropsychological function in schizophrenia. In: *Contemporary Issues in the Treatment of Schizophrenia*, C. L. Shriqui, H. A. Nasrallah, ed. American Psychiatric Press, Washington, DC, 1995, p. 187.

Hoff, A. C., M. Sakuma, M. Wieneke, et. al. Longitudinal neuropsychological follow-up study of patients with first-episode schizophrenia. *Am J Psychiatry* 156:1336, 1999.

Hogarty, G. E, S. J., Kornblith, D. Greenwald, et al. Three-year trials of personal therapy among schizophrenic patients living with or independent of family. I: Description of study and effects of relapse rates. *Am J Psychiatry* 154:1504, 1997.

Holcomb, H. H., N. G. Cascella, G. K. Thaker, et al. Functional sites of neuroleptic drug action in the human brain: PET/FDG studies with and without Haloperidol. *Am J Psychiatry* 153:41, 1996.

Holzman, P., L. Proctor, D. Hughes. Eye-tracking patterns in schizophrenia. *Science* 181: 179, 1973.

Horden, A, M. Sandfer, I. Green, et al. Psychiatric diagnosis. *Br J Psychiatry* 114: 935, 1968.

Huber, G., G. Gross, R. Schuttler. A long term follow-up Study of schizophrenia. *Acta Psychiatr Scand* 52:49, 1975.

Hutton, S. B., B. K. Puri, L. -J., Duncan, et al. Executive function in first-episode schizophrenia. *Psychol Med* 28:463, 1998.

Hutton, S. B., C. Kennard. Oculomotor abnormalities in schizophrenia. *Neurology* 50: 604, 1998.

Igert, C., G. C. Lairy. Intret prognostique de I'EEG au cours deL'evoltitions des schizophrenes. *Electroencephalogr Clin Neurophysiol* 14:183, 1962.

Ingraham, L., S. Kety. Adoption studies of schizophrenia, *Am J Med Genet* 97:18, 2000.

Israel, R. H., N. A. Johnson. Discharge and readmission rates in 4,254 consecutive first admissions of schizophrenia. *Am J Psychiatry* 112:903, 1956.

Ito, H., S. Nyberg, C. Halldin, et al. PET imaging of central 5-HT2A receptors with carbon-11-MDL 100,907. *J Nucl Med* 39:208, 1998.

Jacobsen, L. K., J. N. Giedd, C. Tanrikut, et al. Three-dimensional cortical morphometry of the planum temporale in childhood-onset schizophrenia. *Am J Psychiatry* 154:685, 1997a.

Jacobsen, L. K., J. N. Giedd, A. C. Vaituzis, et al. Temporal lobe morphology in childhood-onset schizophrenia. *Am J Psychiatry* 153:355, 1996.

Jacobsen, L. K., J. N. Giedd, P. C. Berquin, et al. Quantitative morphology of the cerebellum and fourth ventricle in childhood-onset schizophrenia. *Am J Psychiatry* 154: 1663, 1997b.

Jason, G. W., O. Suchowersky, E. M. Pajurkova, et al. Cognitive manifestations of Huntington disease in relation to genetic structure and clinical onset. *Arch Neurol* 54: 1081, 1997.

Jerinigan, T. L., L. M. Katz, J. A. Moses, et al. Computed tomography in schizophrenics and normal volunteers. *Arch Gen Psychiatry* 39:765, 1982.

Jeste, D. V., M. J. Harris, A. Krull, et al. Clinical and neuropsychological characteristics of patients with late-onset schizophrenia. *Am J Psychiatry* 152:722, 1995.

Jeste, D. V., L. McAdams, B. Palmer, et al. Relationship of neuropsychological and MRI measures to age of onset of schizophrenia, *Acta Psychiatr Scand* 98: 156, 1998.

Johnstone, E. C., T. J. Crow, C. D. Frith, et al. Cerebral ventricular size and cognitive impairment in chronic schizophrenia. Lancet 2:924, 1976.

Kahn, E. Organic driveness: a brainstem syndrome and an experience with case reports. *N Engl J Med* 210:748, 1934.

Kane, J. M. Schizophrenia. *N Engl J Med* 334: 34, 1996.

Kantor, R. E., W. G. Herron. *Reactive and Process Schizophrenia*. Science and Behavior Books, Palo Alto, CA, 1966.

Kapur, S., R. Zipursky, C. Jones. A PET study of quetiapine in schizophrenia. *Arch Gen Pstychiatry* 57:553, 2000.

Karp, B., M. Garvey, L. Jacobson, et al. Abnormal neurologic maturation in adolescents with early-onset schizophrenia. *Am J Psychiatry* 158:118, 2001.

Keefe, R., J. Silverman, R. Mohs, et al. Eye tracking attention, and schizotypal symptoms in non-psychotic relatives of patients with schizophrenia. *Arch Gen Psychiatry* 54: 169, 1997.

Kendell, R. Psychiatric diagnosis in Britain and the United States. *Br J Psychiatry* Spec No 9:453, 1975.

Kendell, R., R. E. The major functional psychoses: are they independent entities or part of a continuum? In: *Concepts Of Mental Disorder*, A. Kerr, H. McClelland, eds., Gaskell, London, 1991, 1. 16.

Kendler, K. S., A. M. Gruenberg, M. T. Tsuang, Psychiatric illness in first-degree relatives of schizophrenic and surgical control patients. A family study using DSM-III criteria. *Arch Gen Psychiatry* 42(8):770, 1985.

Kendler, K. S., M. McGuire, A. M. Gruenberg, et al. The Roscommon family study. I. Methods, diagnosis of probands, and risk of schizophrenia in relatives. *Arch Gen Psychiatry* 50:527 and 781, 1993.

Kendler, K. S., Genetic analysis. In: *Genetic Approaches to Mental Disorders*, E. Gershon, C. R. Cloninger, American Psychiatric Press, 1994, p. 99.

Kendler, K. S., S. L. Karkowski, F. A. O'Neill, et al. Resemblance of psychotic symptoms and syndromes in affected sibling pairs from the Irish Study of high-density schizophrenia families: evidence for possible etiologic hetrogeneity. *Am J Psychiatry* 154: 191, 1997.

Kendler, K. S., Molecular genetics of schizophrenia. In: *Neurobiology of Mental Illness*, D. Charney, E. Nestler, B. Bunney, eds. Oxford University Press, New York, 1999, pp. 203–214.

Keshavan, M., G. Hogarty. Brain maturational processes and delayed onset schizophrenia. *Dev Psychopathol* 11:525, 1999.

Kety, S. Genetic aspects of schizophrenia. *Psychiatr Ann* 6:11, 1976.

Kety, S. P. Wender, B. Jacobson, et al. Mental illness in the biological and adoptive relatives of schizophrenic adoptees. *Arch Gen Psychiatry* 51:442, 1994.

Ketter, T. A., B. A. Malow, R. Flamini, et al. Anticonvulsant withdrawal-emergent psychopathology. *Neurology* 44:55, 1994.

Kinney, D., D. Yurgelun-Todd, S. Tramer. Pre-and perinatal complications and risk for bipolar disorder. *J Affect Disord* 50:117, 1998.

Klaf, F. S., J. G. Hamilton. Schizophrenia—a hundred years ago and today. *J Ment Sci* 107:819, 1961.

Klein, D. F., J. M. Davis. *Diagnosis and Drug Treatment of Psychiatric Disorders*. Williams & Wilkins, Baltimore, 1969.

Klemm, E, F. Grünwald, S. Kasper, et al. [^{123}I]IBZM SPECT for imaging of striatal D_2 dopamine receptors in 56 schizophrenic patients taking various neuroleptics. *Am J Psychiatry* 153:183, 1996.

Kraepelin, E. *Dementia Praecox and Paraphrenia*, 8th Ger. ed. Livingstone, Edinburgh, 1925.

Kulynych, J. J., K. Vladar, D. W. Jones, et al. Superior temporal gyrus volume in schizophrenia: a study using MRI morphometry assisted by surface rendering. *Am J Psychiatry* 153:50, 1996.

Kung, L. S. Demorea, L. Siebenson, et al. Synaptic changes in the striatum of schizophrenic cases: a controlled postmortem ultrastructural study. *Synapse* 28:125, 1998.

Lachman, H. M., B. Morrow, R. Shprintzen, et al. Association of codon 108/158 catechol-O-methyltransferase gene polymorphism with the psychiatric manifestations of velo-cardio-facial Syndrome. *Am J Med Genet* 67:468, 1996.

Lacks, P. B., J. Colbert, M. Harrow, J. Levine. Further evidence concerning the diagnostic accuracy of the Halstead Organic Test Battery. *J Clin Psychol* 26:480, 1970.

Larsen, V. Physical characteristics of disturbed adolescents. *Arch Gen Psychiatr* 10:55, 1964.

Lauriello, J., A. Hoff, M. H. Wieneke, et al. Similar extent of brain dysmorphology in severely ill women and men with schizophrenia. *Am J Psychiatry* 154:819, 1997.

Lencer, R., C. Malchow, K. Trillenberg-Krecker, et al. Eye tracking dysfunction in families with sporadic and familial schizophrenia. *Biol Psychiatry* 47: 391, 2000.

Leonard, S., C. Adams, C. R. Breese, et al. Nicotinic receptor function in schizophrenia. *Schizophr Bull* 22:431, 1996.

Levitas, A. Neuropsychiatric aspects of fragile X syndrome. *Sem in Clin Neuropsychiatry* 1:154, 1996.

Lewis, D. A., S. A. Anderson. The functional architecture of the prefrontal cortex and schizophrenia. *Psychol Med* 25:887, 1995.

Liberson, W. T., I. W. Scherer, C. J. Ulett. Further observations on EEG effects of chorpromazine. *Electroencephalogr Clin Neurophysiol* 10:192, 1958.

Liddle, P. F., D. L. Morris. Schizophrenic syndromes and frontal lobe performance. *Br J Psychiatry* 158:340, 1991.

Lipska, B. K., N. R. Swerdlow, M. A. Geyer, et al. Neonatal excitotoxic hippocampal damage in rats causes post-pubertal changes in prepulse inhibition of startle and its disruption by apomorphine. *Psychopharmacology* 122:35, 1995.

Litman, R., D. Pickar. Noradrenergic systems. In: *The New Pharmacotherapy of Schizophrenia*, A. Breier, ed. American Psychiatric Press, Washington DC, 1996, p. 133.

Maier, W., D. Lichtermann, J. Minges, et al. Continuity and discontinuity of affective disorders and schizophrenia. *Arch Gen Psychiatry* 50:871, 1993.

Marsh, L., D. Harris, K. O. Lim, et al. Structural magnetic resonance imaging abnormalities in men with severe chronic schizophrenia and an early age at clinical onset. *Arch Gen Psychiatry* 54:1104, 1997.

May, P.R.A., H. Tuma, W. Dixon, et al. Schizophrenia: a follow-up study of the results of five forms of treatment. *Arch Gen* Psychiatry 38:776, 1981.

Mayer-Gross, W., E. Slater, M. Roth. *Clinical Psychiatry*, 3rd ed. Williams & Wilkins, Baltimore, 1969.

McGuffin, P., M. J. Owen, A. E. Farmer. Genetic basis of schizophrenia. *Lancet* 346:678, 1995.

Muscovitch, A., T. Katzelenbogen. Electroshock therapy, clinical and EEG studies. *J Nerv Ment Dis* 107:517, 1948.

Myers, S., D. Caldwell, G. Purcell. Vestibular dysfunction in schizophrenia. *Biol Psychiatry* 3:255, 1973.

Niswander, G. D., G. M. Haslerud, C. D. Mitchell. Changes in cause of death of schizophrenic patients. *Arch Gen Psychiatry* 9:229, 1963.

Nopoulos, P., I. Torres, M. Flaum, et al. Brain morphology in first-episode schizophrenia. *Am J Psychiatry* 152:1721, 1995.

Nordström, A. L., L. Farde, S. Nyberg, et al. D_1, D_2, and 5-HT_2 receptor occupancy in relation to Clozapine serum concentration: a PET study of schizophrenic patients. *Am J Psychiatry* 152:1444, 1995.

Olney, J. W., N. B. Farber. Glutamate receptor dysfunction and schizophrenia. *Arch Gen Psychiatry* 52:998, 1995.

Onstad, S., I. Skre, S. Torgersen, et al. Twin concordance for DSMIIIR schizophrenia. *Acta Psychiatr Scand* 83:395, 1991.

Ornitz, E. Vestibular dysfunction in schizophrenia and childhood autism, *Compr Psychiatry* 11:159, 1970.

Park, S., P. S. Holzman, P. S. Goldman-Rakic. Spatial working memory deficits in the relatives of schizophrenic patients. *Arch Gen Psychiatry* 52:821, 1995.

Pearlson, G. D., Wong D. F., Tune L. E., et al. In vivo D_2 Dopamine receptor density in psychotic and nonpsychotic patients with bipolar disorder. *Arch Gen Psychiatry* 52: 471, 1995.

Penn D. L., Mueser K. T. Research update on the psychosocial treatment of schizophrenia. *Am J Psychiatry* 153(5):607–617, 1996.

Pettegrew, J. W., M. S. Keshavan, K. Panchalingam. Alterations in brain high-energy phosphate and membrane phospholipid metabolism in first-episode, drug-naïve schizophrenics: a pilot study of the dorsolateral prefrontal cortex by in vivo phosphorus 31 nuclear magnetic resonance spectroscopy. *Arch Gen Psychiatry* 48:563, 1991.

Petty, R. G., P. E. Barta, G. D. Pearlson, et al. Reversal of asymmetry of the planum temporale in schizophrenia. *Am J Psychiatry* 152:715, 1995.

Phillips, L. Case history data and prognosis in schizophrenia. *J Nerv Ment* 117:515, 1953.

Pollin, W., J. Stabenau. Biological, psychological, and historical differences in a series of monozygotic twins discordant for schizophrenia. In: *Transmission of Schizophrenia*, D. Rosenthal, S. Kety, eds. Pergamon, London, 1968.

Pope, H., J. Lipinski, B. Cohen, et. al. Schizoaffective disorder. *Am J Psychiatry* 137: 921, 1980.

Pryor, S., Is platelet release of 2-arachidonoyl-glycerol a mediator of cognitive deficits? *Med Hypothesis* 55:494–501, 2000.

Quitkin, F., A. Rifkin, D. Klein. Neurologic soft signs in schizophrenia and character disorders. *Arch Gen Psychiatry* 33:845, 1976.

Ratakonda, S., J. M. Gorman, S. A. Yale, Amador. X. F. Characterization of psychotic conditions. *Arch Gen Psychiatry* 55:75–81, 1998.

Reichman, W. E., A. C. Coyne, S. Amirneni, et al. Negative symptoms in Alzheimer's disease. *Am J Psychiatry* 153(3): 424–426, 1996.

Remar, E. M., P. B. Hagopian. Changing Clinical Syndromes: Forty-Year Perspective. Presented at 125th Annual Meeting of American Psychiatric Association, Dallas, Texas, May 1972.

Rieder, R., D. Rosenthal, P. Wender, H. Blumenthal. The offspring of schizophrenics. *Arch Gen Psychiatry* 32: 200, 1975.

Rochford, J. M., T. Detre, G. J. Tucker, M. Harrow. Neuropsychological impairments in functional psychiatric diseases. *Arch Gen Psychiatry* 22:114, 1970.

Rodríquez, V. M., R. M. Andreé, M.J.P. Castejón, et al. SPECT Study of regional cerebral perfusion in neuroleptic-resistant schizophrenic patients who responded or did not respond to Clozapine. *Am J Psychiatry* 153:1343, 1996.

Rosenbaum, G. Feedback mechanisms in schizophrenia. In: *Lafayette Clinic Studies on Schizophrenia*. Wayne State University Press, Detroit, 1971, p. 163.

Rosenheck, R., J. Cramer, W. Xu, et al. A comparison of Clozapine and Halperidol in hospitalized patients with refractory schizophrenia. *N Engl J Med* 337:809, 1997.

Russell, A. J., J. C. Munro, P. B. Jones, et al. Schizophrenia and the myth of intellectual decline. *Am J Psychiatry* 154:635, 1997.

Sacker, A., D. Done, T. Crow, et al. Antecedents of schizophrenia and affective illness. *Br J Psychiatry* 166:734, 1995.

Schwab, B., R. E. Drake, E. M. Burghardt. Health care of the chronically mentally ill: the culture broker model. *Community Ment Health J* 42:174, 1988.

Shagass, C. M. Amadea, P. Duerton. Eye-tracking performance in psychiatric patients. *Biol Psychiatry* 9: 245, 1974.

Sharma, R. P., P. G. Janicak, G. Bissette, C. B. Nemeroff. CSF neurotensin concentrations and antipsychotic treatment in schizophrenia and schizoaffective disorder. *Am J Psychiatry* 154:1019, 1997.

Shaywitz, B. A., S. Shaywitz, K. Pugh, et al. Sex differences in functional organization of the brain for language. *Nature* 373:607, 1995.

Shaywitz, S., B. Shaywitz, K. Pugh, et al., Functional disruption in the organization of the brain for reading in dyslexia. *Proc Natl Acad Sci* USA 95:2636, 1998.

Shimkunas, A. M., M. D. Gyntherm, K. Smith. Abstracting ability of schizophrenics before and during phenothiazine therapy. *Arch Gen Psychiatry* 14:79, 1966.

Solomon, P., P. H. Leiderman, J. Mendelson, D. Wexler. Sensory deprivation: a review. *Am J Psychiatry* 114:357, 1957.

Stanley, J. A., P. C. Williamson, D. J. Drost, et al. An In Vivo study of the prefrontal cortex of schizophrenic patients at different stages of illness via phosphorus magnetic resonance spectroscopy. *Arch Gen Psychiatry* 52:399, 1995.

Steiner, W. G., S. L. Pollack. Limited usefulness of EEG as a diagnostic aid in psychiatric cases receiving tranquilizing drug therapy. *Prog Brain Res* 16:97, 1965.

Strakowski, S., P. Keck, K. Sax, et al. Twelve-month outcome of patients with DSM IIIR schizoaffective disorder. *Schizophr Res* 35:167, 1999.

Stromgren, E. Psychogenic psychosis. In: *Themes and Variations in European Psychiatry*, S. Hirsch, M. Shepard, eds. University Press of Virginia, Charlottesville, 1974, p. 97.

Susser, E. S. *Prenatal Exposures in Schizophrenia*. American Psychiatric Press, Washington DC, 1999.

Swain, J. M., E. B. Litteral. Prolonged effect of chlorpromazine: EEG findings in a senile group. *J Nerv Ment Dis* 131:550, 1960.

Swerdlow, N. R., B. K. Lipska, D. R. Weinberger, et al. Increased sensitivity to the sensorimotor gating-disruptive effects of apomorphine after lesions of medial prefrontal cortex or ventral hippocampus in adult rats. *Psychopharmacology* 122:27, 1995.

Szymanski, S., J. A. Lieberman, J. M. Alvir, et al. Gender differences in onset illness, treatment response, course, and biologic indexes in first-episode schizophrenic patients. *Am J Psychiatry* 152:698, 1995.

Tandon, R., J. F. Greden. Cholinergic excess and negative symptoms in schizophrenia. In: *Negative Schizophrenic Symptoms*, J. F. Greden, R. Tandon, eds. American Psychiatric Press, Washington, 1991, p. 61.

Taylor M., R. Abrams. Cognitive impairments in schizophrenia. *Am J Psychiatry* 141: 196, 1984.

Thaker, G., H. Adami, M. Moran, M. Lahti, S. Cassady. Psychiatric illnesses in families of subjects with schizophrenia-spectrum personality disorders: high morbidity risks for unspecified functional psychoses and schizophrenia. *Am J Psychiatry* 150:66, 1993.

Thaker, G., S. Cassiday, H. Adami, et. al. Eye movements in spectrum personality disorders. *Am J Psychiatry* 153:362, 1996.

Tice, L. F. New drugs of 1967. *Am J Pharmacol* 140:4, 1968.

Tienari, P. Psychiatric illness in identical twins. *Acta Psychiatr Scand* Suppl:171, 1963.

Tienari, P., L. C. Wynne, J. Moring, et al. Finnish adoptive family study: sample selection and adoptee DSM-III R diagnoses. *Acta Psychiatr Scand* 101:413, 2000.

Tsuang, M. T., R. Woolson, J. Fleming. Long term outcome of major psychosis. *Arch Gen Psychiatry* 39:1295, 1979.

Tucker, G. J., S. Rosenberg. Computer content analysis of schizophrenic speech. *Am J Psychiatry* 132:611, 1975.

Tucker, G. J., T. Detre, M. Harrow, G. H. Glaser. Behavior and symptoms of psychiatric patients and the electroencephalogram. *Arch Gen Psychiatry* 12:278, 1965.

Tucker, G. J., E. W. Campion, P. A. Kelleher, P. M. Silberfarb. The relationship of subtle neurological impairments to disturbances of thinking. *Psychother Psychosom* 24:165, 1974.

Tucker, G. J., P. M. Silberfarb. Sensorimotor functions and cognitive disturbance in psychiatric patients. *Am J Psychiatry* 132:17, 1975.

Tucker, G. J., R. B. Ferrell, T.R.P. Price. The hospital treatment of schizophrenia. In: *Treatment and Care of Schizophrenia,* A. S. Bellack, ed. Grune and Stratton, Orlando, 1984.

Tucker, G. J., Psychological impact of neurological disease. *Continuum* 3:95, 1997.

Tucker, G. J., Seizure disorders presenting with psychiatric symptomatology, *Psychiatr Clin North Am* 21:625, 1998.

Vaillant, G. E. Prospective prediction of schizophrenic remission. *Arch Gen Psychiatry* 11:509, 1964.

Vega, A., O. A. Parsons. Cross-validation of the Halstead-Reitan tests for brain damage. *J Consult Psychol* 31:619, 1967.

Verdoux, H., J. R. Geddes, N. Takei, et al. Obstetric complications and age at onset in schizophrenia: an international collaborative meta-analysis of individual patient data. *Am J Psychiatry* 154:1220, 1997.

Vita, A., S. Bressi, D. Perani, et al. High-resolution SPECT study of regional cerebral blood flow in drug-free and drug-naïve schizophrenic patients. *Am J Psychiatry* 152: 876, 1995.

Vygotsky, L. S. *Thought and Language.* E. Hanfman, G. Vakar, eds. and trans. John Wiley, New York, 1962.

Walker, E., E. Emory. Infants at risk for psychopathology. *Child Dev* 54:1269, 1983.

Watson, C. G., R. W. Thomas, D. Andersen, J. Felling. Differentiation of organics from schizophrenics at two chronicity levels by use of the Reitan-Halstead Organic Test Battery. *J Consult Clin Psychol* 32:679, 1968.

Weinberger, D. R., D. R., L. B. Bigelow, J. E. Mcinman, et al. Cerebral ventricular enlargement in chronic schizophrenia. *Arch Gen Psychiatry* 37:11, 1980.

Weinberger, D. R., K. F. Berman, R. F. Zec. Physiologic dysfunction of dorsolateral prefrontal cortex in schizophrenia. II. Regional cerebral blood flow evidence. *Arch Gen Psychiatry* 43:114, 1986.

Weinberger, D. R. Schizophrenia as a neurodevelopmental disorder. In: *Schizophrenia,* S. R. Hirsch, D. R. Weinberger, eds. Blackwell Science, Oxford, 1995.

Winokur, G. The schizoaffective continuum: Euclid's second axiom. *Ann Clin Psychiatry* 1:19, 1989.

Winokur, G., Tsuang, M. T. *The Natural History of Mania, Depression, and Schizophrenia.* American Psychiatric Press, Washington DC, 1996.

Woodruff, P.W.R., I. C. Wright, E. T. Bullmore, et al. Auditory hallucinations and the temporal cortical response to speech in schizophrenia: a functional magnetic resonance imaging study. *Am J Psychiatry* 154:1676, 1997.

Woods, B. Is schizophrenia a progressive neurodevlopmental disorder? *Am J Psychiatry* 155:1661, 1998.

Wright, P., N. Takei, L. Rifkin, et al. Maternal influenza, obstetric complications, and schizophrenia. *Am J Psychiatry* 152:1714, 1995.

Wyatt, R. Antipsychotic medications and the long term course of schizophrenia. In: *Contemporary Issues in the Treatment of Schizophrenia,* C. Shriqui, H. Nassrallah, eds. American Psychiatric Press, Washington, DC, 1995, p. 385.

Wynne, L. C. Methodologic and conceptual issues in the study of scbizophrenics and their families. In: *Transmission of Schizophrenia,* D. Rosenthal, S. Kety, eds. Pergamon, London, 1968: p. 185–200.

Yamada, T. Heterogeneity of schizophrenia as demonstrable in EEC. *Bull Osaka Med Sch* 6:107, 1960.

Young, D. A., M. Waldo, J. H. Rutledge III, et al. Heritability of inhibitory gating of P50 auditory-evoked potential in monozygotic and dizygotic twins. *Neuropsychobiology* 33:113, 1996.

Yudofsky, S., R. Hales. *American Psychiatric Press Textbook of Neuropsychiatry,* American Psychiatric Press, Washington DC, 1997.

Zappacosta, B, D. Monza, C. Meoni, et al. Psychiatric symptoms do not correlate with cognitive decline, motor symptoms, or CAG repeat length in Huntington's Disease. *Arch Neurol* 53:493, 1996.

Zornberg, G., S. Buka, M. Tsuang. The problem of obstetrical complications and schizophrenia. *Schizophr Bull* 26:249, 2000.

Chapter Four

DISORDERS OF COGNITIVE FUNCTION

The terms *organic brain syndrome* and *dementia* are applied to those acquired disorders of thinking and cognitive functions where altered structure or function of the brain can be identified. Generally, neurologists care for patients with these disorders. When no lesion or physiologic change is apparent, cognitive dysfunctions are often labeled *functional* or *psychological* disorders. Psychiatrists care for these patients. The inadequacy of this distinction is immediately apparent: any change in behavior must be the result of altered brain activity. In 1994 DSM-IV recognized this arbitrary distinction and did away with the division of behavior disorders into *organic* and *nonorganic* conditions. The section called "Organic Disorders" in previous DSM editions is called "Delirium, Dementia, and Amnestic and Other Cognitive Disorders" in DSM-IV; this category now stands alongside Affective, Anxiety, Schizophrenic Disorders, etc., removing any implication that there is one group of disorders related to the brain and another group that is just psychological (Tucker et al., 1994). To some degree, cognitive, affective, and behavioral symptoms characterize all disorders of the brain. There are cognitive disturbances in most of the major psychiatric disorders (see Chapters 3 and 5). However, the primary symptoms of delirium, dementia, and amnestic disorders are disturbances of cognition. Cognition comes from the Latin *cognitio*, which means *to think*. It refers to how one knows the world, which is achieved by a number of complex functions including orientation to time, place and person; memory; arithmetic ability; abstract thought; the ability to focus and to be logical. While disturbances of orientation, memory and numerical ability are the hallmarks of dementia and delirium, it is important to note that other types of dysfunction are also variably present, often depending on the location or nature of the lesion. Impairment of verbal and spatial abilities is common as well as personality changes and changes in the level of consciousness. Consequently, to make the diagnosis of a dementia, delirium, or amnestic disorder, the clinician must systematically evaluate: *(1)* orientation; *(2)* memory; *(3)* verbal, spatial, and numerical ability; *(4)* level of consciousness; *(5)* perception; *(6)* executive functions and *(7)* changes in personality. Only one of these areas may be involved in the disorder, but more often several are disturbed to varying degrees. Disturbances of executive functions tend to be the earliest signs of brain dysfunction, and often indicate that the frontal lobes are involved. Executive functions are basically those that one needs to live a normal life: the ability to plan and sequence activities, insight, judgment, social awareness and impulse control (Burgess et al., 1998). When there is a disturbance of higher brain function these abilities are commonly impaired whether the disturbance is caused by a neurological or psychiatric illness. The summary statement of the clinician's observations of cognitive functions is what is called the formal mental status examination (Taylor, 1981; Trzepacz and Baker, 1993).

Virtually all brain disorders can cause cognitive dysfunction. The site of the lesions may be related to specific symptoms and if these regional symptoms are prominent, the syndrome will often be labeled by the supposed anatomical site of the lesion, e.g., frontal lobe syndrome, or by the cause of the symptom, e.g., stroke. Such syndromes can be described *(1)* by anatomical site *(2)* by the etiology of the disturbance or *(3)* by its effect on cognitive function. We feel the weakest descriptor is the anatomical one as most behaviors and symptoms are caused by the interaction of many systems in the brain. Discrete symptoms can always be specified when describing those associated with the dementia or delirium or when citing their etiology. One must remember, however, that even though the patient's main symptoms may be hemiparesis and aphasia, and we attribute them to stroke, the patient may also meet the diagnostic criteria for dementia. In order to treat such a patient well, it is important to recognize both the motor/sensory symptoms caused by the stroke and the problems caused by dementia.

The diagnostic process for disorders of higher cortical functioning in both psychiatry and neurology remains clinical. Laboratory tests usually help only to rule out neurological or medical conditions such as thyroid disease or brain tumors (Bruckner-Davis et al., 1995). The main diagnostic instrument is the skill and knowledge of the examiner (Chapter 7).

REGIONAL SYNDROMES

Three major neurological factors shape the clinical manifestations of brain dysfunction: *(1)* the amount of tissue destroyed; *(2)* the location of the lesion in the brain; and *(3)* the nature of the disease process. With the advent of MRI, and particularly with the development of dynamic techniques to study the human brain as it functions (FMRI, PET, SPECT), we have entered a new era of localization. These powerful techniques based primarily on blood flow have yielded much information on where certain functions take place in the brain but not much on how they are carried out. The brain is a dynamic system of many interacting circuits, which makes it difficult to identify the precise site of a dysfunction. Consider as an example the following brain–behavior correlations: lesions in the dorsolateral premotor cortex have been associated with a loss of executive functions; lesions of the orbitofrontal cortex with disinhibition; and lesions of the anterior cingulate cortex with apathy (Cummings and Coffee, 2000). These same areas, however, have been implicated in such complex behavioral conditions as schizophrenia, mania, depression, OCD, personality disorders, and violence. Though it is clear that anatomical specialization exists in the human brain, the most replicable functional imaging results so far relate to behaviors that are relatively simple and discrete as in dyslexia, whereas the most conflicting findings relate to complex behaviors as in schizophrenia and depression. Even the anatomical localization of discrete functions such as language, however, can vary widely from individual to individual (Calvin et al., 1973).

Another obstacle to localization is related to the complex structure of the brain itself. Similar behavioral changes can occur when specific sites are destroyed and when tracts connecting these sites are interrupted. Chapman and Wolff (1959) in their classic study correlated the amount of brain tissue removed during the surgical removal of a tumor with postoperative behavior. When brain damage was not extensive (involving less than 120 gm of cortical tissue), executive functions were found to be impaired even though orientation and memory remained intact. Chapman and Wolff described four areas of dysfunction:

1. Expression of needs, appetites, and drives. There is less seeking of challenges and adventure, less imagination, less desire for human association and sexual activity, along with a passive acceptance of circumstances and a lack of aspiration. When mild, such symptoms mimic depression, and indeed, patients with slight brain damage often are depressed; the depression may be a reaction to or a manifestation of their deficit.
2. Capacity to adapt for the achievement of goals. Brain-damaged individuals have a decreased ability to anticipate either dangerous or propitious circumstances, to plan, arrange, invent, postpone, modulate, or discriminate in achieving goals. Business failure or unwise sexual liaisons, for example,

may occur in the course of advancing disease and may cause great distress to the patient's family, especially when he seems normal in other ways.
3. Socially inappropriate reactions under stress.
4. Incapacity to recover promptly from the effects of stress.

Deficits in the third and fourth categories can lead to the *catastrophic reaction* first noted in war veterans who had apparently recovered from brain injuries. When confronted with an arithmetic problem they once could have solved easily, patients became "dazed, agitated, anxious, started to fumble; a moment before amiable, they became sullen, evasive, and exhibited temper" (Goldstein, 1948). Although all of the above represent classic loss of executive functions caused by tissue loss almost the same clinical picture can be observed in patients who have had discrete surgical lesions of frontal tracts for frontal lobotomies (Shevitz, 1976).

Clinical Symptoms Associated with Frontal Lobe Dysfunction

Though symptoms of brain dysfunction such as those indicated above may appear regardless of the site of the lesion, they are often associated with frontal lobe damage. This has led to the formulation of a frontal lobe syndrome. Mesulam (2000) defines two types of frontal syndromes, but notes that they are umbrella terms covering diffuse sets of dysfunctions:

1. *Frontal abulia*—loss of creativity, initiative, and curiosity with emotional blunting and apathy.
2. *Frontal disinhibition*—impulsivity, loss of judgment, insight and foresight.

The frontal lobes are the largest neocortical region, and much of their tissue, particularly anterior to the motor region, can be removed with little or no disturbance of motor and sensory function. Bilateral frontal lobe damage can cause subtle alterations in the highest integrative functions without causing disorientation or memory disturbance. Lesions of similar extent elsewhere in the neocortex and subcortex, and in regions to which frontal fibers project, may produce the same symptom complex but, in addition, are accompanied by disorders of movement, sensory function, speech, and visual motor function, which often overshadow the disordered thought prominent in frontal lobe lesions.

Though the behavioral changes that are part of the frontal lobe syndrome may not be absolutely specific, it may be worthwhile to describe here those additional changes that characteristically occur when the frontal lobes are damaged. There may be a strong tendency toward inappropriate jocularity (witzelsucht) as well as inappropriate ill humor. Emotional "incontinence" is common, i.e., crying and laughing, which often alternate rapidly. This is provoked by minimal stimuli and often is not related to feelings of sadness or mirth. Indeed, a dulling of subjective emotionality is also characteristic. Dulled responsiveness may lead to poor self-control and an inability to understand the consequences of actions and to orient actions to the social and ethical standards of the community. When lesions are extensive, dulling may give way to torpor and apathy and sometimes to a state of *akinetic mutism*, in which the patient can speak and can move but will often not respond to spoken commands or even to painful stimuli but will tend to lie still, speechless, with open eyes. The patient looks awake and therefore is not considered to be in coma yet has little more cognitive function than a comatose person.

Some adverse reactions to antipsychotic medication may be confused with akinetic mutism. These include catatonic and akinetic reactions (Gelenberg and Mandel, 1977; Van Putten and May, 1978) and the neuroleptic malignant syndrome (NMS) (Lazarus et al., 1989; Koch et al., 2000). Parkinson-like drug reactions are characterized by a mixture of catatonic symptoms (waxy flexibility, reduced responsiveness, slow responses, incontinence of urine) with stiffness, bradykinesia, rigidity, and tremor. The onset is usually gradual and the symptoms may not respond well to anti-Parkinson agents.

The NMS is manifested by the abrupt development of lead-pipe rigidity, "plastic" akinesia, hyperthermia, altered consciousness (mutism, stupor, coma), and autonomic dysfunction (fever, sialorrhea, increased heart rate, incontinence) (Caroff, 1980). The blood creatine phosphokinase (CPK) level is characteristically elevated as a result of muscle breakdown. This can be so severe that renal failure can develop. The incidence of NMS is estimated to occur in 0.5 to 1 percent of those taking neuroleptic medication. Recovery is usually complete within 5 to 10 days after withdrawal of neuroleptics, but there is 20 percent mortality in this condition. It has been reported with all other dopamine receptor blockers and seems to be more frequent in males, especially those over 40 years of age, and in patients with brain damage. The EEG may be indicative of a metabolic encephalopathy. Some patients may appear to be suffering from encephalitis, but the cerebrospinal fluid is normal. The etiology is believed to be similar to that of the hyperthermia noted after the administration of some anesthetics. Other than withdrawal of the medication and supportive therapy, there is at present no specific treatment, although dantrolene and bromocriptine are reportedly helpful (Lazarus et al., 1989).

Motor signs are somewhat more specific for frontal lobe disease. When the motor portions of the frontal lobe are involved, particularly areas 4 and 6 or their many subcortical connections, motor paralysis may develop. In addition, a form of increased muscle tone (*gegenhalten, paratonia*) may develop. This is also called *counterpull* and is manifested by the semivoluntary resistance the patient increasingly offers to passive movement of his limbs. When the examiner attempts to extend the patient's elbow, for example, the patient will resist, and his resistance will increase as the elbow is extended farther. Forced grasping may be seen in response to tactile stimulation of the patient's palm by the examiner's fingers. When the examiner attempts to extend the patient's fingers while disengaging his own from the patient's grip, he may encounter counterpull.

Various forms of gait disorder may result from frontal lobe damage. One type that is quite similar to cerebellar ataxia may be seen in frontal lobe lesions and presumably reflects the many connections of the frontal lobe with the pons and cerebellum. Apraxia of gait may lead to loss of the ability to stand and walk, or even to sit steadily, despite a well-coordinated movement of the limbs. A form of *marche a petit pas* that superficially may resemble the small stepped gait usually associated with Parkinson's disease may be seen. It is widely based, however, and the patient often seems to be uncertain as to where be is going. A peculiar characteristic is the ability of some patients to step over lines and to climb stairs when they cannot walk on a flat, unmarked surface. Freezing in open doorways also occurs. Difficulty with the initiation of gait can be encountered in parkinsonism as well as in gait apraxia, but this symptom of parkinsonism can be treated successfully with L-dopa, whereas frontal gait apraxia does not respond to this medicine. Increased flexor tone caused by frontal lobe damage ultimately may lead to paraplegia in flexion.

Area 8 of the frontal lobes controls voluntary conjugate eye movements. Stimulation of area 8 causes the eyes to deviate conjugately to the opposite side. Destruction of area 8 leads to deviation of the eyes conjugately to the side of the lesion; but this is a temporary phenomenon, seen mainly in the first days and weeks following acute lesions. During convulsive seizures, the head and eyes characteristically turn away from the lesion, and during the postictal phase, they deviate back again toward the lesion. Because the frontal regions devoted to eye movements are so extensive, a good screening test for frontal disease is visual tracking. The patient should be able to follow the examiner's smoothly moving finger along a horizontal plane. If the patient's eye movement is jerky, discontinuous, or if it deviates from the examiner's finger, the presumption of frontal disease is justified. The ability to suppress antisaccades, to look up or down (to raise the outer limbus of the iris more than 5 mm, to lower it more than 7 mm), to maintain fixation for 30 seconds and to stop blinking after the third tap on the bridge of the nose are all frontal tests involving the eyes. The frontal battery should also include the two-and three-stepped Luria tests, the face–hand test, limb placement, grasp, snout, and suck reflexes and a test of word fluency (Chapter 7). Abnormalities on three or more of these tests correlate with abnormalities on the Halstead-Reitan battery (Jenkyn et al., 1977, 1985) and the brain MRI (Bae et al., 1998).

Clinical Symptoms Associated with Parietal Lobe Dysfunction

In general, patients with parietal disease are poor observers, have no awareness of their deficits, and perform variably on psychological tests from day to day. Lesions of the dominant hemisphere usually produce disturbances of speech, and lesions of the nondominant hemisphere produce gnostic deficits, faulty corporeal awareness, and defective visuospatial conceptualization. When such deficits are seen in patients who are not grossly disoriented, or dysmnesic, parietal lobe dysfunction should be suspected. Critchley's classic monograph (1953) described the clinical deficits that occur in parietal lobe disease. His categorization of abnormality is summarized in Table 4–1. Table 4–2 indicates some of the

Table 4–1 Some Neurological Deficits Seen with Parietal Lobe Damage

Tacticle Dysfunction

"Primary": Hemihypalgesia for touch, pain, heat, and cold
"Cortical": Astereognosis; agraphesthesia, extinction on simultaneous bilateral stimulation, two-point discrimination loss, position sense deficit with pseudoathetosis, sensory ataxia

Motility Disturbance

Apraxia for learned activities (following commands) or automatic acts (walking), *gegenhalten*, perseveration, echopraxia
Ataxia
Muscular wasting

Constructional Apraxia

Gerstmann Syndrome

Finger agnosia
Dycalculia
Right-left disorientation
Agraphia

Disordered Body Image

Unilateral neglect
Anosognosia
Denial

Visual Defects

Cortical blindness
Anton's syndrome (blindness with confabulation)
Hemianopia
Distortions: Macropsia, micropsia, obliquity, drifting, alexia

Source: Critchley, 1953.

Table 4–2 Origin of Some "Parietal"-Type Deficits in Single Retrorolandic Lesions

DYSFUNCTION	HEMISPHERE	LOBE(S) MAINLY INVOLVED
Apraxia		
Constructional	R > L 4:1	Parietal
Dressing	R > L 5:1	Parietal
Agnosia		
Somatognosia		
Denial of half of body opposite lesion	R	Parietal
Finger agnosia (bilateral)	L > R 6:1	Parietal, especially supramarginal and angular gyri
Visual Agnosia		
Neglect of space on side opposite lesion	R > L 10:1	Parietal
Nonrecognition of faces	R > L 3:1	Parietal
Nonrecognition of objects, pictures, colors	L	Occipital or post-temporal
Numbers not correctly placed	L > R 3:1	Parietal
Alexia	L	Temporal-occipital parietal
Agraphia	L	Temporal-parietal occipital
Acalculia	L > R 3:1	Temporal or parietal
Aphasia		
Fluent		
Wernicke (poor comprehension, poor repetition)	L	Temporal-parietal
Conduction (good comprehension, poor repetition)	L	Parietal-temporal
Anomic-amnestic (good comprehension, good repetition)	(a) Widespread brain disease (b) Recovery from other forms of aphasia (c) Also L parietal (angular gyrus)	
	L	Posterior-temporal
Nonfluent (motor)	L[a]	Frontal, temporal, parietal, rolandic

Source: Based on Hécaen (1962) and Geshwind (1971).

[a] R in a minority of sinistrals.

variability in the symptoms of single retro-Rolandic lesions that may give rise to parietal symptoms.

Hecaen (1962) and Hecaen and Angelergues (1962) provide a still valid basis for certain generalizations. Dysphasia and dyscalculia are characteristic of posterior left hemisphere lesions but do not occur in all patients. The speech of sinistrals in general is less seriously and less permanently affected by single posterior lesions of either hemisphere. Ideomotor apraxia, when it is the result of a single posterior lesion, is seen only with lesions of the left hemisphere and only in a small minority of these cases. Dressing apraxia and spatial agnosia are most characteristic of right hemisphere disease but affect only a minority of patients. Delerium can result from an infarct in either parietal lobe but is more commonly encountered in right parietal strokes than in left. Sometimes the only clinical clue that indicates focal disease in a delirious patient with a parietal stroke is a field cut to threat on the side opposite the lesion. Like all sensory deficits, this sign is difficult to elicit in a confused patient.

Symptoms characteristic of dementia or frontal disease such as indifference to failure and catastrophic reactions, and confusion can be encountered in many patients with unilateral posterior lesions. The most characteristic and striking feature of parietal lobe disease is that patients have agnosognosia—they do not recognize their sometimes obvious and extensive deficits e.g., hemiplegia, hemisensory deficit, hemianopsia, this feature of parietal disease can complicate their rehabilitation.

Clinical Symptoms Associated with Temporal Lobe Dysfunction

When lesions of the temporal lobes produce cognitive deficits, there may be concomitant paranoia, psychosis, depression, sexual dysfunction, and rarely, episodic violence (Tucker et al., 1986). The language deficits that may occur with posterior left temporal lobe lesions are presented below. The temporal lobe also plays a role in memory functions, though the mind's ability to record, store, and recall events cannot be regarded as localized in that region. Recent memory loss is the hallmark of all neurologic disorders that cause severe cognitive dysfunction, whether they are induced by focal or diffuse disease. There is no doubt, however, that the medial temporal lobe and the rest of the limbic system play an especially important role in memory function.

Memory loss (amnesia) has four clinical characteristics) *(1)* impaired ability to learn new material, *(2)* normal immediate recall (digit span, etc.), *(3)* preserved ability to retrieve some old, over-learned material, *(4)* intact intelligence, naming, and personality (Benson and McDaniel, 1991). In humans, limited bilateral lesions in regions of the limbic system can produce a severe, permanent disturbance of recent memory. This has been repeatedly noted after bilateral hippocampal destruction or after unilateral lesions in patients whose other hippocampus was impaired. That both of the hippocampuses are important for recent memory has been further emphasized by the observation that bilateral destruction of the amygdala, another limbic structure, does not cause any memory deficit. The fornix, however, must play some role in memory, given that its bilateral destruction makes the mental recording of ongoing events and their subsequent recall difficult, but the extent of memory deficit after sectioning of the fornices is not as great as that caused by hippocampal lesions (Ojemann, 1966).

Lesions in other areas of the brain can also disrupt memory function. Destruction of both the dorsomedian thalamic (DMT) and medial pulvinar nuclei produces severe recent memory deficits even when the hippocampus is intact. Dorsomedian thalamic lesions have been identified as the major anatomical correlate of recent memory loss in Wernicke-Korsakoff encephalopathy. Lesions in the mammilary bodies had previously been regarded as the locus of amnesia in that condition (Victor et al., 1971). Stimulation of the lateral surface of the temporal lobes, especially the superior temporal gyrus, in neurosurgical patients under local anesthesia, evokes remote memories, chiefly auditory and visual, apparently of long forgotten events. Usually these events were trivial and not of obvious psychodynamic significance (Penfield and Perot, 1963). Removal of the stimulated regions has not obliterated such memories, however, so it would be incorrect to conceive of the temporal cortex as a unique memory storage center.

OTHER SYMPTOMS OF CORTICAL DYSFUNCTION

Aphasia

The division of the aphasia into anterior (Broca or expressive) and posterior (Wernicke or receptive) types has prevailed for over 100 years. Geshwind (1971) proposed dividing aphasias into nonfluent and fluent. He considered pathology around the Sylvian fissure to be the primary source of most aphasia and identified nonfluent aphasia with precentral lesions and fluent aphasia with postcentral pathology. Benson (1979) agreed with this but said that this division characterized only approximately one-third of aphasic patients. He stressed that repetition is impaired in patients with perisylvian lesions, whereas repetition is normal or superior in patients whose aphasia derives from zones adjacent to the perisylvian language areas. One of Benson's greatest contributions is his delineation of extrasylvian (transcortical) aphasias (Benson and Ardila, 1996).

New methods are available for determining the site and extent of brain lesions that cause aphasia. Computed tomography and MRI using T-1 and T-2 sequences started the modern era of brain localization. To these have been added the fluid attenuated inversion recovery (FLAIR) MRI technique and diffusion weighted images (DWI). Functional MR, SPECT, and PET have shown much more extensive deficits in some patients than static imaging tests such as CT and MRI (Mettler et al., 1981). In general, the classical concepts regarding the cerebral sources of aphasia based on gross pathology have been confirmed (Kreisler et al., 2000), but there is considerable variation among individuals. Some of the variation is related to the freshness and type of damage and some to premorbid factors such as handedness, asymmetries in the size of the anterior and posterior halves of the two hemispheres (Bear et al., 1986), and individual variations in brain organization, some of which may have experiential roots (Rapin and Allen, 1988). Subcortical structures (thalamus and basal ganglia) and white matter tracts that connect portions of the cortex that support speech can all cause aphasic disorders when they are damaged.

Either hemisphere can support language despite the genetic program that normally establishes speech in the left hemisphere of most individuals. Unilateral lesions sustained early in life do not prevent the development of language (Annett, 1973). Even left hemispherectomy in children for control of epilepsy does not permanently prevent the development of language (Basser, 1962). Unilateral lesions on either side in children cause transient but not permanent aphasia. On the basis of intracarotid amytal injections in epileptics prior to surgery, Milner (1974) reported that if left-sided lesions are perisylvian, the right hemisphere is likely to have become dominant for language, whereas if lesions are extrasylvian, dominance remains in the left hemisphere.

The secondary, pathological lateralization of language to the right hemisphere in left hemisphere damaged children is evidence of the interhemispheric plasticity in the organization of a child's brain with respect to language. Recovery of speech in left hemisphere–damaged adults may also derive from a reorganization of language sources in the right hemisphere as well as within the left hemisphere (Kinsbourne, 1971; Knopman et al., 1984; Ohyama et al., 1996). Impressive evidence of right hemispheric participation in adult language function has been presented by Kinsbourne (1971); he studied three right-handed men who suffered left hemispheric strokes that caused aphasia and found that all three were able to speak a little at the time of testing and that one had shown considerable improvement. The speech in all three, however, was markedly impaired. Intracarotid injections of amytal caused complete speech arrest when the right carotid was injected but not when the left carotid was injected. It thus appears that whatever speech these patients retained or recovered after they sustained left hemispheric damage originated not in the remaining undamaged portion of the left hemisphere but in the right hemisphere

The dysphasic language in adults with left hemispheric lesions supposedly originates in the remaining intact portions of the left hemisphere. On the basis of the Kinsbourne study, it appears likely that dysphasic language is largely right hemispheric and that recovery from aphasia depends largely on how completely the right hemisphere can redevelop language skills. The participation of the right hemisphere in dysphasic speech may well be the reason why various forms of aphasia correlate incompletely with the anatomical locus of the lesion (Mazzocchi and Vignolo, 1979).

The contribution of the minor hemisphere to speech has been investigated by Gazzaniga and Sperry (1967) in patients whose cerebral hemispheres were functionally separated by commissural section. Testing each hemisphere independently, they found that information perceived by the minor (right) hemisphere could not be communicated in speech or writing and that complex calculation likewise appeared to be solely a function of the major (left) hemisphere. Nonetheless, the minor hemisphere showed considerable ability to comprehend written and spoken language, though less than the major hemisphere. These experiments suggest that in individuals with intact left hemispheric speech function, the right hemisphere may make some contribution to the understanding of language but is incapable of producing language.

Two opposing theories about aphasia had arisen by the beginning of the twentieth century, and they are still maintained. According to one theory, language is a property of cortical centers that have a particular functional significance. Destruction of these centers, the association fibers between them, or the projection fibers from them, it is believed, will produce predictable forms of aphasia. According to the other theory, the locus of the lesion is less important in determining the speech deficit than the adequacy of the remaining circuits.

The classic work of Penfield and Roberts (1959) provides evidence that supports the second theory. During operations on epileptic patients whose seizures had been impossible to control with medication alone, they stimulated and excised virtually all areas of the cortex thought to have a role in speech. Stimulation in either hemisphere produced vocalization and arrest of speech. It never resulted in actual speech or even words, but only grunts or the enunciation of syllables. In these and other studies that followed, such "speech areas" as the temporal and parietal regions, the supplementary motor area, and Broca's area have been removed. Excision of each area produced only temporary aphasic disturbances as long as the rest of the brain was intact.

What leads to the dominance of one hemisphere, how dominance is maintained, and how recovery from aphasia occurs are not known. Nor is it known whether the change in the language potential of the minor hemisphere that is thought to occur in childhood is the result of inactivity of that hemisphere or whether the dominant zone has some active role in the change. The mechanism of dominance may be analogous to the one demonstrated by Wiesel and Hubel (1965) for the visual cortex. If one eye of a newborn kitten is occluded for 2 to 3 months, the visual cortex becomes unresponsive to impulses from that eye permanently, but it is normally responsive to impulses from the unoccluded eye. When both eyes are occluded for 2 or 3 months and then tested, most of the visual cortical cells that still respond register visual impulses from both eyes.

Thus, it appears that the seeing eye of the monocularly occluded cat either preempts all the dendritic connections of the visual cortex or inhibits (suppresses) impulses that come from the occluded eye.

The development of right-handedness is part of the process by which the left hemisphere becomes dominant for speech and other functions. The fact that major speech functions reside in the left hemisphere of most sinistrals indicates that the two functions—handedness and speech—are independent. Yet the state of left-handedness implies that the right hemisphere is not completely subordinate to the left. In sinistrals, hemispheric speech dominance is less complete than in dextrals. This is manifested by the less serious and less permanent nature of speech deficits that result from either left or right hemispheric lesions in sinistrals. This is because the speech potential of the right hemisphere of sinistrals has not been permanently rendered ineffective by the dominant left hemisphere. Thus, both hemispheres are closer to being equipotential for language function in sinistrals. The time-course of recovery from aphasia after a destructive lesion has been sustained reflects the time necessary for the reorganization of remaining circuits for the development of speech functions, not just the recovery time for cells damaged but not destroyed. If reorganization supports restoration of speech, theoretically, it is conceivable that learning and practice can aid the redevelopment of language skills in previously underused circuits and that speech therapy could have a positive impact. This expectation has been realized in several group studies (Basso et al., 1979; Wertz et al., 1986).

Some remission in the symptoms of acquired aphasia is typically seen in patients with nonprogressive brain diseases, such as cerebrovascular disorders. Significant spontaneous recovery is often thought to occur even 3 to 6 months after onset. Available data suggest that most spontaneous recovery occurs mainly in the first month after the onset of aphasia (Pashek and Holland, 1988). Some improvement may continue for the next few months. The most important factors in recovery are early age of onset, left-handedness, and lack of bilateral or widespread brain damage. A variety of systematic rehabilitation procedures for aphasia have been developed. These have been summarized and discussed by Benson and Ardila (1996).

Progressive aphasia is a manifestation of dementia of various types that starts as aphasia without other signs of dementia and evolves over several years to a more general decline in cognitive capacity. It has been seen in Alzheimer's, Pick's, and Creutzfeld-Jakob diseases. Other neurobehavioral symptoms can be the presenting ones in these disorders with alexia, visual agnosia, or apraxia preceeding general dementia by several years. Progressive aphasia is therefore not a disease but a manifestation of any one of several dementing diseases (Benson and Ardila, 1996).

Like speech, there are other cortical functions that are unequally represented in various brain regions. Apraxia, agnosia, acalculia, agraphia, and alexia may result from retrorolandic lesions. Like aphasia, apraxia, and agnosia in sinistrals are generally less severe and less permanent than in dextrals (Hecaen and Angelergues, 1962).

Apraxia

Apraxia can be defined as an inability to carry out a voluntary act that the patient should know how to do, the nature of which the patient understands, in the absence of paralysis, sensory loss, or ataxia. In dextrals, apraxia of both sides of the body is likely to result from lesions in the posterior left hemisphere, especially the supramarginal gyrus of the parietal lobe. Certain forms of apraxia are more likely to result from right parietal lesions; these include dressing apraxia and constructional apraxia (loss of the ability to copy a two-dimensional figure).

Agnosia

Agnosia is the failure to perceive the nature and meaning of a sensory stimulus when the sensory pathways conveying it are intact. Visual agnosia is present, for example, when a patient is unable to recognize an object he clearly sees. The inability to recognize objects, pictures, and colors is almost always the result of a lesion in the posterior temporal—parietal regions but lesions in these regions do not always give rise to this form of agnosia. When present, visual agnosia is usually associated with other deficits of mental and cognitive function including the nonrecognition of faces (prosopagnosia) and hemianopsia (Benson and Greenberg, 1969; Rubens and Benson, 1971; Bender and Feldman, 1972). It is likely to be associated with a right parietal lesion, though only a minority of patients with right parietal lesions manifest this sign (Hecaen, 1962; Meadows, 1974). Probably some patients with left hemisphere disease would have this symptom but language disturbance prevents its detection.

Auditory agnosia, *pure word deafness*, describes the inability to understand words that can be heard. The pathology involves the primary auditory cortex (Heschel's gyrus) and/or its connection to the thalamus (Benson and Ardila, 1996).

Alexia and Agraphia

Rare syndromes like alexia without agraphia attest to the specialization of some cortical functions within specified brain regions. In this syndrome, patients can write—their names, for example—and then cannot read what they have written. There is usually a lesion in the splenium of the corpus callosum and a right hemianopsia-producing lesion in the left occiput. Even more rarely, hemianopsia is not present but the lesion in the splenium and adjacent white matter interrupts the connections of the visual cortex with the dominant angular gyrus (parietal lobe) so that the information that reaches the visual cortex cannot be transmitted to where it is interpreted and from which writing originates. If there is a lesion in the left angular gyrus there is alexia with agraphia (and usually a hemianopsia). Agraphia is an element of the Gerstmann syndrome.

The Gerstmann syndrome (1940) has four components, right-left disorientation, finger agnosia (the inability to name the fingers), acalculia, and agraphia. When all four components co-occur, there is usually a lesion in the left angular gyrus (Benson and Ardila, 1996). Each of the individual components alone or in combination with one or two of the others can be encountered with pathology elsewhere in the brain. The left angular gyrus is not a center for these functions, though it is an important component in the circuitry that supports them. Agraphia and acalculia may result from left temporal lobe lesions and acalculia from right hemispheric lesions (Hecaen, 1962). This information is summarized in Table 4–2.

DYSFUNCTIONS ASSOCIATED WITH SEVERING THE CORPUS CALLOSUM—SPLIT BRAINS

The theory that supple widespread neuronal circuits exist for all the higher functions is supported by the innovative experiments on commissurotomized patients. The nature of the functional differences between the left and right hemispheres has been explored by psychological testing of epileptic patients in whom commissurotomy was performed as a reasonable measure of last resort to control their seizures. In the initial postoperative period, such patients characteristically appear somewhat dull; there is temporal confusion, but orientation and speech are intact. Patients restrict their physical activity and have to be urged to perform the simplest body functions. As they begin to move about, a degree of spatial disorganization becomes apparent. The patient often settles into a repetitive pattern of behavior, such as closing a door with the right hand and opening it with the left, which stops only when he is distracted from the activity (Wilson et al., 1977). By flashing pictures, objects, written material, and numbers in a single visual field or by presenting objects for touch by one hand, the examiner can test each hemisphere independently. Material presented to the subject's right visual field or right hand registers in the left hemisphere. A picture of an orange, for example, can be flashed to the right visual field. The patient can then correctly retrieve by touching with his right hand an orange from a series of test objects. The subject would say in a normal fashion that the stimulus had been an orange.

If another object, such as a key, were projected to the left visual field, it would register in the right hemisphere. This information could not be conveyed to the left hemisphere because of the callosotomy. The patient claims that he has seen nothing (in other words, the left hemisphere "is talking"). The patient would be unable to use his right hand to retrieve the key from a group of test objects but with his left hand, the patient could retrieve the key. If the patient were asked what has been retrieved with his left hand, he would reply that be didn't know. Once again, this represents the "left hemisphere talking." The left hemisphere neither "saw" the visual stimulus nor had direct access to the tactile information. Because the right hemisphere performs consistently and well in such tests over a longer period of time, one assumes that it "knows" and is "aware" of the test stimulus but isn't able to "talk" about it (Gazzaniga and Smylie, 1984).

Anterior section of the corpus callosum frequently results in transient hemiparesis of the nondominant leg and temporary difficulties in initiating speech. Posterior section is followed by disconnection symptoms such as those in the example above. Visual and tactile stimuli presented to the nondominant hemisphere cannot be verbally identified because of disconnection from the language-dominant hemisphere. Total callosotomy additionally interrupts interhemispheric communication between the motor regions. This results in deficits in bimanual coordination and apraxia of the nondominant hand to verbal commands. Some of the symptoms subside, probably because of increased use of ipsilateral sensory and motor pathways. The residual symptoms are not disabling given that unrestricted visual scanning of the environment ensures bilateral representation of sensory experience. Cognitive functions are frequently improved by callosotomy (perhaps by lowering AED requirements), although preexisting lateralized deficits may be exacerbated. Language deficits are observed mainly in patients with crossed dominance. Studies in children reveal that callosotomy performed before puberty is not followed by permanent disconnection deficits. This may be attributable to the greater neural plasticity of the immature brain (Sauerwein and Lassonde, 1997).

In many ways the right hemisphere is identical in function to the left; reaction times are the same, intermodal transfers from vision to touch and from touch to vision are as efficient in both, and the ability to respond emotionally to provocative stimuli is equal in both but not the same. The right hemisphere is a bit disinhibited, more amused by earthy humor, for example. The left hemisphere is more proper and respectful of social conventions. The right hemisphere can "learn" any of a number of visual and tactile problems with the same rapidity as the left hemisphere. In short-term memory experiments, the right hemisphere functions as well as the left and its ability to control the left half of the body is equal to that of the left hemisphere in controlling the right. Stereognostic recognition for the left hand is present and intact in the right hemisphere, as it is for the right hand in the left hemisphere.

The major differences between the right and left hemispheres are seen in the analysis of language, speech, arithmetic, and morality. The left hemisphere is capable of speech but the adult right hemisphere is not. The left hemisphere has the capacity for complicated mathematical computations, but the right hemisphere is very poor at arithmetic. In some tasks, mainly those involving spatial patterns, relations, and transformations, the right hemisphere is superior to the left. For example, the right hemisphere has a greater capacity than the left for drawing block designs and for copying test figures. In addition, the right hemisphere apparently processes information by direct perceptual processing and does not depend on verbal reasoning processes for solving problems. It solves spatial problems directly and rapidly. In contrast, the left hemisphere solves similar problems slowly; the process is accompanied by a great deal of talking about the problem. It has been suggested that the left and right hemispheric modes of reasoning might interfere with each other if they were both located in the same hemisphere. If so, this would give an evolutionary rationale for the development of cerebral dominance in human beings (Sperry, 1974).

In young patients who have had commissurotomies and in patients who were born with the congenital absence of the corpus callosum, the interhemispheric differences noted in commissurized adults have disappeared. The functions normally associated with either the left or the right hemisphere may become established in both hemispheres. In independent tests of each hemisphere in such patients, it has been determined that the right hemisphere can produce spoken language, writing, and calculations as well as the left, and the left can perform spatial tasks as well as the right. In both young commissurotomized patients and patients with congenital agenesis of the corpus callosum, there is a tendency for language facility to develop normally but for nonverbal functions to be somewhat impaired (Sperry, 1974). This indicates plasticity of the nervous system and argues against the identification of a cerebral structure, even a hemisphere, with a particular function. It supports the view that the specific tasks of the "dual processor," language and nonverbal tasks, can be subserved by more than one neuronal circuit (Gazzaniga, 2000).

There is much less evidence relating lateralized hemispheric dysfunction to psychiatric illness, despite what might be called a clinical renaissance of cerebral localization in psychiatry. There have been approximately 40 studies of schizophrenia alone, most of which advance the hypothesis that some form of left hemisphere hyper- or hypoactivity is present. These theories have little factual basis and often depend on unreliable or untested indicators of cerebral dominance and cerebral activity. For example, lateralized amplitude of EEG activity or initial eye movements to the right or left are proposed as indicators of hemispheric dominance, but their correlation with other standards of dominance or with normal functioning has not been established (Marin and Tucker, 1981; Taylor and Abrams, 1984). Current evidence suggests that the major psychoses are characterized by bilateral rather than by lateralized dysfunction and that they possibly involve certain amine pathways.

DIFFUSE DISORDERS OF COGNITIVE FUNCTION—DELIRIUM AND DEMENTIA

Delirium is an excellent example of how the primary cognitive disorders differ from regional syndromes. Delirium demonstrates how the nature of the disease process is critical to the character of the brain syndrome rather than the anatomical site or size of the lesion. Brain syndromes of acute onset are often characterized by delirium. Delirium (Table 4–3) is a cognitive disorder of acute onset most often caused by toxic or metabolic causes. In delirium one can see all the symptoms of cognitive dysfunction, especially disorientation and alterations in level of consciousness, but also fear, irritability, and visual/tactile hallucinations.

The mechanisms underlying delirium are unclear. There is some indication that it is a disturbance of subcortical function affecting the ascending reticular formation. This pathway is intimately related to the ability to focus attention (Trzepacz et al., 1989; Figel et al., 1990, 1991).

There are two kinds of delirium (Meagher et al., 2000): an agitated or hyperactive type and a hypoactive or somnolent type. The agitated type is characteristically seen in such conditions as delirium tremens (alcohol withdrawal), fever, and anticholinergic overdose. The patient is overactive, often difficult to restrain, and tremulous. Hepatic coma often provides a good example of a somnolent delirium; the patient is difficult to arouse and when aroused seems quite confused and may often have myoclonus or asterixis. No clear neurotransmitter system has been implicated in either type of delirium, although anticholinergic agents will certainly make most delirious states worse. Flumazeil, a benzodiazepine antagonist, has been reported as being effective in temporarily reducing delirium in hepatic coma and in other delirious states, which may implicate the GABA system in some types of delirium (Bostwick and Masterson, 1998).

Delirium is the brain's acute or subacute response to a significant somatic stress. Other names that have been used for the condition are *acute brain failure*,

Table 4–3 Summary of Diagnostic Criteria for Delirium Based on DSM-IV

Disturbance of consciousness (defined as reduced ability to focus, sustain, or shift attention)
A change of cognition or the development of a perceptual disturbance that is not accounted for by a preexisting, established, or evolving dementia
Develops over a short period time (usually hours to days) and tends to fluctuate
Evidence that the disturbance is caused by a medical disorder or drug

acute confusional state, and *toxic-metabolic encephalopathy*, and they imply the cataclysmic nature of the stress. Toxic and metabolic disturbances can clearly cause delirium, but in other cases it may simply reflect the severity of illness. There are distinct risk factors for delirium; it is more common in the very young and the old, (particularly when febrile or overmedicated); when there is evidence of brain damage particularly dementia; and with the use of medications, particularly anticholinergics, meperidine, and benzodiazepines (Schor et al., 1992; Marcantonia et al., 1994, a, b). In the elderly, delirium is a poor prognostic sign. Francis et al. (1990) studied 229 patients 70 years of age or older who had been admitted to a general hospital. Twenty-two percent became delirious during the hospital stay; risk factors for the development of delirium were abnormal sodium levels, severity of illness, dementia, fever or hypothermia, psychoactive drug use, and azotemia. Patients with three or more of these risk factors had a 60 percent chance of developing delirium. The patients with delirium had a higher mortality rate, stayed longer in the hospital, and were more likely to be transferred to chronic care facilities. Even those who do not meet the full diagnostic criteria for delirium but develop, during hospitalization, some of the symptoms, such as disorientation, clouding of consciousness, or perceptual disturbances (illusions or delusions), are as much at risk for a poor outcome as if they met the full diagnostic criteria (Levkoff et al., 1996).

Delirium can be mistaken for depression in hospitalized patients because of the patient's often slowed, disorganized responses and inattentive manner. Psychiatric consultation services often find that 25%–40% of the referrals for depression turn out to be delirious reactions (Nicholas and Lindsey, 1995; Armstrong et al., 1997). Another factor that makes the diagnosis easy to miss is delirium's fluctuating course; a patient can perform quite well on formal mental status testing in the morning and be quite confused at night. As delirium is often a response to another condition, the accurate recognition of delirium is the first critical step in the effective care of the patient. Infection, often of the urinary tract, can cause delirium especially in mildly to moderately demented patients. Delirium clears in such cases when the infection resolves.

Delirium is almost the only disorder in DSM-IV that is consistently associated with a laboratory abnormality. The EEG in delirium is usually abnormal and this abnormality usually ceases when the delirium ceases. In most cases of delirium the EEG will show a diffuse bilateral slowing. At times there may be evidence of fast-wave activity superimposed on the basic slowing. The pathophysiology of the EEG changes is unclear although they are generally felt to reflect some change in metabolic activity, perhaps related to the cholinergic system. Anticholinergic agents can produce both delirium and EEG changes (Tune and Bylsma, 1991).

The treatment of delirium should be directed at the underlying causal condition but symptomatic measures can help too. These involve attempts to orient the patient, keep the room lighted at night, and, as a last resort, restrain him or her. Benzodiazepines and haloperidol in sedating regular dose schedules (oral, IM, or IV) have all been useful in the acute management of delirious patients. Often these medications are used in heroic doses, particularly in intensive care units where the agitated delirious patient can interfere with the treatment of the primary condition by pulling out IVs or trying to get out of bed (Frye et al., 1995).

Dementia is a disorder of varied etiologies that consists of multiple cognitive deficits and often motor and speech disturbances without a disruption of attention as in delirium (Table 4–4). Delirium is an acute disorder of the brain and dementia is most often a chronic disorder. When the term *acute* is used with de-

Table 4–4 The Differential Diagnosis of Dementia

Degenerative	*Neoplastic*
Alzheimer's disease	Gliomas[a]
Pick's disease	Meningiomas[a]
Huntington's chorea	Secondary tumors[a]
Mechanical	*Infectious*
Trauma[a]	Lues[a]
Occult hydrocephalus[a]	Abscess[a]
Subdural hematoma[a]	Chronic meningitis[a]
	Subacute sclerosing panencephalitis
Metabolic	Creutzfeldt-Jacob disease
Hypothyroidism[a]	
Hyponatremia[a]	*Exogenous Poisoning*
Hypercalcemia[a]	Metals[a]
Hypoglycemia[a]	Bromides[a]
Porphyria[a]	Alcohol[a]
Hypoxia[a]	Barbiturates[a]
Wilson's disease[a]	Belladonna alkaloids[a]
Uremia[a]	Organic phosphates[a]
Hepatic coma[a]	Hallucinogens[a]
Carbon dioxide narcosis[a]	Psychotropics[a]
Vascular	*Vitamin Deficiency*[a] especially:
Arteriosclerosis	B_1[a]
Collagen disease[a]	B_6[a]
	B_{12}[a]
	Niacin[a]
	Folate[a]

[a] Potentially reversible by medical or surgical means.

mentia, it implies a reversible cognitive disturbance, but in general the term dementia means stasis or inexorable progression. Until recently, almost all dementias were attributed to Alzheimer's or cerebrovascular diseases (multi-infarct dementia [MID]). With increased research on aging, many other forms of dementia have been recognized and some are fairly common. Pick's or frontotemporal atrophy (FTA) and Lewy body dementia (LBD) are two common types of dementia. The risk of dementia is approximately 1 percent at the age of 60 years and reaches 30 to 50 percent by the age of 85. With increased standardization of diagnostic criteria (Table 4–5) it has become clear that approximately 70 percent of dementia is caused by Alzheimer's disease; MID accounts for approximately 15 percent; FTA for approximately 5 percent (Eldmacher and Whitehouse, 1996). We expect the rates of MID, FTA, and LBD to rise as diagnostic sophistication increases and the comorbidity of these conditions becomes clearer.

As the population ages, clinicians will be confronted with disorders of cognition with increasing frequency. Recently, the American Academy of Neurology has published comprehensive practice guidelines, supported by extensive data, for the diagnosis and management of cognitive disorders. The first guideline refers to patients with symptoms of mild cognitive impairment, e.g., isolated memory impairments, without any other symptoms of dementia (Petersen et al., 2001). These patients are at high risk for dementia and should be followed regularly with standardized neuropsychological tests. The guideline for the diagnosis of dementia notes that in addition to neuropsychological testing, screening for treatable causes of dementia such as depression, hypothyroidism, and vitamin deficiencies is critical (Knopman et al., 2001). The evidence-based review of the management and treatment of dementia showed only a small benefit for the use of cholinesterase inhibitors, primarily in mild to moderate dementia, and indicated that vitamin E might delay worsening of symptoms. Good support was found for the active treatment of both depression (SSRIs) and agitation and psychosis (atypical antipsychotics) in patients with dementia. Psychoeducational

Table 4–5 Summary of DSM-IV Criteria for Dementia of the Alzheimer's Type

Multiple cognitive deficits manifested by both memory impairment (impaired ability to learn new information or to recall previously learned information) and one (or more) of the following:
- aphasia
- apraxia
- agnosia

Disturbance of executive functions
Significant impairment of in social or occupational functioning
Gradual onset and continuing decline

efforts for the families of cognitively impaired patients delayed nursing home placements (Doody et al., 2001).

Alzheimer's Disease

Alzheimer's disease (AD) is a progressive, partly treatable condition of unknown etiology that is often fatal within seven years of diagnosis. Described 100 years ago, it is surprising there is still controversy as to whether it is a genetic condition and what is the nature of the basic defect. Neurofibrillary tangles and neuritic plaques in the cerebral cortex characterize the neuropathology. It is probably familial in approximately 10 percent of cases (Heston, 1979). It is common knowledge that the brain shrinks in the course of aging and it is commonly assumed that the loss of cortical neurons is even greater in AD. Using a computerized method of image analysis that permits the high speed counting of large numbers of cells, Terry (1979) compared the brains of 20 clinically and histologically diagnosed cases of AD with brains from 20 normal individuals who died between the ages of 70 and 90 years. He found that the AD brains showed no significant loss of small neurons, no significant increase in glia, and no significant shrinking of neuronal or neuropil size. However, subsequent studies showed a 40 percent decrease in the number of large neurons throughout the neocortex (Terry and Katzman, 1983). The qualitative changes in neurons are as significant as the quantitative loss of cells. The microscopic hallmarks of AD are neuritic plaques (often containing amyloid), masses of ring-shaped silver-staining material in the cortex, and neurofibrillary tangles, intraneuronal fibers that stain with silver. A correlation exists between the numbers of these lesions and the psychometric deficiency (Blessed et al., 1968). Some cases of AD, especially familial ones, show "lawless" secondary growth of dendrites with bizarre clusters of spine-rich dendrites (Scheibel, 1979). Other signs of dendritic abnormality in AD have been reported (Buell and Coleman, 1979).

These neuropathologic changes appear to be quite relevant to the pathogenesis of Alzheimer's disease. Patients with Down syndrome, almost all of whom will develop dementia, also develop the same plaques, neurofibrillary tangles and amyloid deposits that are found in Alzheimer's disease if they live to be 30 years old (Schupf et al., 2001). The gene for amyloid production is located on chromosome 21, which has also been implicated as one of the chromosomes associated with early-onset Alzheimer's disease and Down syndrome (van Duijn et al., 1995; Blacker and Tanzi, 1998). Although the role of amyloid deposits is unclear, some have suggested that in both conditions the disease progression may relate to continued deposition and degradation of amyloid (Hyman et al., 1993). Other chromosomes that have been implicated in early onset Alzheimer's disease are 14 and 1; but all of these currently identified chromosomes can only account for approximately 50 percent of the cases of early onset Alzheimer's disease.

Every person has two genes that produce a certain type of apolipoprotein (APOE) and there are four types of such genes (1,2,3,4). One gene comes from each parent. Most people who have *APOE-4* from both parents will develop Alzheimer's disease by the age of 70. With two *APOE-3* genes the risk of Alzheimer's disease is much less. With one *APOE-3* and one *APOE-4*, the risk is intermediate (Roses, 1997; Blacker and Tanzi, 1998). The presence of *APOE-4* also lowers the age of onset of Alzheimer's disease. It is clear that there are other genetic factors not yet understood in the majority of Alzheimer's disease cases.

The new imaging techniques, though not being diagnostic of Alzheimer's disease have helped us understand the disease process. As people age, MRIs have shown an increased likelihood of white matter and perivascular hyperintensities called leukoaraiosis. These hyperintensities are some of the MRI manifestations of small vessel disease and correlate with increased ventricular volume, higher systolic blood pressures, lower frontal lobe metabolism, lower scores on neuropsychological tests of frontal lobe functions (DeCarli et al., 1995) and "frontal" signs on neurological examination (Blake et al., 1995; Bae and Pincus, 1998). Similar correlations of leukoaraiosis on MRI have been noted in patients with late-life onset of depression (Cahn et al., 1996; Salloway et al., 1996). Many of these changes are at subcortical locations that support the premotor frontal cortex, reflecting their role in frontal lobe function.

Biochemical studies of AD have indicated that there are no major deficits in several neurotransmitters, including norepinephrine, 5-hydroxytryptamine, dopamine, and gamma-aminobutyric acid (GABA), but that acetylcholine is seriously impaired. The major enzymes responsible for acetylcholine synthesis and hydrolysis, choline acetyltransferase, and actylcholinesterase, are markedly reduced. A presynaptic acetylcholine deficiency in AD is thought to exist, as there is no loss of postsynaptic acetylcholine receptors in the brains of AD patients (Davies, 1979). The loss of cholinergic neurons is specific rather than generalized; those of the basal nucleus of Meynert are heavily affected whereas those of the candate, putamen, and anterior horn cells are not. Cohen et al. (1995) has also shown that older adults have decreased choline uptake from the blood stream into the brain. The cholinergic system role in Alzheimer's disease is as yet unclear. Medications that inhibit acetylcholinesterase, (tacrine, donepezil, metrifonate, galantamine), all induce minor improvement in the cognitive symptoms of Alzheimer's disease, but do not alter the course of the illness (Knapp et al., 1994; Morris et al., 1998; Rogers, et al., 1998; Wilcock et al., 2000).

One of the major changes in the DSM-IV classification of Alzheimer's disease was the recognition that Alzheimer's disease involves not only memory loss but significant behavioral symptoms as well. Along with the primary symptoms, AD patients can have depression, delusions, and other conditions. Mega et al. (1996) studied a group of 50 Alzheimer's disease patients with mild, moderate, and severe cognitive impairments and compared them to age-matched controls. Eighty percent of the Alzheimer's disease patients had behavioral changes; the most common behavioral changes were apathy (72%), agitation (60%), anxiety (48%), irritability (42%), dysphoria and aberrant motor behavior (38%), disinhibition (36%), delusions (22%), and hallucinations (10%). Agitation, dysphoria, apathy, and aberrant motor behavior were significantly correlated with increasing cognitive impairment. Aggressive behavior has also been found to be more common in the Alzheimer's disease patients who are psychotic (Aarsland et al., 1996). Incontinence and aggression are the most common reasons for institutionalization of AD patients. One of the remarkable phenomena observed in AD patients is that the personality is often preserved even when cognitive processes are quite impaired. Many patients can carry on very appropriate conversations in social situations but when questioned about things that require memory functions, one suddenly becomes aware of how impaired they are. There is no way to predict the rate of progression of the dementing process of Alzheimer's disease. Clinically the Alzheimer's disease patient can remain relatively stable for years, but when cognitive functions begin to slip, the rate of change usually accelerates. The development of extrapyramidal symptoms, psychosis, or myoclonus signal deterioration (Chen et al., 1991; Stern et al., 1996).

Problems with memory often begin several years before the family consults a physician. There is often a disparity between the family assessment and the patient's self-assessment. When a patient complains of memory loss and the family does not agree, the patient's complaints are usually benign. If the patient does not acknowledge a problem but the family does, it is very likely that the patient is ill. From that point on the usual survival is approximately 8 to 10 years. Once the Alzheimer's patient is placed in an institution, the average survival time for men is approximately 2.1 years and for women approximately 4.5 years (Heyman et al., 1997). In general, dementia severity, general debility, vascular disease, sensory impairments, and aphasia seem to predict increased mortality (Bracco et al., 1994; Bowen et al., 1996).

Factors that may reduce the risk of Alzheimer's disease or slow the rate of decline are just beginning to emerge. Groups of patients who have used medications such as estrogen (Tang et al., 1996), anti-inflammatory agents (McGeer et al., 1996), and selegiline or alpha-tocopherol (Sano et al., 1997), all have had a lower prevalence of AD than comparable groups that have not. Ginko biloba is comparable to cholinesterase inhibitors in salutary effect (Wettstein, 2000). Many studies now show that patients with greater cognitive reserve (higher education levels and occupations that require more cognitive effort) seem to develop Alzheimer's disease less frequently and even when they do the cognitive impairments for the same amount of tissue damage are not as great (Stern et al., 1994, 1996; De Ronchi et al., 1998). Conversely, a history of learning disabilities has been associated with higher rates of dementia (Cooper, 1997).

Vascular Dementia

Vascular dementia (formerly called multi-infarct dementia) can result from discrete, small infarcts, caused by hyalinization of small vessels and from more severe strokes, intracerebral hemorrhages, emboli, and varied types of vasculitis. Although the course has been classically described as fluctuating with a stepwise progression, it can also be insidious; consequently the history of other medical conditions and the evaluation of the cardiovascular system, especially blood pressure is crucial. Sultzer et al. (1993) studied 28 pairs of patients (1 with vascular dementia and 1 with Alzheimer's disease) and found that the patients with vascular dementia had more severe motor retardation, depression, and anxiety when the levels of cognitive impairment were similar, but in spite of these research findings the clinical differentiation of the individual patient is still difficult. Risse et al. (1990) highlighted the difficulty of the clinical differential diagnosis of dementia in a study of 25 patients who met antemortem criteria for the diagnosis of Alzheimer's disease. At autopsy only 68 percent met neuropathological criteria for the diagnosis of Alzheimer's disease. Those that did not meet criteria at autopsy had dementias of diverse etiologies, e.g., corticostriatal degeneration, Parkinson's disease with Lewy bodies, and Pick's disease. The now-famous "Nuns Study" in which serial psychological tests were performed in life and an autopsy after death showed that AD patients without vascular disease had better cognitive function than those with AD alone and infarcts alone (Snowden et al., 1997).

Pick's Disease and Dementia of the Lewy Body Type

Current histopathologic techniques and imaging methods have delineated two seemingly distinct types of dementia: Pick's disease or frontotemporal atrophy and Lewy body dementia (LBD). Pick's disease produces prominent degeneration in the frontotemporal areas and at times there is also degeneration of anterior spinal neurons, the basal ganglia, or both. Inclusion bodies that have biochemical similarity are found in both of these frontotemporal degenerations, however it is more the localization of the degenerations that unites these syndromes. Both of these frontotemporal dementias have been linked to a genetic abnormality on chromosome 17 (Kertesz and Munoz, 1998).

It has been found recently that 15%–25% of demented elderly patients have Lewy bodies in their brain stems and cortexes. In most of the neuropathological studies of patients with Lewy body dementia there are some neuropathological findings that are similar to the neuropathologic findings in vascular and Alzheimer's dementia, but there are some dementia cases that have just Lewy bodies. As Lewy bodies have been found primarily in patients with Parkinson's disease the relationship of Lewy bodies to all of these conditions is as yet unclear (Klatka et al., 1996; McKeith et al., 1996). The clinical course of Lewy body dementia is interesting as there are prominent psychiatric symptoms in additon to cognitive changes. In Lewy body dementia there is rapid fluctuation in cognitive functions, particularly attention and alertness; recurrent well formed and detailed visual hallucinations; delusions and depression and motor features of parkinsonism (Klatka et al., 1996).

Human Immunodeficiency Virus-1 Dementia

Another recently described but fairly common cause of dementia is that associated with acquired immunodeficiency syndrome (AIDS) infections. In the course of human immunodeficiency virus-1 (HIV-1) infections, dementia is quite common, particularly late in the course of the illness, but when the dementia symptoms occur early in the course of the HIV-1 infection it seems to be a bad prognostic sign and often heralds a rapidly deteriorating course (Martin, 1994; Wilkie, et al., 1998).

Occult Hydrocephalus

Of the chronic conditions causing dementia, one of the most difficult to diagnose is occult hydrocephalus. Accuracy of diagnosis is important because this condition can be reversed by a relatively simple neurosurgical procedure, the placement of a ventriculoperitoneal shunt. Occult hydrocephalus is usually confused with one of the nontreatable causes of chronic dementia, such as AD or vascular dementia. The classical patient is a middle-aged or elderly person with gait disturbances, incontinence, and dementia whose ventricles are large and whose cerebrospinal fluid pressure, measured at lumbar puncture, is normal (Adams, 1975). In some patients, a previous history of head trauma, subarachnoid hemorrhage, meningeal inflammation, or tumor suggests the possibility of a deficit in the absorption or circulation of cerebrospinal fluid. But in most cases where the diagnosis of occult hydrocephalus is considered, the patient has become progressively demented over a period of months or years without any such history. At an early stage these patients sometimes consult a psychiatrist for symptoms like apathy, psychomotor retardation, and forgetfulness, which may easily be mistaken for a depressive reaction (Price and Tucker, 1977). Characteristically, a gait disturbance (apraxia) appears first and is more severe than the accompanying mental changes. This contrasts with Alzheimer's disease, which begins with dementia and does not impair gait until a relatively late stage of illness. Urinary incontinence and personality change have led us, heuristically, to describe such patients as "wobbly, wet, and weird." Magnetic resonance imaging and CT scanning have not been very useful tools for distinguishing hydrocephalus ex vacuo (in which brain cell loss has resulted in large ventricles) from hydrocephalic dementia. Enlarged ventricles and atrophy of the cortical gyri may be seen in both conditions. Evidence of enlarged ventricles, when unassociated with widening of the cortical sulci, as demonstrated by computerized axial tomography and when the cerebrospinal fluid pressure is normal, may suggest occult hydrocephalus (Gawler et al., 1976). But this too is not likely to avoid misdiagnosis.

Direct continuous monitoring of the intraventricular pressure via a catheter placed in one of the lateral ventricles for periods of 24 to 72 hours in patients suspected of being hydrocephalic has revealed intermittent increases above the normal range in some patients, particularly during REM sleep when the cerebral blood flow is increased. Some of these patients have subsequently benefited dramatically from shunting. Transient improvement after removal of 15 to 20 ml of cerebrospinal fluid may predict improvement with shunting (Fisher, 1982), but this test is unreliable. The time between lumbar puncture and improvement, if any, and the period of time needed for observation have not been established. The choice of patients for shunting relies on the art of medicine, which is to say that no firm criteria have been established. In general, the patients who have most consistently benefited from shunting have been those with demonstrable pathology whose symptoms have developed subacutely. Examples are patients with parasellar or posterior fossa tumors or malformations, and those who have had meningitis, subarachnoid hemorrhage, or head trauma. The shunting procedure, which sounds simple, is fraught with hazards and failures. Blocked shunts, subdural hematomas, and infection justify a conservative approach to this condition, which is not easily diagnosed (Clarfield, 1989).

CEREBRAL WHITE MATTER DYSFUNCTION AND COGNITIVE CHANGES

The primary symptoms of grey matter diseases, memory loss, and seizures, are not as common in white matter diseases where motor-sensory functions are more prominent than cognitive loss. Although patients with multiple sclerosis often have significant depression and cognitive impairment it is primarily a disorder of the white matter of the brain and as such represents another interesting model of the commonality, complexity, and ubiquity of behavioral symptoms associated with neurological disorders. Almost half the volume of the cerebral hemisphere is white matter (Filley, 1998). Cerebral white matter is mostly comprised of the tracts that connect the nerve cell bodies or gray matter. Each axon that traverses the brain and comprises part of the white matter is an extension of a nerve cell, the body of which is in the gray matter. Consequently it is often difficult to speak of a pure white matter disorder, because the cell bodies of which the white matter are extensions may also be dysfunctional when their axons or the myelin that covers the axons is dysfunctional. The major white matter tracts are those that connect and transmit sensory and motor information, commissure fibers that connect the two cerebral hemispheres, and short and long association fibers that connect portions of the cerebral hemispheres. The most common disease of white matter is multiple sclerosis. Multiple sclerosis is an inflammatory disorder of the myelin sheaths that causes waxing and waning sensory and motor symp toms. Associated with multiple sclerosis (MS) are frequent mood and cognitive changes (Klonoff et al., 1990; Nyenhuis et al., 1995; Sadovnick et al., 1996). As one would expect from a disorder that affects pathways, almost half of which connect with the frontal lobes, the cognitive changes are primarily in the area of poor concentration and inattention with consequent secondary problems in memory and learning. These cognitive changes are similar to those demonstrated by Parkinson's and Huntington's disease patients. They represent changes more in the efficiency of mental functioning than actual loss of function (Caine et al., 1986). There is little loss of language function in MS. Depression and lability of affect are common in MS. Patients also have significant elevations in cortisol and CRF, just as has been noted in depressed patients who do not have MS (Fassbinder et al., 1998). The cognitive symptoms of white matter, frontal, and subcortical dementias can be very similar.

DEPRESSION IN DEMENTIA

Demented patients often appear to be depressed. Depressed patients can also appear to be demented. Confusion, psychomotor retardation, and general apathy are commonly observed in depressed patients. These symptoms often connote brain damage, but clinicians have been reluctant to regard them as symptoms of brain dysfunction because they are reversible. With the increasing use of neuropsychological tests in psychiatry, however, it has become clear that most psychiatric syndromes, particularly schizophrenia and affective disorders, have manifestations that are characteristic of neurological impairment. To explain these reversible symptoms of dementia in psychiatric patients, the term *pseudodementia* has been used. (McAllister, 1983). There are no validated diagnostic criteria for *pseudo-dementia*, but Caine (1981) has stipulated the following characteristics: *(1)* A patient with a primary psychiatric diagnosis is intellectually impaired. *(2)* The features resemble, at least in part, a clear cognitive deficit. *(3)* The intellectual disorder is reversible. *(4)* The patient does not appear to have any significant neuropathology. Some have added various other discriminating features such as: the patient often acts as a caricature of a demented patient and frequently answers, "I don't know," to many of the questions that one would think he should be able to answer (Wells, 1979). Also, the EEG is usually normal in pseudodementia. Neuropsychologists can help to differentiate dementia from depression (Lezak, 1995).

The cognitive symptoms associated with depression may be a bad prognostic sign both for the future development of dementia and the irreversibility of the cognitive symptoms noted during the depression (Emery and Oxman, 1992; Alexopoulus et al., 1993). The often high levels of cortisol secretion in depressive disorders suggest a possible pathophysiologic mechanism (Nelson and Davis, 1997); in animals, prolonged elevated glucocorticoid secretion causes hippocampal damage. Thus, the prolonged stress of a depressive illness with its concomitant stimulation of glucocorticoids could lead to some of the cognitive changes associated with the illness. Another possible mechanism is suggested by animal studies showing that stress can increase dopaminergic (D1) activity in the premotor frontal cortex and also affect cognitive function (Arnsten and Goldman-Rakic, 1998). Methylphenidate is an underused remedy for the negative symptoms: inactivity, social withdrawal, inattentiveness, daytime somnolence, and loss of initiative of depression with dementia (Galynker et al., 1997).

NEUROPSYCHOLOGICAL TESTING

When dementia is moderate or severe, neuropsychological testing usually serves to confirm the physician's clinical impression, but in cases of mild or minimal dementia, psychological tests can provide clinical information that is not readily apparent to a careful interviewer (Lezak, 1995; Chen et al., 2000). Neuropsychological testing can give information about the localization of a lesion and, when repeated at intervals, can provide precise information as to the progression or regression of a disease process. This can be quite useful for treatment planning (Report Academy of Neurology, 1996). It is not easy to differentiate depression in the elderly from Alzheimer's or other dementias by neuropsychological tests. The response of deficits to successful antidepressant treatment is the only certain way (Robbins et al., 1996).

COGNITIVE SYNDROMES IN CHILDHOOD

Children have a different response to brain damage than adults, especially at an early age. Lateralization and dominance with regard to speech, reading, writing, and praxis are not fully established until several years after birth. After early unilateral injury to either hemisphere, these functions become established on the healthy side and surgical removal of the damaged tissue produces no further deficit. Thus, unilateral brain damage in children is less likely to cause permanent loss of speech or the other lateralized functions. Large unilateral injuries in infants, however, tend to produce a more widespread deficit in intellectual abilities than do similar injuries in adults. It is not clear why this is so. The older a child at the time of injury, the more likely he is to suffer impairment resembling that of an adult with a similar lesion. The classical cortical dysfunctions that may result from single lesions in adults are seen only in young children who have sustained bilateral cortical damage because these functions have not yet become lateralized. These dysfunctions include dyscalculia, right–left confusion, finger agnosia, constructional apraxia (Hansen, 1963), and aphasia (Landau et al., 1960).

In infancy there is an exuberant development of synaptic connections that peaks around age two. This probably underlies the greater reorganizational capacity of the immature brain to recover functionally after focal injury.

Early Childhood Autism

Disorders of speech are the hallmark of early childhood autism, a behavioral syndrome first described by Kanner (1957) and often in the past mislabeled "childhood schizophrenia." The diagnostic criteria for schizophrenia in children are the same as the criteria for adult schizophrenia, with emphasis on hallucinations and delusions. In children schizophrenia is referred to as early-onset schizophrenia. DSM-IV has placed autism within a group of disorders that represent serious developmental problems, called pervasive developmental disorders (PDD); all the disorders involve severe social and communicative impairments and often stereotyped behaviors, interests, and activities.

Although almost all the pervasive developmental disorders entail impaired speech functions, one does not. Asperger's syndrome can include all the symptoms of autism but without the speech delays or mental retardation. Another PDD is disintegrative disorder (Heller's syndrome), development is normal from between 2 and 10 years but then the child undergoes a severe regression and develops autism. All of this suggests a spectrum of autistic conditions rather than a single entity. Autism still remains the most common PDD. Using the DSM-IV diagnostic criteria for autism, its prevalence is approximately 1 per 1000 (Rapin, 1997).

The syndrome of autism includes speechlessness and an inability to make meaningful patterns out of auditory or visual stimuli. Typically, it begins in the first few years of life. Characteristically, feeding difficulties and excessive screaming mark the first year of life. Motor developmental milestones are usually somewhat delayed but within the normal range. Social withdrawal, odd behavior, and peculiar affect are usually quite noticeable by the second or third year of life. Autistic children have a marked inability to form human relationships and give a sharp impression of extreme solitariness. The severity of these symptoms varies, and those children who develop speech by 5 years of age have a fair chance of achieving independence in later life. Nearly all those who do not speak by this age require permanent care. Autism is often seen in children who also show strong evidence of neurological abnormality; it may be associated with phenylketonuria, tuberous sclerosis, and infantile spasms during the first year of life. Many autistic children have multiple cognitive deficits and perhaps half have electroencephalographic abnormalities or a history of seizures or both (Rutter, 1966; Rapin, 1998).

About the only feature that childhood autism shares with schizophrenia is the term "autism," itself one of Bleuler's fundamental symptoms. Otherwise, the two conditions are very different in age of onset, symptomatology, sex distribution (1:1 schizophrenia; 4 boys: 1 girl in childhood autism, PDD, Asperger's), and the social and intellectual status of the patient's family (high in autism and tending toward low in schizophrenia) (Kolvin et al., 1971). The only autistic syndrome that is more common in girls is Rett's disorder (stereotyped hand movements, poor coordination, language delay, social isolation, onset 6–48 months after normal development).

The prevalence rate of autism is 4 per 10,000 population. Only 9.7 percent of 207 families with one autistic child had more than one (Ritvo et al., 1989). There is no increase in the prevalence of schizophrenia in the families of autistic children, though anxiety and depression are more prevalent than in the general population.

The bulk of evidence seems to suggest that autism is not a disease entity itself but rather a behavioral syndrome of childhood that can result from many different disorders of the central nervous system that cause bilateral dysfunction and defective speech. In these terms, it is not difficult to understand why autistic children often have varying deficits in comprehension, symbolic thinking, and the formation of abstract concepts that reflect varying degrees of central nervous system dysfunction and the diseases that cause it. This could easily explain why the pattern of cognitive functioning is often uneven, with "islets of intelligence."

One strange aspect of autism is the occasional appearance of an isolated, unusual, and highly developed skill in an autistic child. Such is the case of the *idiot-savant*, who can tell on what day of the week any date will fall, though he is otherwise incapable of doing simple arithmetic and generally functions at a grossly retarded level. Similarly isolated and abnormally developed skills relating to music, memory, factual knowledge of history or science, or ability to read have been described in children who lack any developmental delay but have features of autism: eccentric, mirthless, flat personalities, unable to adapt socially. This is Asperger's syndrome. The abilities demonstrated are especially striking because they contrast so vividly with the individuals' low social capabilities. Recent studies have shown that approximately 75 percent of the patients with autism are mentally retarded. By adulthood at least one-third of those with autism will have at least two unprovoked seizures (Rapin, 1997).

Little is known about the etiology of autism though there seems to be a very high concordance in monozygotic twins (90%), but only 5–10% concordance in dizygotic twins (Bailey et al., 1995). The cerebellar cortex, the parietal lobes, and the corpus callosum have been implicated in a number of studies using MRI but not confirmed in others (Courchesne et al., 1988; Garber et al., 1989; Egaas et al., 1995; Hendrew et al., 1997; Piven et al., 1997). The neuropathologic studies of the brains of autistic children also point to the cerebellum, describing a paucity of Purkinje and granular cells. The brains also tend to be larger (Rapin, 1997).

The identification of the cerebellum as the site of abnormality in autism, about as clear a disorder of cerebral gray matter as exists (seizures and cognitive deficits), reveals much about the deficiency of the investigative tools available to us. The light microscope and MRI miss the neuropil, the site of synapses. We have no information about the number and quality of synapses in autism and we have every right to expect that they are abnormal. The cerebellum has no cognitive role, or a very minor one (Fiez, 1996). It is difficult to believe that it is truly the source of the behavioral abnormalities autism presents.

There is a little evidence that disturbed serotonin metabolism may play a role in autism. Increased levels of whole-blood and platelet serotonin as well as increased serotonin transporter levels have been reported (Marazziti et al., 2000). Tryptophan depletion and the use of agents that block serotonin uptake seem to improve many of the symptoms of autism (Longhurst et al., 1997); however, these effects may be related to nonspecific actions of medication rather than indicating a causal role for serotonin. These disparate findings would suggest that autism results from some generalized developmental process that affects information processing and language function. Some cases may have genetic determinants, others may be acquired, the result perhaps of prenatal influences that cannot be identified.

Attention-Deficit Hyperactivity Disorder

Attention-deficit hyperactivity disorder (ADHD) is the latest name to be applied to this condition; other terms have been minimal brain damage (MBD), attention-deficit disorder (ADD), hyperkinetic syndrome, and hyperkinesis. In part the names keep changing because the classification changes, and in part because theories about etiology change. Minimal brain damage was dropped because the relation to brain damage was unclear, although the World Health Organization (ICD-10) retains the diagnostic requirement of a history of perinatal or traumatic neonatal events. DSM-IV requires that the symptoms must appear before the age of 7 years and that the impairments must be significant in two or more settings (e.g., home and school). The symptoms must be present for at least 6 months. They are divided into two categories. The first is *inattention*: the subject fails to give close attention to details (makes careless mistakes); has difficulty sustaining attention; does not seem to listen when spoken to directly; does not follow through; has organizational difficulties; avoids or dislikes tasks requiring attention; often loses things; is easily distracted; or forgetful (six or more of the above symptoms are necessary). The second type is *hyperactivity–impulsivity symptoms*: fidgets and squirms; often unexpectedly leaves his seat; runs and climbs excessively; has trouble playing quietly; is constantly "on the go"; blurts out answers before questions are completed; has trouble awaiting turn; often interrupts and intrudes (six or more of the above symptoms are necessary). This division leads to three types of ADHD, an inattentive type, a hyperactive–impulsive type and a mixed type. Using the criteria in DSM-IV, the prevalence in this country runs approximately 3%–5% (3:1 greater in males), which is much higher than the prevalence in Europe (Arnold and Jensen, 1995). As diagnostic criteria have become clearer, it has also become evident there are significant comorbid conditions; 25%–30% of children with ADHD have learning disabilities; conduct and/or oppositional disorder, mood, anxiety disorders, or Tourette's syndrome. There is also increasing evidence that ADHD persists into adolescence (50%–80%) and adulthood (30%–50%) with significant psychiatric comorbidity of substance abuse, antisocial personality, mood and anxiety disorders (Zametkin, 1995; Murphy and Barkley, 1996; McCann and Roy-Byrne, 2000; Pliszka, 2000). The diagnosis of comorbid conditions is essential to effective treatment.

Many neurological conditions such as head trauma, seizures, and infection can manifest symptoms similar to ADHD (Zametkin and Ernst, 1999). Most children with ADHD show no signs of major neurological deficit, but many have minor signs. These include clumsiness; impaired succession movements; excessive synkinesis; motor impersistence; mild involuntary movements of a choreiform nature; inability to perform tandem gait, to stand on either foot, to hop, or in children more than 7 years of age, to skip. Stereognosis, graphesthesia, and two-point discrimination may also be impaired.

Other forms of childhood psychopathology can be mistaken for ADHD (Zametkin and Ernst, 1999). Depression, especially in the agitated form, could interfere with attentiveness and cause a child to be moody, irritable, hostile, overactive, unable to concentrate at home or school, and contribute to awkward socialization. Such a child could be forgetful and distractible. Mania expressed at age 6 could also produce the picture of a driven, hyperactive child, with poor concentration and easily distracted, who says and does unwelcome things. Obessive-compulsive disorder and other anxiety disorders (see pp. 203–205, 231–232) often cause poor concentration (Spencer et al., 1998), as may schizophrenia.

It is clear that the diagnosis of ADHD requires a careful evaluation. Many questions have been raised about the over diagnosis of this condition in both children and adults. This is based on the increased prescriptions for stimulants (Klein, 1995; Safer et al., 1996). Whether this represents an increasing awareness of the condition or an overuse of medication is still not clear (Elia et al., 1999; Zametkin and Ernst, 1999). This increased awareness is also apparent in the general population and it is a frequent self-diagnosis that brings parents and adults to consult physicians. Careful monitoring of the effectiveness of the medication can help in diagnosis, as in the correctly diagnosed patient the results of treatment are often dramatic (Elia et al., 1999).

Significant evidence has accumulated to show that there is a genetic element in some cases of ADHD. The relative risk for ADHD in the relatives of ADHD patients is 2%–10%. Although estimates from twin studies demonstrate that there is an 80 percent heritability of ADHD (Farone et al., 1998, 1999). There is some data to indicate familial subtypes where Attention-deficit hyperactivity disorder is comorbid with bipolar disorder and in others there is comorbidity with antisocial behavior (Farone et al., 1998). Molecular genetic studies have begun to focus on polymorphisms of the dopamine transporter gene (which inactivates dopamine) in ADHD patients (McCraken et al., 2000).

Magnetic resonance imaging studies of ADHD have found changes in the caudate, the corpus callosum, and the cerebellar regions; leading to postulations of a subcortical-cerebello-thalamo-premotor frontal circuit causing the motor and executive deficits noted in ADHD (Matochik et al., 1994; Baumgardner et al., 1996; Castellanos et al., 1996; Filipek et al., 1997; Mataro et al., 1997; Berquin et al., 1998). Functional imaging studies of ADHD have indicated frontal and striatal dysfunction (Zametkin et al., 1990; Ernst et al., 1994; Lou et al., 1998; Gustafsson et al., 2000; Krause et al., 2000).

Treatment. Over the years the stimulants, dextroamphetamine and methylphenidate, have become the standard treatment, each achieving efficacy rates of 70 percent for the symptoms of ADHD (Elia et al., 1999; Vitiello et al., 2001). In children with ADHD these drugs do not cause euphoria and rarely cause addiction. Transient tics have been noted with their use. Desipramine, imipramine, and bupropion have been tried, but the therapeutic effect was not sustained in long-term use (Biederman et al., 1989; Singer et al., 1995; Connors et al., 1996). The anticholinergic and cardiac effects of the TCAs limit their use in children. Sudden deaths have been reported with the use of TCAs, and they should be considered only if the stimulants do not work (Elia et al., 1999). Clonidine has also been found to be effective in ADHD (Elia et al., 1999). Psychoeducational efforts, behavior modification and social skills training are important components of the treatment of ADHD (Zametkin and Ernst, 1999).

Attention-deficit hyperactivity disorder in adults. Adult ADHD has received much attention in the media and it has become a popular self-diagnosis. One study (Roy-Byrne et al., 1997) of 143 adult patients referred to a specialty clinic for evaluation of ADHD found that only 32 percent met the diagnostic criteria, although another 36 percent had some ADHD symptoms without meeting the diagnostic criteria. The patients who did not meet the diagnostic criteria for adult ADHD usually had no documented history of childhood ADHD and often had severe comorbid substance abuse disorder (Biederman et al., 1995; Roy-Byrne et. al., 1997; Mannuzza and Klein, 2000). Mannuzza et al. (1991) followed up 91 white males with a childhood diagnosis of ADHD at a mean age of 25 years and found that although 30%–50% continued to have some symptoms, only approximately 10 percent had clinical symptoms that interfered with their ability to function. Comorbid substance abuse is a significant factor in the cause of adult ADHD (Biederman et al., 1993; Murphy and Barkely, 1996). Although there are many fewer controlled studies of the treatment of adult ADHD, the same drugs as used for children, seem effective in adults (Cox et al., 2001; Wilens et al., 2001).

CONCLUSION

In this chapter we discuss what appear to be a diverse group of disorders. But what defines them primarily is that they all represent disturbances of cognition. Certainly any disturbance of the brain will cause cognitive changes. Seizure disorders manifest cognitive changes; in fact the postictal state is an excellent example of delirium, but seizure disorders are episodic disturbances of brain function and the cognitive changes are usually transient and not the prominent clinical features. Depression can have cognitive changes but what defines a depression is the alteration of mood. Schizophrenia also shows cognitive disturbances but again this is not the defining diagnostic characteristic. The disorders discussed in this chapter, e.g., Alzheimer's disease, delirium, autism, etc. have distinct natural histories but they all have as their most prominent characteristic a disturbance of cognition, e.g., difficulties in orientation, attending to stimuli, executive functions, etc.

REFERENCES

Aarsland, D., J. L. Cummings, G. Yenner, et al. Relationship of aggressive behavior to other neuropsychiatric symptoms in patients with Alzheimer's disease. *Am J Psychiatry* 153: 243, 1996.

Adams, R. D., et al. Recent observations on normal pressure hydrocephalus. *Schweiz Arch Neurol Neurochir Psychiatr* 116: 7, 1975.

Alexopoulus, G., B. Meyers, R. Young, et al. The course of geriatric depression with irreversible dementia: a controlled study. *Am J Psychiatry* 150: 1693, 1993.

Annett, M. Laterality of childhood hemiplegia and the growth of speech and intelligence. *Cortex* 9: 3, 1973.

Armstrong, S. C., K. L. Cozza, K. S. Watanabe. The misdiagnosis of delirium. *Psychosomatics* 38: 433, 1997.

Arnold, E., P. Jensen. Attention-deficit disorders. In: *Comprehensive Textbook of Psychiatry/VI*, H. Kaplan, B. Sadock, eds. Williams and Wilkins, Baltimore, 1995, p. 2295.

Arnsten, A.F.T., P. S. Goldman-Rakic. Noise stress impairs prefrontal cortical cognitive function in monkeys: evidence for a hyperdopaminergic mechanism. *Arch Gen Psychiatry* 55: 362, 1998.

Bae, C., J. H. Pincus, M. E. Quig, et al. Neurologic signs predict periventricular white matter lesions on MRI. Abstract American Academy Neurology Meeting, April 28, 1998. *Neurology* 50:A448, 1998.

Bailey, A., A. Le Couteur, I. Gottesman. et al. Autism as a strongly genetic disorder: evidence from a British twin study. *Psychol Med* 25: 63–77, 1995.

Basser, L. S. Hemiplegia of early onset and the faculty of speech with special reference to the effects of hemispherectomy. *Brain* 85: 427, 1962.

Basso, A. E. Capitani, L. A. Vignolo. Influence of rehabilitation on language skills in aphasic patients. *Arch Neurol* 36: 190, 1979.

Baumgardner, T. L., H. S. Singer, M. B. Denckla, et al. Corpus callosum morphology in children in Tourette syndrome and attention deficit hyperactivity disorder. *Neurology* 47: 477, 1996.

Bear, D., D. Schiff, J. Saver, et al. Quantitative analysis of cerebral asymmetries: Fronto-occipital correlation, sexual dimorphism and association with handedness. *Arch Neurol* 43: 598, 1986.

Bender, M. B., M. Feldman. The so-called "visual agnosias." *Brain* 95:173, 1972.

Benson, D. F., A. Ardila. *Aphasia: A Clinical Perspective*. Oxford University Press, New York, 1996.

Benson, D. F., J. P. Greenberg. Visual form agnosia: a specific defectin visual discrimination. *Arch Neurol* 20: 82, 1969.

Benson, D. F. *Aphasia, Alexia, and Agraphia*. Churchill Livingston, New York 1979.

Benson, D. F., K. D. McDaniel. Memory disorders. In: *Neurology in Clinical Practice*, Vol 2, W. G. Bradley, R. B. Daroff, G. M. Fenichel, C. D. Marsden, eds. Butterworth-Heinemann, Boston, 1991, p. 1389.

Berquin, P. C., J. N. Giedd, L. K. Jacobsen, et al. Cerebellum in attention-deficit hyperactivity disorder. A morphometric MRI study. *Neurology* 50: 1087, 1998.

Biederman, J., R. Baldessarini, V. Wright, et al. A double blind placebo controlled study of desiramine in the treatment of ADD. *J Am Acad Child Adolesc Psychiatry* 28: 903, 1989.

Biederman, J., S. Farrone, T. Spencer, et al. Patterns of comorbidity, cognition, and psychosocial functioning in adults with ADHD. *Am J Psychiatry* 150: 1792, 1993.

Biederman, J., Wilens T., E. Mick, et al. Psychoactive substance use disorders in adults with attention deficit hyperactivity disorder (ADHD): effects of ADHD and psychiatric comorbidity. *Am J Psychiatry* 152: 1652, 1995.

Blacker D., R. E. Tanzi. The genetics of Alzheimer disease. *Arch Neurol* 55: 294, 1998.

Blake, P., J. Pincus, C. Buckner. Neuorlogic abnormalities in murderers. *Neurology* 45: 1641, 1995.

Blessed, G., B. E. Tomlinson, M. Roth. The association between quantitative measures of dementia and of senile changes in the cerebral gray matter of elderly subjects. *Br J Psychiatry* 114: 797, 1968.

Bostwick, J. M., B. J. Masterson. Psychopharmacological treatment of delirium to restore mental capacity. *Psychosomatics* 39: 112, 1998.

Bowen, J. D., A. D. Malter, L. Sheppard, et al. Predictors of mortality in patients diagnosed with probable Alzheimer's disease. *Neurology* 47: 433, 1996.

Bracco, L., R. Gallato, F. Grigoletto, et al. Factors affecting course and survival in Alzheimer's disease. A 9-year longitudinal study. *Arch Neurol* 51: 1213, 1994.

Brucker-Davis F., M. C. Skarulis, M. B. Grace, et al. Genetic and clinical features of 42 kindreds with resistance to thyroid hormone. The National Institutes of Health Prospective Study. *Ann Intern Med* 123: 572, 1995.

Buell, S. J., P. D. Coleman. Dendritic growth in the aged human brain and failure of growth in senile dementia. *Science* 206: 854, 1979.

Burgess, P., N. Alderman, J. Evans. The ecological validity of test of executive function, *J Int Neuropsychologic Soc* 4: 547, 1998.

Cahn, D. A., P. F. Malloy, S. Salloway, et al. Subcortical hyperintensities on MRI and activities of daily living in geriatric depression. *J Neuropsychiatry* 8: 404, 1996.

Caine, E. Pseudodementia. *Arch Gen Psychiatry* 38: 1359, 1981.

Caine, E., K. A. Bamfor, R. B. Schiffer, et al. A controlled neuropsychological comparison of Huntington's disease and multiple sclerosis. *Arch Neurol* 43: 249, 1986.

Caroff, S. N. The neuroleptic malignant syndrome. *J Clin Psychiatry* 41: 79, 1980.

Castellanos, F., J. Giedd, W. Marsh, et al. Quantitative brain MRI in ADHD. *Arch Gen Psychiatry* 53: 607, 1996.

Chapman, L. F., H. C. Wolff. The cerebral hemispheres and the highest integrative functions of man. *Arch Neurol* 1: 357, 1959.

Chen, J.-Y., Y. Stern, M. Sano, R. Mayeux. Cumulative risks of developing extrapyramidal signs, psychosis, or myoclonus in the course of Alzheimer's disease. *Arch Neurol* 48: 1141, 1991.

Chen, P., G. Ratcliff, S. Belle, et al. Cognitive tests that best discriminate between presymptomatic AD and those who remain nondemented. *Neurology* 55: 1847–1853, 2000.

Clarfield, A. NPH: saga or swamp. *JAMA* 262: 2592, 1989.

Cohen, B. M., P. F. Renshaw, A. L. Stoll, et al. Decreased brain choline uptake in older adults. *JAMA* 274: 902, 1995.

Connors, C., C. Casat, C. Gualtieri, et al. Bupropion in ADHD. *J Am Acad Child Adol Psychiatry* 35: 1314, 1996.

Cooper, S.-A. High prevalence of dementia among people with learning disabilities not attributable to Down's syndrome. *Psychol Med* 27: 609, 1997.

Courchesne, E., Yeung-Courchesne, G. A. Press, et al. Hypoplasia of cerebellar vermal lobules VI and VII in autism. *N Engl J Med* 318: 1348, 1988.

Cox, D. J., R. L. Merkel, B. Kovatchev, et al. Effect of stimulant medication on driving performance of young adults with attention deficit hyperactivity disorder: a preliminary double-blind placebo controlled trial. *J Nerv Ment Dis* 189: 63, 2001.

Critchley, M. *The Parietal Lobes*. Edward Arnold, London, 1953.

Cummings, J. L., C. E. Coffey. Neurobiological basis of behavior, In *American Psychi-*

atric Press Textbook of Geriatric Neuropsychiatry. American Psychiatric Press, Washington, DC 2000, p. 81.

Davies, P. Biochemical changes in Alzheimer's disease-senile dementia. In: *Congenital and Acquired Cognitive Disorders*, R. Katzman, ed. Raven Press, New York, 1979.

DeCarli, C., D.G.M., Murphy, M. Tranh, et al. The effect of white matter hyperintensity volume on brain structure, cognitive performance, and cerebral metabolism of glucose in 51 healthy adults. *Neurology* 45: 2077, 1995.

De Ronchi, D., L. Fratiglioni, P. Russi, et al. The effect of education on dementia occurrence in an Italian population with middle to high socioeconomic status. *Neurology* 50:1231, 1998.

Doody, R., J. Stevens, C. Beck, et al. Practice parameter: management of dementia. *Neurology* 56:1154, 2001

Egaas, B., E. Courchesne, O. Saitoh. Reduced size of corpus callosum in autism. *Arch Neurol* 52:794, 1995.

Eldmacher, D. S., P. J. Whitehouse. Evaluation of dementia. *New Engl J Med* 335:330, 1996.

Elia, J, P. Ambrosini, J. Rapoport. Treatment of ADHD. *New Engl J Med* 340:780, 1999.

Emery, V. O., T. E. Oxman. Update on the dementia spectrum of depression. *Am J Psychiatry* 149:305, 1992.

Ernst, M, L. L. Liebenauer, C. King. Reduced brain metabolism in hyperactive girls. *Am Acad Child Adolesc Psychiatry* 33:858, 1994.

Farone, S. V., J. Biederman, D. Mennin, et al. A prospective four-year follow-up study of children at risk for ADHD: psychiatric, neuropsychological, and psychosocial outcome. *J Am Acad Child Adolesc Psychiatry* 35:1449, 1996.

Farone, S. V., J. Biederman, D. Mennin, et al. Bipolar and antisocial disorders among relatives of ADHD children: parsing familial subtypes of illness. *Am J Med Genet* 81:108, 1998.

Farone, S. V., J. Biederman. The neurobiology of ADHD In *Neurobiology of Mental Illness*, D. Charney, E. Nestler, B. Bunney, eds. Oxford University Press, New York, 1999, pg. 788.

Fassbender, K., R. Schmidt, R. Mossner, et al. Mood disorders and dysfunction of the hypothalamic-pituitary-adrenal axis in multiple sclerosis. *Arch Neurol* 55:66, 1998.

Fiez, J. Cerebellar contributions to cognition. *Neuron* 16:13, 1996.

Figiel, G. S., C. E. Coffey, W. T. Djang. Brain magnetic resonance imaging findings in ECT-induced delirium. *J Neuropsychiatry* 2:53, 1990.

Figiel, G. S., M. A. Hassen, C. Zorumski, et al. ECT-induced delirium in depressed patients with Parkinson's disease. *J Neuropsychiatry* 3:405, 1991.

Filipek, P., R. Semrud-Clikeman, R. Steingard, et al. Volumetric MRI analysis comparing subjects having ADHD with normal controls. *Neurology* 48:589, 1997.

Filley, C. M. The behavioral neurology of cerebral white matter. *Neurology*. 50:1535, 1998.

Fisher, C. M. Hydrocephalus as a cause of disturbances of gait in the elderly. *Neurology* 32:1358, 1982.

Francis, J., D. Martin, W. N. Kapoor. A prospective study of delirium in hospitalized elderly. *JAMA* 263:1097, 1990.

Frye, M. A., M. F. Coudreaut, S. M. Hakeman, et al. Continuous droperidol infusion for management of agitated delirium in an intensive care unit. *Psychosomatics* 36:301, 1995.

Galynker, I., C. Ieronimo, C. Miner, et al. Methylphenidate treatment of negative symptoms in patients with dementia. *J Neuropsychiatry Clin Neurosci* 9:231, 1997.

Garber, H. J., E. R. Ritvo, L. C. Chiu, et al. A magnetic resonance imaging study of autism: normal fourth ventricle size and absence of pathology. *Am J Psychiatry* 146(4):532, 1989.

Gawler, J., G. H. DuBoulay, J. W. Bull, et al. Computerized tomography: a comparison with pneumoencephalography and ventriculography. *J Neurol Neurosurg Psychiatry* 39:203, 1976.

Gazzaniga, M. S., C. S. Smylie. Dissociation of language and cognition. A psychological profile of two disconnected right hemispheres. *Brain* 107:145, 1984.

Gazzaniga, M. S., R. W. Sperry. Language after section of the cerebral commissures. *Brain* 90:131, 1967.

Gazzaniga, M. S., Cerebral specialization and interhemiospheric communication. *Brain* 123:1293, 2000.

Geldmacher, D. S., P. J. Whitehouse. Evaulation of dementia. *N Engl J Med* 335:330, 1996.

Gelenberg, A. J., M. R. Mandel. Catatonic reactions to bigb-potency neuroleptic drugs. *Arch Gen Psychiatry* 34:947, 1977.

Gerstmann, J. Syndrome of finger agnosia, disorientation for right and left, agraphia, and acalculia. *Arch Neurol Psychiatry* 44:398, 1940.

Geshwind, N., A. M. Galaburda. Cerebral lateralization. Biological mechanisms, associations, and pathology: a hypothesis and a program for research. *Arch Neurol* 42: 428, 521, 634, 1985.

Golden, C. J. A standardized "version of Luria's neuropsychological tests." In: *Handbook of Clinical Neuropsychology,* S. Filskov, T. Ball, eds. John Wiley, New York, 1981, p. 608.

Goldstein, K. *After-Effects of Brain Injuries in* War: *Their Evaluation and Treatment.* Grune & Stratton, New York, 1948.

Gustafsson, P., G. Thernlund, E. Ryding, et al. Associations between cerebral blood flow measured by SPECT, EEG, behavior symptoms, cognition and neurological soft signs in children with ADHD. *Acta Paediatr* 89:830, 2000.

Hansen, E. Reading and writing difficulties in children with cerebral palsy. In: *Minimal Cerebral Dysfunction*, R. C. MacKeith, M. Bax, eds. 1963 (No. 10, N.Y. Little Club Clinics in Developmental Medicine), p. 58.

Hecaen, H. Clinical symptomatology in right and left hemisphere lesions. In: *Interhemispheric Relations and Cerebral Dominance*, V. B. Mountcastle, ed. Johns Hopkins University Press, Baltimore, 1962, p. 215.

Hecaen, H., P. Angelergues. L'aphasie, l'agnosie chez les gauchers: modalites et frequence des trouble selon l'hemisphere atteint. *Rev Neurol* 106:510, 1962.

Hendren, R. L., I. De Backer, G. J. Pandina. Review of neuroimaging studies of child and adolescent psychiatric disorders from the past 10 years. *J Am Acad Child Adolesc Psychiatry* 39:815, 1997.

Heston, L. L. Genetic relationships to Down's syndrome and hematologic cancer. In: *Congenital and Acquired Cognitive Disorders*, R. Katzman, ed. Raven Press, New York, 1979.

Heyman, A., B. Peterson, G. Fillenbaum, C. Pieper. Predictors of time to institutionalization of patients with Alzheimer's disease: the CERAD experience, Part XVII. *Neurology* 48:1304, 1997.

Hyman, B. T., K. Marzloff, P. V. Arriagda. The accumulation of senile plaques or amyloid burden in Alzheimers disease. *J Neuropathol Exp Neurol* 52:648, 1993.

Jenkyn, L. R., D. B. Walsh, C. M. Culver, et al. Clinical signs in diffuse cerebral dysfunction. *J Neurol Neurosurg Psychiatry* 40:956, 1977.

Jenkyn, L. R., A. G. Reeves, T. Warren, et al. Neurologic signs in senesance. *Arch Neurol* 42:1154, 1985.

Kertesz, A., D. Munoz. Pick's disease, frontotemporal dementia, and Pick complex. *Arch Neurol* 55:302, 1998.

Kinsbourne, M. The minor cerebral hemisphere as a source of aphasic speech. *Arch Neurol* 25:302, 1971.

Klatka, L. A., E. D. Louis, R. B. Schiffer. Psychiatric features in diffuse Lewy body disease: a clinicopathologic study using Alzheimer's disease and Parkinson's disease comparison groups. *Neurology* 47:1148, 1996.

Klein, R. The role of methylphenidate in psychiatry. *Arch Gen Psychiatry* 52:429–433, 1995.

Klonoff, H., C. Clark, J. Oger, et al. Neuropsychological performance in patients with mild multiple sclerosis. *J Nerv Ment Dis* 179:127, 1991.

Knapp, M. J., D. S. Knopman, P. R. Solomon, et al. A 30-week randomized controlled trial of high-dose tacrine in patients with Alzheimer's disease. *JAMA* 271:985, 1994.

Knopman, D. S., A. B. Rubens, O. A. Selnes, et al. Mechanisms of recovery from aphasia: evidence from serial xenon 133 cerebral blood flow studies. *Ann Neurol* 15: 530, 1984.

Knopman, D. S, S., DeKoskey, J. Cummings, et al. Practice parameter: diagnosis of dementia. *Neurology* 56:1143, 2001.

Koch, M., S. Chandragiri, S. Rizvi, et al. Catatonic signs in NMS. *Compr Psychiatry* 41:73, 2000.

Kolvin, I., C. Ounsted, L. M. Richardson, R. F. Garside. III. The family and social background in childhood psychoses. *Br J Psychiatry* 118:396, 1971.

Krause, K., S. Dresel, J. Krause, et al. Increased striatal dopamine transporter in adult patients with ADHD. *Neurosci Lett* 285:107, 2000.

Kreisler, A., O. Godefroy, C. Delmaire, et al. The anatomy of aphasia revisited. Neurology, 54:1117, 2000.

Landau, W. M., R. Goldstein, F. R. Kleffner. Congenital aphasia: a clinicopathologic study. *Neurology* 10:915, 1960.

Lazarus, A., S. Mann, S. Caroff. *The Neuroleptic Malignant Syndrome and Related Conditions*, American Psychiatric Press, Washington, DC, 1989.

Levkoff, S. E., B. Liptzin, P. D. Cleary, et al. Subsyndromal delirium. *Am J Geriatr Psychiatry* 4:320, 1996.

Lezak, M. *Neuropsychological Assessment*, 3rd ed. New York, Oxford University Press, 1995.

Longhurst, J., M. Potenza, C. McDougle. Autism. *New Eng J Med* 337:1555, 1997.

Lou, H., J. Andresen, B. Steinberg, et al. The striatrum in a putive cerebral network activated by verbal awareness in normals and in ADHD children. *Eur J Neurol* 5:67, 1998.

Mannuzza, S., R. Klein, K. Addalli. Young adult mental status of hyperactive boys and their brothers. *J Am Acad Child Adol Psychiatry* 30:743, 1991.

Mannuzza, S., K. Klein. Long term prognosis in ADHD. *Child Adolesc Psychiatry Clin N Am* 9:711, 2000.

Marazziti, D., F. Muratoni, A. Cesari, et al. Increased density of the platelet serotonin transporter in autism. *Pharmacopsychiatry* 33:165, 2000.

Marcantonio, E. R., L. Goldman, C. M. Mangione, et al. A clinical prediction rule for delirium after elective noncardiac surgery. *JAMA* 271:134, 1994a.

Marcatonio, E. R., G. Juarez, L. Goldman, et al. The relationship of postoperative delirium with psychoactive medications. *JAMA* 272:1518, 1994b.

Marin, R., G. J. Tucker. Psychopathology and hemispheric dysfunction. *J Nerv Ment Dis* 169:546, 1981.

Martin, A. Clinically significant cognitive dysfunction in medically asymptomatic human immunodeficiency virus infected individuals. *Psychosom Med* 56:18, 1994.

Mataro, M. Garcia-Sánchez, C. Junqué, et al. Magnetic resonance imaging measurement of the caudate nucleus in adolescents with attention-deficit hyperactivity disorder and its relationship with neuropsychological and behavioral measures. *Arch Neurol* 54: 963, 1997.

Matochik, J., L. Liebenauer, C. King, et al. Cerebral glucose metabolism in adults with attention deficit-hyperactivity disorder after chronic stimulant treatment. *Am J Psychiatry* 151:658, 1994.

Mazzocchi, F., L. A. Vignola. Localization of lesions in aphasia: clinical-CT correlation in stroke patients. *Cortex* 15:627, 1979.

McAllister, T. Pseudodementia. *Am J Psychiatry* 140:528, 1983.

McCann, B., P. Roy-Byrne. ADHD and learning disability in adults. *Semin Clin Neuropsychiatry* 5:191, 2000.

McCracken, J., S. Smalley, J. McGough, et al. Evidence of linkage of a tandem duplication polymorphism upstream of the dopamine D4 receptor gene (DRD4) with ADHD. *Mol Psychiatry* 5:531, 2000.

McGeer, P. L., M. Schulzer, E. G. McGeer. Arthritis and anti-inflammatory agents as possible protective factors for Alzheimer's disease: a review of 17 epidemiological studies *Neurology* 47:425, 1996.

McKeith, I. G., D. Galasko, K. Kosaka, et al. Consensus guidelines for the clinical pathological diagnosis of dementia with Lewy bodies (DLB): report of the consortium on DLB international workshop. *Neurology* 47:1113, 1996.

Meadows, J. C. The anatomical basis of prosopagnosia. *J Neurol Neurosurg Psychiatry* 37:489, 1974.

Meagher, D., P. Trzepacz. Motoric subtypes of delirium. *Semin Clin Neuropsychiatry* 5: 13, 2000.

Mega, M. S., J. L. Cummings, T. Fiorello, J. Gornbein. The spectrum of behavioral changes in Alzheimer's disease. *Neurology* 46:130, 1996.

Mesulam, M., *Principles of Behavioral and Cognitive Neurology*, 2nd Ed. Oxford University Press, New York, 2000, p 42.

Mettler, E. J., C. G. Wasterlain, D. E. Kuhl, et al. FDG positron emission computed tomography in a study of aphasia. *Ann Neurol* 10:173, 1981.

Milner, B. Hemispheric specialization: scope and limits. In: *The Neurosciences: Third Study Program*, F. O. Schmitt, F. G. Worden, eds. MIT Press, Cambridge, MA, 1974, p. 75.

Morris, J. C., P. A. Cyrus, J. Orazem, et al. Metrifonate benefits cognitive, behavioral, and global function in patients with Alzheimer's disease. *Neurology* 50:1222, 1998.

Murphy, K., R. A. Barkley. Attention deficit hyperactivity disorder adults: comorbidities and adaptive impairments. *Compr Psychiatry* 37:393, 1996.

Nelson, J. C., J. M. Davis. DST studies in psychotic depression: a meta-analysis. *Am Psychiatry* 154:1497, 1997.

Nicholas, L. M., B. A. Lindsey. Delirium presenting with symptoms of depression. *Psychosomatics* 36:471, 1995.

Nyenhuis, D. L., S. M. Rao, J. M. Zajecka, et al. Mood disturbance versus other symptoms of depression in multiple sclerosis. *JINS* 1:291, 1995.

Ohyama, M., M. Senda, S. Kitamura et al. Role of the nondominant hemisphere and undamaged area during word repetition in poststroke aphasics. A PET activation study. *Stroke* 27:897, 1996.

Ojemann, R. G. Correlations between specific human brain lesions and memory changes: a critical study of the literature. *Neurosci Res Prog Bull* 4:1, 1966.

Pashek, G. V., A. L. Holland. Evolution of aphasia in the first year post onset. *Cortex* 24:411,1988.

Penfield, W., P. Perot. The brain's record of auditory and visual experience. *Brain* 86: 595, 1963.

Penfield, W., L. Roberts. *Speech and Brain Mechanisms*. Princeton University Press, Princeton, 1959.

Petersen, R., J. Stevens, M. Ganguli, et al. Practice parameter: early detection of dementia: mild cognitive impairment. *Neurology* 56: 1133, 2001.

Piven, J., K. Saliba, J. Bailey, S. Arndt. An MRI study of autism: the cerebellum revisited. *Neurology* 49:546, 1997.

Pliszka, S. Pattterns of psychiatric comorbidity with ADHD. *Child Adolesc Psychiatr Clin N Am* 9:525, 2000.

Price, T. R., G. J. Tucker. Psychiatric and behavioral manifestations of normal pressure hydrocephalus. *J Nerv Ment Dis* 164:51, 1977.

Rapin, I. Autism. *New Eng J Med* 337:97, 1997.

Rapin, I., Progress in the neurobiology of autism. *CNS Spectrums* 3:50, 1998.

Rapin, I., D. A. Allen. Syndromes in developmental dysphasia and adult aphasia. In Language, Communication and the Brain. Editor Fred Plum, Assoc for Research in Nerv and Mental Dis 66:57, 1988.

Report of the Therapeutics and Technology Assessment Subcommittee of the American Academy of Neurology. Assessment: neuropsychological testing. *Neurology* 47:592, 1996.

Risse, S. C., M. A. Raskind, D. Nochlin, et al. Neuropathological findings in patients with clinical diagnoses of probable Alzheimer's disease. *Am J Psychiatry* 147:168, 1990.

Ritvo, E. R., B. J. Freeman, C. Pingre, et al. The UCLA-University of Utah epidemiologic survey of autism prevalence. *Am J Psychiatry* 146:194, 1989.

Robbins, T. W., R. Elliott, B. J. Sahakian. Neuropsychology—dementia and affective disorders. *Br Med Bull* 52:627, 1996.

Rogers, S. L., M. Farlow, R. Doody. A 24–233k double blind, placebo controlled trial of Donepezil in patients with Alzheimer's disease. *Neurology* 50:136, 1998.

Roses, A. A model for susceptibility polymorphisms for complex diseases: APOE and AD. *Neurogenetics* 1:3, 1997.

Roy-Byrne, P., L. Scheele, J. Brinkley, et al. Adult attention-deficit hyperactivity disorder: assessment guildelines based on clinical presentation to a specialty clinic. *Compr Psychiatry* 38:133, 1997.

Rubens, A. B., D. F. Benson. Associative visual agnosia. *Arch Neurol* 24:305, 1971.

Rutter, M. Behavioural and cognitive characteristics of a series of psychotic children. In:

Early Childhood Autism: Clinical, Educational and Social Aspects. J. K. Wing, ed. Pergamon, London, 1966, p. 51.

Sadovnick, A. D., R. A. Remick, J. Allen, et al. Depression and multiple sclerosis. *Neurology* 46:628, 1996.

Safer, D., J. Zito, E. Fine. Increased methylphenidate usage for ADHD in the 1990's. *Pediatrics* 98:1084, 1996.

Salloway, S., P. Malloy R. Kohn, et al. MRI and neuropsychological differences in early- and late-life—onset geriatric depression. *Neurology* 46:1567, 1996.

Sano, M., C. Ernesto, R. G. Thomas, et al. A controlled trial of selegiline, alpha-tocopherol, or both as treatment for Alzheimer's disease. *N Engl J Med* 336:1216, 1997.

Sauerwein, H. C., M. Lassonde. Neuropsychological alterations after split-brain surgery. *J Neurosurg Sci* 41:59, 1997.

Scheibel, A. Dendritic changes in senile and presenile dementias. In: *Congenital and Acquired Cognitive Disorders*, R. Katzman, ed. Raven Press, New York, 1979.

Schor, J. D., S. E. Levkoff, L. A. Lipsitz. Risk factors for delirium in hospitalized elderly. *JAMA* 267:827, 1992.

Schupf, N., D. Kapell, B. Nightingale, et al. Specificity of the five fold increase in AD in mothers of adults with Down's Syndrome. Neurology 57:979, 2001.

Shevitz, S. A. Psychosurgery: some current observations. *Am J Psychiatry* 133:266, 1976.

Singer, H., J. Brown, S. Quuaskey, et al. The treatment of ADHD in Tourette's. *Pediatrics* 95:74, 1995.

Snowden, D., L. Greiner, J. Mortimer, et al. Brain infarction and the clinical expression of AD. The Nun study. *JAMA* 277:813, 1997.

Spencer, T., J. Biederman, T. Wilens, Growth deficits in children with ADHD. *Pediatrics* 102:501, 1998.

Sperry, R. W. Lateral specialization in the surgically separated hemispheres. In: *The Neurosciences, Third Study* Program, F. O. Schmitt, F. G. Warden, eds. M.I.T. Press, Cambridge, MA, 1974, p. 5.

Stern, R. A., S. G. Silva, N. Chaisson, D. L. Evans. Influence of cognitive reserve on neuropsychological functioning in asymptomatic human immunodeficiency virus-1 infection. *Arch Neurol* 53:148, 1996.

Stern, Y., B. Gurland, T. Tatemichi, et al. Influence of education and occupation on the incidence of Alzheimer's disease. *JAMA* 271:1004, 1994.

Stern, Y., X. Liu, M. Albert, et al. Modeling the influence of extrapyramidal signs on the progression of Alzheimer disease. *Arch Neurol* 53:1121, 1996.

Sultzer, D. L., H. S. Levin, M. E. Mahler, et al. A comparison of psychiatric symptoms in vascular dementia and Alzheimer's disease. *Am J Psychiatry* 150:1806, 1993.

Tang, M.-X., D. Jacobs, Y. Stern, et al. Effect of oestrogen during menopause on risk and age at onset of Alzheimer disease. *Lancet* 348:429, 1996.

Taylor, M., *The Neuropsychiatric Mental Status*. SP, New York, 1981.

Taylor, M., R. Abrams. Cognitive impairment in schizophrenia. *Amer J Psychiatry* 141: 196, 1984.

Terry, R. Ultrastructural changes in Alzheimer's disease and quantitative studies. In: *Congenital and Acquired Mental Disorders*, R. Katzman, ed. Raven Press, New York, 1979.

Terry, R., R. Katzman. Senile dementia of the Alzheimer type. *Ann Neuro* 14:497–506, 1983.

Trzepacz, P. T., R. J. Sclabassi, D. H. Van Thiel. Delirium: a subcortical phenomenon? *J Neuropsychiatry* 1(3):283–290, 1989.

Trzepacz, P., R. Baker. *The Psychiatric Mental Status Examination*. Oxford University Press, New York, 1993.

Tucker, G., T. Price, V. Johnson, et al. Phenomenology of temporal lobe dysfunction. *J Nerv Ment Dis* 174:348–356, 1986.

Tucker, G., E. Caine, M. Popkin. Introduction to section II. Delirium, dementia, amnestic and other cognitive disorders. In: *DSM IV Sourcebook*, Vol. 1, T. Widiger, A. Frances, H. Pincus, et al, eds. The American Psychiatric Association Press, Washington, DC, 1994, pp. 243–276.

Tune, L. E., F. W. Blysma. Benzodiazepine induced and anticholinergic induced delerium in the elderly. *Int Psychogeriatr* 3:397, 1991.

Van Duijn, C. M., L. M. Havekes, C. Broeckhoven, et al. Apolipoprotein E genotype and association between smoking and early onset Alzheimer's Disease, *BMJ* 310(6980): 627, 1995.

Van Putten, T., P.R.A. May. "Akinetic depression" in schizophrenia. *Arch Gen Psychiatry* 35:1101, 1978.

Victor, M., R. D. Adams, G. H. Collins. The Wernicke-Korsakoff syndrome: a clinical and pathological study of 245 patients, 82 with post-mortem examinations. *Contemp Neurol Ser* 7:1, 1971.

Vitiello, B., J. B. Severe, L. L. Greenhill, et al. Methylphenidate dosage for children with ADHD over time under controlled conditions: lessons from the MTA. *J Am Acad Child Adolesc Psychiatry* 40:188, 2001.

Wells, C. E. Pseudodementia. *Amer J Psychiatry* 136:895, 1979.

Wertz, R. T., D. G. Weiss, J. L. Alten, et al. Comparison of clinic, home and deferred language treatment for aphasia. A Veterans Administration Cooperative study. *Arch Neurol* 43:653, 1986.

Wettstein, A. Cholinesterase inhibitors and Gingko extracts-are they comparable in the treatment of dementia? *Phytomedicine* 6:393, 2000.

Wiesel, T. N., D. H. Hubel. Extent of recovery from the effects of visual depreivation in kittens. *J Neurophysiol* 28:1060, 1965.

Wilcock, G., S. Lilienfeld, E. Gaens. Galantamine in AD. *BMJ* 321:1445, 2000.

Wilens, T., T. Spencer, J. Biederman, et al. A contolled trial of bupropion for ADHD in adults. *Am J Psychiatry* 158: 282, 2001.

Wilkie, F. L., K. Goodkin, C. Eisdorfer, et al. Mild cognitive impairment and risk of mortality in HIV-1 infection. *J Neuropsychiatry* 10:125, 1998.

Wilson, D. H., A. G. Reeves, M. Gazzaniga, et al. Cerebral commissurotomy for control of intractable seizures. *Neurology* 27:708, 1977.

Zametkin, A. J., T. E. Nordahl, M. Gross, et al. Cerebral glucose metabolism in adults with hyperactivity of childhood onset. *N Engl J Med* 323:1361, 1990.

Zametkin, A. J. Attention Deficit Disorder. JAMA 273:1811, 1995.

Zametkin, A. J., M. Ernst, Problems in the management of ADHD, *Eng J Med* 340:40, 1999.

Chapter Five

MOVEMENT, MOOD, AND OBSESSIVE-COMPULSIVE DISORDERS

At first glance, movement, mood, and obsessive-compulsive disorders seem a strange assortment of conditions to group together, but there is commonality in the anatomical and neurochemical findings and treatment of these disparate conditions. Symptoms coexist in varying combinations in diseases such as depression, obsessive-compulsive disorder (OCD), Tourette's syndrome, Parkinson's disease, and Huntington's disease. Although the actual pathologic mechanisms have not been clarified in each type of disorder, the catecholamine and indoleamine systems of the brain have been implicated in all of them. Anatomic evidence indicates that the corpus striatum, globus pallidus, and their connections with the frontal lobes and thalamus are important to the pathophysiology of movement disorders, mood disorders, subcortical dementia, obsessive-compulsive disorder, psychosis, and sleep disorders. There is also considerable overlap in the pharmacological treatment of these conditions, and this area is a common clinical and theoretical meeting ground for psychiatrists and neurologists.

PARKINSON'S DISEASE

There are three major symptoms of Parkinson's disease (PD): *tremor, bradykinesia, and postural instability. Rigidity*, a physical sign, is also characteristic.

All these are the result of dopamine deficiency. The *tremor* of parkinsonism occurs mainly when the patient is resting or holding sustained postures. It is dampened during voluntary movements. For this reason, of the three cardinal symptoms, tremor interferes least with normal motor functioning. The tremor of Parkinson's disease is absolutely characteristic, and there is only one other condition that can be confused with it, and that is the extrapyramidal side effects of dopamine receptor blocking drugs. Most of these are neuroleptics, but metoclopramide (Reglan) and prochlorperazine (Compazine), common remedies for nausea, also can produce all symptoms of PD, including resting tremor.

Bradykinesia is best defined as slowness in carrying out motor acts, in initiating and sometimes in arresting movements. It can seriously impair functioning and makes it difficult for a patient to be dexterous both in fine and gross motor acts, though when it is mild, the disability it imposes is often misunderstood, by patients and physicians, to be the result of normal aging or arthritis. Bradykinesia causes PD patients to delay a few seconds before they can begin walking. This is especially noticeable when they first rise from a seated position or when they change the direction of gait. Sometimes freezing occurs under these circumstances. Some patients experience freezing in doorways. This feature, really a form of gait apraxia, is also seen in patients with frontal lobe dysfunction who do not have dopamine deficiency. Patients with PD may lose associated or spontaneous movements such as swinging arms while walking. The gait of a typical PD patient is small-stepped and narrow-based. Patients with degeneration of nerve cells that are outside the dopamine system tend to have a gait that is small-stepped but broad-based.

Postural instability is the most disabling symptom. An inability to adjust rapidly to postural changes may result in frequent falling and serious injury. Sometimes patients take several short, hesitant, "stuttering" steps (marche a petit pas, festinating) when they start walking or when they turn, and falling that is caused by this can be the cause of serious injuries.

Other clinical features of PD that relate to the three cardinal symptoms are expressionless features, a feeling of weakness and of being slowed, flattening and weakness of the voice, diminished dexterity, micrographia, and cogwheel rigidity. Patients can have tremor without the other symptoms of PD. They may also have bradykinesia and/or postural instability without tremor. Symptoms can be unilateral, confined to the arms or to the legs without involvement of the rest of the body or may be generalized. Patients whose symptoms commence with tremor have the best prognosis: 80 percent do not become demented or incapacitated motorically. Dementia and irreversible motor symptoms eventually develop in most of those who never have the typical resting tremor (Rajput et al., 1993).

Mostly sporadic, PD is rarely inherited as an autosomal dominant. When this is the case, the onset of the disease can be quite early, in the second or third decade. Ordinary PD begins at age 59 on average, and it affects approximately 1 percent of the population over the age of 60.

While the term *Parkinson's disease* should be reserved for conditions that result from deficiency of dopamine in the brain, it is applied in practice to both those patients who have pure dopamine deficiency and those who have motor symptoms (bradykinesia, postural instability) that do not result from dopamine deficiency but from the degeneration of other portions of the extrapyramidal system. When most of the motor symptoms, but not all, reverse with dopamine replacement therapy, the syndrome may be called *Parkinson's Plus* The word "plus" indicates the involvement of cells outside the dopaminergic system.

Many degenerative diseases primarily affect regions of the nervous system that lie outside the dopaminergic system. By also affecting dopamine neurons, such diseases can also cause a clinically significant degree of dopamine deficiency. In these cases, we can treat the symptoms that result from dopamine deficiency, but the primary symptoms, the ones that arise outside the dopamine system, are usually untreatable. Striatonigral degeneration (SND), olivopontocerebellar atrophy (OPCA), progressive supranuclear palsy (PSP), multisystem atrophy (MSA), Lewy body dementia (LBD), multi-infarct dementia (MID) are all diseases that result from the loss of neurons outside the dopamine system but often produce some degree of dopamine deficiency, and hence can lead to the symptoms of parkinsonism. Only the symptoms that derive from dopamine deficiency can be treated with dopamine replacement. When tremor occurs in these conditions, it is usually an intention tremor, not a resting tremor.

Thus, there are four kinds of degenerative conditions that are loosely called "Parkinson's." One is pure dopamine deficiency. This is true PD. It is eminently treatable and has the best prognosis. The second is Parkinson's Plus, i.e., mostly dopamine deficiency mixed with symptoms that arise from disease of the nervous system beyond dopamine deficiency. The third (SND, OPCA, PSP, MSA, LBD, MID, etc.) looks like PD in the sense that there is bradykinesia and postural instability, but these symptoms are only slightly relieved by dopamine replacement therapy as they mostly derive from lesions outside the dopamine system. The same untreatable diseases can also cause Parkinson-like motor disablility and death without ever causing clinically significant dopamine deficiency and dopamine replacement therapy is completely ineffective (Table 5–1).

We do not know if non-Parkinson diseases that can produce dopamine deficiency are separate entities or rather different points in the same spectrum, but lumping all of them under the heading "parkinsonism" has muddied the understanding of the course of illness and the effect of therapy. For example, dementia is feared as the inevitable consequence of PD, though it is unusual in pure dopamine deficiency but common in the others. L-dopa has been mistakenly blamed for the ultimate loss of responsiveness to dopamine replacement therapy and partly for this reason L-dopa is witheld when it would be the most effective

Table 5–1 Parkinsonism

		RESPONSE TO L-DOPA		
DISEASE CATEGORY[a]	SYMPTOMS	EARLY SMOOTH	MODERATE "WEARING–OFF"	END "ON–OFF"
Dopamine Deficiency Only				
(Parkinson's disease)	Resting tremor Bradykinesia Postural instability	Complete resolution of symptoms		
Mainly Dopamine Deficiency				
(Parkinson's Plus)	Resting tremor Bradykinesia Postural instability	Symptom resolution, some residual		
Some Dopamine Deficiency				
(Striatonigral degeneration, multisystem atrophy, progressive supranuclear palsy, Lewy body dementia corticobasilar degeneration, etc.)	Bradykinesia Postural instability Intention tremor Dementia	Little symptom resolution		
No Dopamine Deficiency				
(Same diseases as under *Some Dopamine Deficiency*)	Bradykinesia Postural instability Intention tremor Dementia	No symptom resolution		

[a]There is a tendency for each disease category to progress to the next category over the years.

therapy. The cause of L-dopa unresponsiveness, if it occurs, is likely to be the evolution of dopamine deficiency into one of the other, more malignant forms of parkinsonism. Alternatively, periodic nonresponsiveness could just represent sensitivity to dietary protein in the "on–off" phase of dopamine deficiency. The term *end stage Parkinson's* has developed two meanings. One use of the term describes a patient with no clinically significant dopamine deficiency but with other brain involvement who is curled into a ball in flexion, helpless, and demented. Dopamine replacement therapy has no beneficial effect but only makes the patient hallucinate more. The other meaning of the term "end stage Parkinson's," refers to a patient who has essentially no dopaminergic neurons left but no other brain involvement. Properly treated for dopamine deficiency, he or she can function normally, motorically, and intellectually, indefinitely.

Pathogenesis

Dopaminergic neurons are shaped like a tree. The trunk is the cell body, the root system is comprised of the dendrites which receive impulses from other neurons, and the leaves are the axon terminals through which each cell communicates its messages to other nerve cells. Each cell has thousands of connections with other nerve cells. The dopaminergic axons project from the substantia nigra in the midbrain up to the caudate, putamen, and globus pallidus, to the diencephalon, to portions of the frontal lobe, and to the limbic system. Dopamine is synthesized, stored, released, and taken up again (reuptake) by the very dopaminergic axon terminal that released it. Reuptake of released dopamine is the main mechanism of dopamine-inactivation. Insufficient dopamine can cause slowness of thinking as well as movement (Lees, 1994). In addition to dyskinesia, excessive dopamine can cause racing thoughts, mania, delusions, confusion, and visual hallucinations. Presumably, the cognitive manifestations of dopamine deficiency and overdosage are mediated through dopaminergic projections to the frontal lobe, basal ganglia, diencephalon, and limbic system.

There is some regional variation in the location of lesions that correlates roughly with clinical type. The akinetic-rigid forms of dopamine deficiency correlate with greater dopaminergic cell loss in the ventrolateral part of the substantia nigra. The neurons in this area project primarily to the dorsal putamen. The akinetic-rigid forms of PD are more likely to be associated with dementia and to show behavioral–cognitive toxicity with dopamine replacement therapy.

Cell loss in the medial part of the substantia nigra seems to have a better prognosis and correlates better with the tremor of PD. The dopaminergic neurons of this area project to the caudate nucleus and anterior putamen. In the Parkinson-like syndromes such as MSA there is cell loss in the lateral substantia nigra and transsynaptic degeneration of striatonigral efferents (that remain intact in uncomplicated dopamine deficiency (true PD). There is loss of dopamine receptors as well in the PD-like syndromes that may well explain dopamine unresponsiveness (Jellinger, 1999).

L-dopa

The response to dopamine replacement is the most important criterion for differentiating true PD from the more malignant degenerative conditions that can mimic it. Obviously, to treat dopamine deficiency one would hope to use dopamine, but dopamine cannot pass through the blood–brain barrier. Its immediate metabolic precursor, dopa, does pass through the blood–brain barrier, and in the brain it is decarboxylated to dopamine. Dopa is administered orally in the levo form as levodopa or L-dopa. We can reduce the amount of L-dopa needed to provide a good therapeutic response by combining L-dopa with another drug called carbidopa. This is a dopa decarboxylase inhibitor that reduces the decarboxylation of L-dopa to dopamine before dopa can reach the brain, thus permitting more of the administered dose of L-dopa to reach the brain.

The effect of L-dopa on end-stage PD patients is remarkable. When it was first introduced in the 1960s, totally incapacitated patients, who had been in nursing homes for years, could rise again and resume normal motor function. L-dopa is one of the most dramatically effective medications in the history of medicine. It does not lose efficacy with time unless the disease evolves into one of the more malignant, degenerative forms.

It is curious that dopamine can be generated from dopa in severe PD to provide even a short period of normal functioning. After all, if the dopamine neurons have died, where does dopamine synthesis occur? The answer is not known, but presumably dopamine is generated anywhere a molecule encounters a decarboxylating enzyme that can metabolize it. Then the newly generated dopamine diffuses to its postsynaptic receptors (Melamed et al., 1980). The decarboxylating step is nonspecific and not rate-limiting and can be accomplished in the virtual absence of dopaminergic neurons. Thus, administered L-dopa can overcome the inadequacy of dopamine synthesis.

Normally, the inactivation of dopamine after it has interacted with its postsynaptic receptor depends on its reuptake and storage by the dopaminergic neurons. Their loss reduces the brain's capacity to inactivate and store dopamine. The loss of the inactivation mechanism allows higher and more prolonged elevations of dopamine in the immediate vicinity of the dopaminergic receptors following levodopa administration. This predisposes to toxicity manifested as dyskinesia and hallucinations.

Stages of Parkinson's Disease

Three stages of dopamine deficiency can be differentiated by the patient's response to administered L-dopa: early, moderate, and end-stage (Table 5–1).

Stage I—early dopamine deficiency—mildly symptomatic. There is more than an 80 percent reduction of dopaminergic cells (Hornykiewicz, 1974) but considerable storage capacity remains so that a patient might be given a dose of replacement dopa three times a day, once a day, or even every other day with good effect and without causing much variation in the patient's motor function. Once dopamine is released, the remaining dopaminergic neurons can take it up, thereby inactivating it. Extra dopamine can be stored within the dopaminergic neurons. At this stage patients cannot tell when a particular dose of L-dopa begins to work or how long the good effect of L-dopa lasts. Their symptoms of parkinsonism may not recur until they have ceased taking L-dopa for 2 to 3 days. Since most doctors prescribe L-dopa on a three doses per day schedule, compliant patients in this stage of illness experience a smooth response to L-dopa that is not linked to the timing of the doses. This happy state lasts for 5 to 10 years. Dopamine deficiency advances more quickly when it begins early (fourth or fifth decade) than if it begins in the seventh or eighth decade. In general, the older the patient at the onset of the symptoms of dopamine deficiency, the longer the first stage of illness lasts.

There is little clinical evidence that treatment with L-dopa hastens the degenerative process in Parkinson's but much has been made of this possibility. The hypothesis that L-dopa is harmful stems in large part from the preclinical observation that the metabolism of L-dopa can generate free radicals. These chemical reactions have been emphasized repeatedly and support the hypothesis that the oxyradicals generated from administered L-dopa attack subcellular organelles and cell membranes and hasten cell death, thereby accelerating the progression of PD. Explanations of how L-dopa–accelerated degeneration could occur have substituted for evidence that this happens (Olanow et al., 1998). Fahn (1996), who reviewed this subject and argued in support of the preclinical studies that indicated L-dopa toxicity, also cited animal studies that had failed to find evidence of such toxicity. Agid (1998) reviewed the literature and found the preclinical evidence to be confusing and not compelling with regard to the existence of dopaminergic toxicity. Weiner (2000) reviewed all the clinical evidence and concluded that, after all these decades of L-dopa use in PD, there is still no convincing evidence that L-dopa in therapeutic doses is toxic at all or that it accelerates PD progression. Even though L-dopa is tried and true, cheap, effective, and safe, many neurologists prefer not to use L-dopa until it is absolutely necessary, or try to use as little as possible, substituting other less effective, more toxic, more expensive drugs (Frucht et al., 1999; Rascol et al., 2000; Parkinson Study Group, 2000). Yet, there is no evidence that any other compound is superior to L-dopa in slowing the course of PD. L-dopa has dramatically improved the symptoms of PD and its use early in the course of PD may actually lengthen patients' lives (Diamond et al., 1987).

Stage II—moderate dopamine deficiency—wearing-off—fluctuations of motor activity. This phase of PD is characterized by the *wearing-off* phenomenon, motor fluctuations that are closely related to the time of L-dopa administration. The wearing-off phenomenon probably reflects disease progression and a decreasing ability of the brain to store dopamine. There is much evidence to support the hypothesis that presynaptic failure of dopamine storage explains the wearing-off phenomenon and that it is not the result of progressive insensitivity or down-regulation of dopamine receptors (Greene, 1988; Sage and Mark, 1994). The evidence that diminished storage capacity of dopaminergic neurons rather than receptor down-regulation is responsible for wearing off includes the following: *(1)* Patients with wearing-off retain the capacity to respond clinically to L-dopa. *(2)* More frequent dosing of L-dopa is effective in controlling the phenomenon. *(3)* After an intravenous L-dopa infusion is stopped, fluctuating patients sustain the anti-Parkinson effect of the medication for a shorter period of time than do stable patients. (Fabbrini et al., 1988; Mouradian et al., 1988). This is what would be expected if the brain's capacity to retain dopamine were reduced and the capacity to respond to dopamine were retained. *(4)* Positron emission tomography studies with (F)-6-fluorodopa in patients with PD have shown less of an accumulation of fluorodopa and its metabolites in the basal ganglia of fluctuating patients than in stable patients (Leenders et al., 1986a, b), presumably because there is reduced capacity to store the dopamine that is derived from the labelled L-dopa. (5) Deprived of dopaminergic afferents, rat basal ganglia exhibit a diminished capacity to store dopamine (Spencer and Wooten, 1984.) *(6)* During off periods, patients retain the capacity to respond to injections of apomorphine, a dopamine agonist. This indicates that the dopamine receptors are functioning normally. (Guttman et al., 1986; Stibe et al., 1988; Wooten, 1988) *(7)* There are normal to increased levels of dopamine receptor binding sites in the basal ganglia of patients with PD (Leenders et al., 1986a, b).

These observations indicate that postsynaptic receptors are available for dopaminergic stimulation, but the presynaptic storage of dopamine is defective. The hallmark of the wearing-off effect is the patient's capacity to tell how long it takes from the time he swallows a dose of L-dopa to the time that dose becomes effective in relieving his symptoms (usually about 30 minutes). The patient can also tell how long the therapeutic effect of a particular dose lasts (usually about 3 hours).

Stage III—end stage of dopamine deficiency. This is the final phase of the disease when virtually no dopamine storage capacity is left. Rapid shifts occur clinically between *on* and *off* periods. The on state refers to mobility, the off state to immobility. A constant delivery of L-dopa to the striatum is essential to support continuous dopamine synthesis in the brain that has become totally depleted of its dopaminergic neurons (Sage and Mark, 1994). In the normal brain and even in the moderately affected parkinsonian brain, an excess of dopamine is stored in the presynaptic neurons and is available for release should the delivery of L-dopa to the brain be temporarily interrupted. In Stage I and II patients, the stores of dopamine can support movement for a little while if the next L-dopa dose is delayed in entering the brain. In Stage III patients, periods of bradykinesia or freezing ("off periods") occur abruptly if L-dopa is delayed in crossing the blood–brain barrier.

There is strong evidence that peripheral pharmacokinetic factors contribute to the complex fluctuations in Stage III patients. A delay in the entry of L-dopa into the brain may result from slow gastric emptying L-dopa is absorbed in the small intestine). This can be ameliorated by placing a tube into the duodenum and delivering L-dopa directly in that manner (Sage et al., 1989).

A more important cause of delay between the time of administration of L-dopa and the onset of its beneficial effect is lag in the transit of L-dopa from the circulating plasma, across the blood–brain barrier, into the brain (Nutt et al., 1984). High concentrations of circulating large neutral amino acids (LNAA) in the plasma is the most common reason for this lag. These amino acids are derived from dietary protein and they compete with L-dopa for the carrier that brings both L-dopa and LNAA into the brain (Juncos et al., 1987).

The deleterious effect of dietary protein on movement is experienced only in Stage III PD. Immobility in response to high levels of plasma LNAA does not occur in normals or in earlier stages of PD's even though elevated plasma levels of LNAA always slow and reduce the entry of L-dopa into the brain (Leenders et al., 1986a, b). Because in Stage III PD there is no dopamine stored in the brain, the patient experiences apparently unpredictable episodes of L-dopa–resistant bradykinesia whenever the plasma LNAA concentration rises above the level that prevents L-dopa from crossing into the brain. Freezing of motor functions can be sudden. Like cars that have just run out of gas, patients stop moving. It is seldom possible to raise the blood levels of L-dopa high enough to overcome the effect of elevated plasma concentrations of LNAAs without also causing severe dyskinesia when the LNAA levels diminish. The combination of high plasma concentrations of both L-dopa and LNAA is probably responsible for the phenomenon called peak dose bradykinesia.

There is a simple explanation for the mysterious sensitivity to L-dopa of Stage III Parkinson's disease patients who develop dyskinesia at lower doses than patients at earlier phases of the disease (Trendelenburg, 1966; Mouradian et al., 1989). The complete loss of the presynaptic dopaminergic cells in the Stage III patient results in the loss of the modulating dopamine inactivation-storage sequence. Without the inactivating reuptake mechanism and storage, dopamine remains too long at the receptor. This unmodulated increase in dopamine concentration at the postsynaptic receptors results in symptoms of overdosage (dyskinesia, hallucinations) because there is no place to store excess dopamine. Therefore, as the disease advances, patients are increasingly subject to developing alternating periods of being off (Parkinsonian) and on (dyskinetic). It is somewhat counter-intuitive but true that patients seem to become more sensitive to L-dopa as their disease progresses, responding to slight overdosage with marked dyskinesia and/or hallucinations. At the same time, patients experience periods of apparent unresponsiveness to administered L-dopa. The therapeutic window between underdosage and overdosage in Stage III is very narrow, and the threshold dose to produce dyskinesias is much lower in patients with end-stage dopamine deficiency than it is in patients with early dopamine deficiency (Mouradian et al., 1989).

Protein Redistribution Diet

Mena and Cotzias (1975) first suggested that plasma LNAAs, derived mainly from dietary protein, antagonize the clinical effectiveness of oral L-dopa. When Stage III PD patients receiving L-dopa were studied on a high-protein diet, they all remained bradykinetic. On the following day, while they consumed a low protein diet, they became mobile, even dyskinetic, while receiving the same doses of L-dopa. The LNAA level bore an inverse relationship to the clinical status of each patient. The level began to rise within 1 hour after the first high protein meal. When the LNAA plasma level increased to 2.5 times fasting levels, all patients became immobile. When the LNAA plasma level dropped, bradykinesia lessened or patients became dyskinetic (Pincus and Barry, 1987a, 1987b, 1987c, 1988).

Since the publication of the first of these reports, the basic findings have been confirmed independently by many groups (Eriksson et al., 1988; Riley and Lang, 1988; Tsui et al., 1989; Bracco et al., 1991). The longest follow-up periods are now 14 years. There has been no tendency for the diet to become less effective over time as a means of maximizing the efficacy of L-dopa (Karstaedt and Pincus, 1992).

Pharmacological Treatment

There are a number of other antiparkinson agents that are commonly prescribed. These fall into different categories depending on their mechanism of action: dopamine uptake inhibitiors, dopamine agonists, monaminoxidase inhibitors, and catechol O-methyltransferanse inhibitors.

Belladonna compounds—Trihexyphenidyl (Artane) and benztropine (Cogentin)—may be mildly effective in Stage I PD. Belladonnas reduce tremor and some of the other Stage I symptoms. They are relatively ineffective in relieving the Parkinson's symptoms of patients with Stage II and Stage III PD. Yet they are much more effective in reversing all the symptoms of neuroleptic drug-induced parkinsonism that results from dopamine receptor blockade.

Belladonnas inhibit dopamine reuptake (Coyle and Snyder, 1969). By blocking the inactivation of released dopamine, the belladonna compounds can overcome some symptoms of patients with mild, Stage I PD. Dopamine reuptake inhibition is not an effective mechanism for relieving the symptoms of advanced PD because there are few dopaminergic neurons left on which such medications can act (Taylor et al., 1991).

The balance theory. The belladonna drugs are anticholinergic and many neurologists mistakenly attribute their anti-Parkinson activity to their anticholinergic action, envisioning such compounds as restoring a balance between acetylcholine and dopamine. The concept is that acetylcholine and dopamine are normally in balance. In PD, there is thought to be an imbalance between the two transmitters because dopamine is depleted and acetylcholine is normal. By reducing acetylcholine levels, according to the balance theory, a new, lower balance can be achieved with dopamine. Consequently, motor activity will return to normal. The balance theory fails to explain the mechanism by which drugs with anticholinergic effects have an impact on PD.

A brief review of the pharmacology of three classes of anticholinergic drugs indicates that anticholinergic activity is irrelevant to PD. Neuroleptics, such as chlorpromazine, are strongly anticholinergic but cause parkinsonian symptoms. Belladonna compounds, like trihexyphenidyl and benztropine, are powerful anticholinergic agents but relieve parkinsonian symptoms. Tricyclic antidepressants (TCA), like amitriptyline, do not affect PD symptoms at all, even though they are strongly anticholinergic. The interaction of drugs with dopaminergic systems is the only explanation for the differential effects of these classes of drugs on PD. Neuroleptics block dopamine receptors and therefore induce parkinsonism or worsen its symptoms. Belladonna compounds block dopamine reuptake and therefore slightly improve some symptoms of PD in the early stage, whereas TCAs have no effect on the dopaminergic systems. Tricyclic antidepressants block serotonin and norepinephrine uptake. They are antidepressants with no effect on the motor symptoms of PD. The balance theory recurs in discussions of chorea, psychosis, and the interaction of drugs. It is woefully inadequate to explain the phenomena to which it has been applied.

Amantadine probably inhibits the dopamine uptake mechanism (Brown and Redfern, 1976; Metman et al., 1998, 1999) and is mildly effective in relieving bradykinesia and tremor in mild Parkinson's disease as it prolongs the duration of action of released dopamine. It is relatively ineffective in relieving the symptoms of severe Parkinson's disease where there are few dopaminergic cells left on which to act. Amantadine also effectively reduces L-dopa–induced dyskinesia and is useful in late stage Parkinson's disease for this purpose. This effect is counter-intuitive and was first reported 34 years after the introduction of amantadine for the treatment of Parkinson's disease. This is an example of how physicians often do not see what they do not expect to see. No convincing theory for amantadine's efficacy in treating dyskinesia has yet been offered, though inhibition of NMDA (glutamate) receptors has been proposed as a mechanism (Kornhuber et al., 1995; Verhagen et al., 1998).

Dopamine agonists including the oldest such agent, bromocriptine (Parlodel), and three newer ones, pergolide (Permax), ropinerole (Requipp), and pramipexole (Mirapex) directly activate dopamine receptors. They are not taken up by presynaptic cells, need not be released at a particular time, and require no inactivation mechanism. Theoretically, they should be very effective in late PD, but unfortunately, they are poor substitutes for dopamine and are much less effective in relieving PD symptoms. They are used most effectively in early PD. Because of their ineffectiveness compared with L-dopa, they also cause less dyskinesia. Bromocriptine is inferior to the others. No study has compared the three newer agonists. All are prone to causing unacceptable cognitive side effects and somnolence, a potentially serious problem for automobile drivers (Lachenmayer, 2000).

The *monamine oxidase inhibitor (MAOI)*, selegiline (Deprenyl, Eldepryl), inhibits beta MAO. This produces a minimal symptomatic benefit by increasing the intracellular dopamine concentration in patients with some dopamine neurons left. The drug is now being used clinically in an attempt to prevent PD from getting worse, but the research on which this is based has been severely criticized (Landau, 1990).

Catechol-O-methyltransferase inhibitors (COMTIs) inhibit the enzyme catechol-O-methyltransferase that is responsible for the degradation of L-dopa. By reducing L-dopa breakdown, COMTIs elevate blood levels of L-dopa and prolong this elevation. The use of tolcopone with L-dopa has allowed patients with fluctuating responses to L-dopa to take L-dopa less frequently (Martinez-Martin and O'Brien, 1998). The deaths from severe liver failure of several patients who were taking tolcopone has dampened enthusiasm for this drug despite the advantages it provides. Encapone (Comtan) has largely replaced tolcapone as a COMTI. Encapone is effective and safe but has a relatively short half-life and must be taken up to eight times a day.

Surgical Treatments

Transplants. Transplantation of fetal cells is based on the concept that the embryonic cells can grow in the striatum and begin to produce dopamine. There have been some reports of clinical benefit and also reports of disabling dyskinesias (Olanow, 2001). However, the transplant would only function as a biological dopamine pump. It could be efficacious only in simple dopamine deficiency and could not relieve symptoms that L-dopa failed to reverse. If L-dopa relieved a patient's symptoms, there should be no need for the transplant.

Pallidotomy/thalamotomy. These procedures relieve dopa-induced dyskinesia, permitting the use of more L-dopa for the treatment of PD symptoms, without resort to a protein redistribution diet. Though the positive effects of thalamotomy have not been fully explained, the procedure is based on evidence that the globus pallidus is over active in PD. Ominously, word fluency, the only function commonly tested that is mediated by the frontal-basal ganglia-dorsal thalamic circuit, has been significantly and permanently affected by pallidotomy (Junque et al., 1999). Major complications have occurred in up to one third of operated patients (Shannon et al., 1998).

Brain stimulation. A permanent in-dwelling electrode placed into the subthalamic nucleus or elsewhere bilaterally and stimulated can reduce tremor and some of the more disabling symptoms of PD. It is a reversible procedure and therefore safer than pallidotomy in the sense that the stimulator can be turned off and the electrodes removed. Neuropsychological testing of executive functioning preoperatively and then postoperatively has not been performed systematically. Tests of posterior brain function have been carried out with generally good results after surgery. Careful neuropsychological testing during stimulation has not been reported yet.

Psychiatric Symptoms in Parkinson's Disease

Depression. There is great variability in the reported incidence of depression in PD. The mean incidence is often cited as 40 percent, but the reported rates vary from 4 to 70 percent in different studies (Cummings, 1992). In part this variability may reflect the difference between samples of specialized clinical populations and community-based surveys. In a recent community-based survey of patients with PD only 7.7 percent of 245 patients with PD met the criteria for major depression (Tandberg et al., 1996). This is a figure that reflects incidence. There is a lifetime prevalence of 6 percent of major depression in community samples (Blazer et al., 1994), which would make the incidence of depression in PD not necessarily more frequent then one would expect in a normal population.

In some measure, the widely varying reports of the incidence and prevalence of depression in PD patients can be explained by the overlapping character of the physical symptoms of PD and depression. For example, slowing of psychomotor functions, problems with eating and sleeping, a negative self-image and a gloomy outlook about the future may all be taken as signs of depression on some standardized depression interviews and rating scales. When a PD patient complains of such symptoms as feeling weak, lacking energy, and feeling useless, it is likely that the symptoms result from PD rather than depression. Thus, symptom checklists for depression may contain a bias towards depression in PD patients. Taylor et al. (1988) confirmed that the depressive symptoms of which PD patients complain are not typical of depression. Depressed PD patients rarely mentioned guilt or self-deprecatory feelings, crying, or anger. Yet there is considerable support for the concept that patients with PD are predisposed to milder depression. The more severe the motor and cognitive symptoms of PD, the more likely the patient is to experience some symptoms of depression (Kuzis et al., 1997; Lauterbach et al., 1997; Tandberg et al., 1997).

Depression, however, is not a simple reaction to having PD. Some PD patients can be very mildly affected motorically but have severe depression, and patients with severe PD may have no depression at all. It is conceivable that depression in PD is a manifestation of Parkinson's Plus; as such, it would be closely related to the underlying neuropathological process rather than to environmental or psychological factors. A Mini-Mental Status Examination score below 24, indicating dementia, increases the probability of major depression in PD patients by a factor of 6.6 (Tandberg et al., 1997).

L-dopa does not relieve depression in PD. It does not significantly increase brain levels of norepinephrine, its major metabolite (Maricce et al., 1995). However, levels of the norepinephrine metabolite, methoxyhydroxyphenethyleneglcol (MHPG), are elevated diffusely in the central nervous system after treatment with L-dopa. This indicates an increase in norepinephrine turnover. Exogenous L-dopa in cats decreases norepinephrine levels in the hypothalamus. This may be the result of a dopamine-induced increase in norepinephrine release. L-dopa has long been known to induce manic episodes in manic-depressive patients (Murphy et al., 1971). Generally, the depression can be relieved by SSRIs, and are preferred, as the anticholinergic side effects of many of the tricyclic antidepressants may lead to delirium (Lieberman, 1998). The depressive symptoms most likely result from some abnormality of the serotonin or norepinephrine systems, since the original papers describing catecholamine and indolamine abnormalities in PD described 50 percent or so depletions of norepinephrine and serotonin along with even more marked reductions in dopamine

Electroconvulsive therapy (ECT) has been used effectively to treat depression in PD patients and may also reduce some of the PD symptoms for a period of days. Improved PD symptoms may reflect increased brain levels of anti-Parkinson medications produced by ECT, for ECT transiently makes the blood–brain barrier more permeable.

Anxiety versus akathisia. Although it has always been difficult to separate anxiety symptoms from depressive symptoms, a 38 percent incidence of anxiety disorders has been found in a small group of well-studied Parkinson's disease patients (Stein et al., 1990; Menza et al., 1993a, b, 1995). This compares to an 11 percent incidence in patients with chronic medical conditions. In our experience, anxiety attacks in PD almost never respond to antidepressants. Anxiety attacks in PD usually represent episodes of akathisia (restlessness) and reflect inadequate amounts of dopamine in the brain. Patients with akathisia complain of shakiness that is internal and cannot be seen by observers. They wish to move about and sometimes ask family members to move their extremities, lest they become frozen. Some complain that they cannot take a deep breath and fear they are going to die. It is easy to misunderstand these symptoms, and not a few patients have been mistakenly and ineffectively treated with antianxiety drugs to relieve episodes. If the patient is inadequately treated with L-dopa, he or she may have constant anxiety, that actually represents akathisia. This can be debilitating to the patient and to the care giver. Undiagnosed, the constantly complaining patient with akathisia may seem to the physician to represent excessively dependent, neurotic, annoying behavior. Limiting protein intake, taking L-dopa regularly on schedule, and using sedative medications after the single high-protein meal are useful management techniques. Sleep abolishes almost all movement disorders including akathisia.

Painful dystonia. Another motor symptom in PD that may lead to an inappropriate consideration of an anxiety or psychosomatic diagnosis is dystonic cramps. These too reflect deficiency of brain dopamine levels. Approximately 25 percent of PD patients who are in the second or third stages of disease develop dystonia. Dystonia refers to an abnormality of posture caused by an abnormal, involuntary contraction of a skeletal muscle. There is often a writhing, athetoid component, and sometimes an action tremor. It is not always painful, but usually the cramp caused by dopamine deficiency is painful. This too reflects deficiency of brain dopamine levels. Though it can affect any skeletal muscle of the body, including the eyes (oculogyric crisis), dopamine-responsive dystonia has a predilection for the feet and toes, which twist and curl, painfully. The cramp often occurs just after or just before the patient takes his medication. This has been called "beginning-of-dose" and "end-of-dose" dystonia. These are equivalent terms. Many patients feel that L-dopa has caused the cramp. Medical personnel can be fooled by this report. In fact, the previous dose of L-dopa is wearing off and the dose that has just been administered (or that is about to be administered) has not yet taken effect. It is the lack of L-dopa, not its use, that is the problem. Dystonia may occur at night when the patient awakens in a relatively unmedicated state. Sleep prevents dystonic cramping. Patients awaken and then develop cramps. Sedatives can help by reducing mid-night awakenings. Taking L-dopa throughout the night on a regular schedule can also prevent dystonic symptoms. This is not very disruptive for those patients who have two or three nocturias. All odd pains in PD patients who are being treated with L-dopa are possible examples of dystonias. Normal GI tests and other negative investigations into the origin of such pains can lead to a mistaken psychiatric diagnosis.

Psychosis. With so many drugs being used to treat PD, it is often difficult to differentiate drug-induced delirium from psychosis caused by structural brain disease. L-dopa can cause delirium, psychosis, and mania (Cummings, 1991;

Sanchez-Ramos et al., 1996). PD patients seem unusually susceptible to confusion and hallucinations postoperatively. Sixty percent of PD patients, undergoing nonbrain surgery, experienced confusion and hallucinations postoperatively. There was no difference whether the anesthesia was general or spinal (Golden et al., 1989). There is also an increased incidence of visual hallucinations in forms of mixed PD-like Lewy body dementia that is unrelated to medication and correlates significantly with the severity of the illness, e.g., presence of dementia, advanced age, and history of depression (Stern et al., 1993; Klatka et al., 1996).

All drugs used to treat PD can produce nightmares, agitation, delirium, loose associations, visual and auditory hallucinations, delusions, and inappropriate affect. The atropine-like compounds are probably most likely to produce this kind of mental change, especially in older patients, and must be used very cautiously at low doses in PD patients if they are used at all. For this reason, it is wise to start atropine-like medications or any other anti-Parkinson agents with relatively small doses to be sure that the patient can tolerate the drug. Because all these medications potentiate dopamine in some way, they can all cause toxic psychosis that shares certain features with schizophrenia, mania, or other psychiatric disorders (Doraiswamy et al., 1995). Most patients who develop hallucinations and delusions while receiving anti-Parkinson medications have some degree of underlying dementia. The new atypical antipsychotics such as clozapine (Clozaril) and quetiapine (Seroquel) have proven effective, without causing increased motor symptoms, in the treatment of both delirium and psychosis in PD (Rabey et al., 1995; Sajatovic and Ramirez, 1995; Lieberman, 1998). Dose reduction of the anti-Parkinson dugs, especially L-dopa, should be tried first.

Usually, PD symptoms in psychotic patients reflect the effects of neuroleptics not idiopathic PD. In those patients unfortunate enough to have PD and mania or schizophrenia, L-dopa and other anti-Parkinson medications must be used with great caution in small, gradually increasing doses. L-dopa can precipitate manic episodes in bipolar patients and can worsen the schizophrenic symptoms of schizophrenics.

Dementia. In the last decade, Lewy body disease has been identified as a new degenerative dementia. It overlaps with Alzheimer's and Parkinson's diseases clinically and pathologically. Lewy body disease shows parkinsonian features, often starting in apparently benign fashion with a typical resting tremor that may respond to medical treatment at first. Within months there is progression of the motor symptoms, and they are dominated by postural instability and bradykinesia. Treatment with dopamine replacement fails to reverse these more disabling motor symptoms and induces or worsens hallucinations and confusion. Early in the course of illness, there is a relatively rapidly developing cognitive impairment with significant fluctuation in alertness and a psychosis with recurrent, complicated visual hallucinations and delusions.

The neuropathological hallmark is the presence of intracytoplasmic inclusions, Lewy bodies. These are identical to the inclusions that are typically seen in PD. The distribution of these Lewy bodies, unlike that in typical PD where they are limited to the substantia nigra, is widespread throughout the neocortical and paralimbic regions. They coexist with plaques that are typical of Alzheimer's disease (Klatka et al., 1996).

There are many causes of Parkinson-like symptoms other than dopamine deficiency. Cerebrovascular disease and neural degenerative disorders can produce bradykinesia, postural instability, and rigidity. However, the resting tremor that is improved by voluntary movement is virtually pathognomonic of dopamine deficiency or dopamine receptor blockade and is generally a good prognostic sign.

Marder et al. (1995) found that the risk for the development of dementia in a group of PD patients was twice that of a matched group without PD. The degree of dementia correlated with the severity of the extrapyramidal symptoms. Aarsland et al. (1996) found that 25 percent of the Parkinson's patients they studied had dementia. The dementia was associated with depressive symptoms, older age of onset, postural instability, and akinesia.

Etiology of Neurodegenerative Disorders

The etiology of PD may be quite similar to that of other degenerative disorders that involve cognitive decline. Many of these also cause bradykinesia, rigidity, and postural instability. Many degenerative conditions of the brain, including PD, are sporadic, but when they are genetic, they are transmitted as autosomal dominants. These include Alzheimer's, disease frontotemporal atrophy (Pick's disease), Creutzefeld-Jakob disease (CJD), spino-cerebellar atrophies (SCA), and Huntington's disease (HD). In each of these diseases, there seems to be an abnormality of a single protein, not necessarily the same protein in each disease, that is a normal constituent of nerve cells. The abnormal protein contains a subtle defect; sometimes only a single amino acid is out of place.

If a protein looked like a string of pearls, perfect except for one marred pearl, the problem would be relatively minor. However, proteins are constructed more like slinky toys. If a middle portion were twisted, the whole toy would become useless. Proteins are usually tightly wound in a three dimensional structure. They are constantly broken down and then resynthesized. Because of their distorted shape, the abnormal proteins in the above-mentioned diseases cannot be hydrolyzed by their usual enzymes and hence accumulate within the cell. The accumulation of the abnormal protein, or parts of it, leads to the death of the cell.

In PD, an abnormal form of the intracellular protein, alpha-synuclein, has been found in dying dopaminergic neurons. The accumulation of this abnormal synuclein appears to cause the intracytoplasmic inclusions (Lewy bodies) that characterize the degenerating nerve cells in PD and LBD. In MSA, synuclein deposition is seen in neurons of the hypothalamus and sympathetic nervous system also (Crowther et al., 2000). It is not clear if LBD, MSA, and PD are the same disease with different patterns of deposition of synuclein or etiologically if they distinct disorders (Spillantini and Goedert, 2000). Fragments of synuclein exist in the plaques of patients with Alzheimer's disease (Duda et al., 2000). It is not yet clear whether all these diseases have a similar pathogenesis, but the idea that PD and certain syndromes related to it may have a similar etiology with the accumulation of an abnormal protein might explain the large overlap among these conditions. (Goedert, 1999)

An abnormal gene for the manufacture of alpha-synuclein appears to be responsible for the rare cases of PD that are inherited by autosomal dominant transmission. The abnormal gene has been identified and the abnormal protein product of that gene has been characterized. The abnormal alpha-synuclein can be identified microscopically in brain tissue and it seems identical to that seen in sporadic PD (Gomez-Tortosa et al., 1998). Yet in sporadic PD, patients have a normal gene for the production of alpha-synuclein. How the brain cells of genetically normal patients can make the abnormal form of alpha-synuclein is a puzzling subject of current research, and one hypothesis is that a form of prion disorder akin to the one that causes CJD and mad cow disease may be responsible (Johnson, 2000). Another idea is that the abnormality resides in the catabolic enzymes that are supposed to break down the affected proteins but cannot do the job.

There may be a similar pathogenesis in HD and SCAs. The accumulation and deposition of protein filaments in HD and some SCAs are the result of trinucleotide repeats (Price et al., 1998). The genes that are located in the nuclei of nerve cells direct the protein synthesis that occurs in these cells. Each gene uses the nucleic acids of its DNA to direct the manufacture of a protein. There is a genetic code for each amino acid that comprises a protein. The trinucleotide sequence, cytosine-arginine-guanidine (CAG) in the DNA codes for the amino acid, glutamine, in the protein. If the CAG sequence repeats with too frequently in the DNA, the resulting protein will have too many glutamine molecules. If there are too many glutamine repeats, a genetic disease results. The location of the gene that contains these trinucleotide repeats determines the disease. The number of CAG repeats determines the severity of the illness.

It has been known for a few years that HD is caused by CAG repeats at a particular locus in chromosome 9. As an animal model of HD, knockout mice were prepared. These were developed with the same genetic defect as humans with HD. The mice became ill with an ultimately fatal, degenerative neurological disorder. When they were sacrificed and examined, intracellular inclusions were discovered in the mouse brains that had never been described in the brains of humans who died with Huntington's disease. Human specimens were then restudied. Neuronal intranuclear inclusions that resembled the inclusions seen in the mice were found in the brains of humans who had died of HD and SCAs, which are also caused by expanded glutamine repeats. The inclusions in HD had been overlooked for years because no one expected to see them (Davies et al., 1999).

In other degenerative disorders, including Alzheimer's and Pick's diseases, the accumulation of abnormal proteins in filaments presumably causes the affected nerve cells to degenerate. In Alzheimer's disease the filaments involved have been shown to consist of the microtubule-associated protein, tau. Mutations in the gene for tau have also been identified as the genetic causes of some forms of Alzheimer's disease and also frontotemporal dementia (Pick's disease) (Goedert and Spillantini 2000). Another view, however, is that the accumulation of abnormal protein found in the plaques (amyloid precursor protein) causes Alzheimer's disease (Goedert et al., 1998; Lorenzo et al., 2000).

ACUTE DRUG-INDUCED MOVEMENT DISORDERS

Parkinsonism and many related movement disorders (dystonias, tics, dyskinesias) can acutely be induced by drugs (Armon et al., 1996; Gorell et al., 1988). The drugs that can induce parkinsonism, chiefly antipsychotics such as chlorpromazine (Thorazine) and haloperidol (Haldol), have their primary pharmacological action at the dopamine receptors, competitively blocking them. Dopamine synthesis is faster after administration of these drugs. This has been interpreted as compensation for the receptor blockade. Though the use of neuroleptics is associated with an increase in the total brain level of dopamine, the crucial action of neuroleptics is to reduce dopamine concentration at the postsynaptic receptor site. Antipsychotics can cause pronounced dystonia. Drug-induced, acute PD-like symptoms and dystonia can almost always be overcome by the administration of the dopamine uptake inhibitors diphenhydramine (Benadryl), belladonna compounds, or amantadine. If neuroleptics must be administered on a long-term basis, control of the acute drug-induced movement disorders can usually be maintained by the use of a belladonna compound. Dopamine receptor blockers can also acutely induce tics and dopamine receptor agonists, like L-dopa, can acutely cause dyskinesia.

Tardive Movement Disorders

The term *dyskinesia* should be restricted to chorea induced by a drug. Acute dyskinesia can be caused by too much L-dopa. After months of treatment with dopamine receptor blockers, however, a similar movement disorder known as tardive dyskinesia can develop. The major components of tardive dyskinesia are abnormal movements of the cheek, face, and tongue such as smacking, chewing, tongue thrusting, lateral jaw movements, or sucking. Choreoathetoid movements of the extremities and vocalization have also been observed. Most of these symptoms are worsened under emotional stress or during other body movements (Klawans and Barr, 1982; Koller, 1983). How blockage of dopamine receptors over time can lead to dyskinesia is not clear as dyskinesia presumably arises from too much dopamine or too great a sensitivity to it.

Drug use is not the only factor in the development of tardive dyskinesia. A review by Kane et al. (1986) revealed an average 5 percent prevalence of spontaneous dyskinesias in 19 different samples of untreated psychiatric patients (all diagnoses) as compared with a 20 percent incidence in populations treated with neuroleptics. Fenton et al. (1997) compared a group of neuroleptic-naive schizophrenic patients to a large group of other psychiatric patients and found that spontaneous dyskinesias were more common among the schizophrenics, implying that these dyskinesias may be related specifically to the pathophysiology of schizophrenia. Many of the characteristic facial movements of tardive dyskinesia were noted in schizophrenics before the advent of phenothiazines (Stevens, 1974). It is possible that tardive dyskinesia could be related to the soft neurological signs found in untreated schizophrenics. These signs include choreiform movements that reflect neurological dysfunction in schizophrenics. Granacher (1981) cautioned against too hastily attributing abnormal movements in a patient taking an antipsychotic drug to tardive dyskinesia, as one may overlook the onset or existence of other movement disorders. The reported incidence in patients receiving phenothiazine chronically varies from 2.9 to 41 percent, probably because of variation in the criteria for diagnosis. Kane et al. (1986) have estimated the cumulative annual risk of tardive dyskinesia in those taking antipsychotics to be approximately 5 percent per year, and in older patients the risk seems to be greater (Caligiuri et al., 1997). When the neuroleptics are used intermittently, there seems to be a much higher incidence of tardive dyskinesias than when they are used continuously. Bipolar patients seem unusually sensitive to the development of tardive dyskinesia, particularly when they are used intermittently (Post and Weiss, 1996; van Harten et al., 1998). The complexity of the neurotransmitter interaction is also highlighted by the fact that tardive dyskinesia has been seen with the use of tricyclic antidepressants (TCA) and with selective serotonin uptake inhibitors (SSRI) (Durif et al., 1995; Vandel et al., 1997). One encouraging aspect of tardive dyskinesia that has begun to emerge is that the symptoms seem to decrease over time after discontinuing or decreasing the dose of medication (Glazer et al., 1990; Koshino et al., 1991). Currently, discontinuation of the dopamine receptor blocker is the main treatment for drug-induced tardive dyskinesia and all other movement disorders related to the use of dopamine receptor blockers. Substitution for D-2 blockers of atypical antipsychotics like quetiapine and clozapine is probably the best course of action for controlling the psychosis. It sometimes seems to improve the tardive movement disorder as well.

DYSTONIA

Dystonia, sustained muscle contractions that frequently cause repetitive writhing movements and abnormal postures, often associated with intention tremor, is often confused with dyskinesia (see Painful Dystonia, above) (Fahn, 1984). Both can result from long exposure to antipsychotics. Difficult as it can be to differentiate dystonia from dyskinesia, the distinction is important, especially in PD. Dyskinesia is worsened by L-dopa and is relieved by withholding L-dopa. Dystonia results from inadequate dopamine replacement therapy. Dystonia in PD is painful, occurs around the time of dosing, and troubles the patient more than the care giver. Related or not to dopamine deficiency, dystonia can be relieved by belladonna drugs but sometimes requires enormous doses. Dystonia can be induced acutely by antipsychotic drugs; it can be tardive or it can arise from a disorder of the nervous system that is unrelated to medication.

The classification of dystonias cannot rest on the basis of neuropathologic findings because in most cases of idiopathic dystonia the neuropathologic findings have been negative. Patients with progressive generalized dystonia, curled into pretzel-like distortions, may literally die of inanition caused by their disease. Yet neuropathologists describe the brains of such patients after autopsy either as normal or as nonspecifically abnormal (Zeman, 1970; Gibb et al., 1988).

The physical examination is normal too, except for the dystonia itself. There are no Babinski signs. With laboratory testing there are no abnormal blood results, and the EEG and MRI are normal. The tools of diagnosis are exclusively clinical, i.e., bedside observation. As a consequence the term *dystonia* has had a checkered history. The subject has been reviewed in an extremely clear fashion by Cunningham-Owens (1990) who pointed out that Wilson defined dystonia as any variability in muscle tone whereas Denny-Brown defined it as fixed abnormalities of posture, and Hammond described gross muscle spasms and distortions of normal posture. Marsden called athetosis distal dystonia, but Wilson called dystonia proximal athetosis.

Oppenheim gave the condition a formal name, *dystonia musculorum deformans*. Most references to dystonia are a shorthand for this longer phrase, which embraces its most common form, a disorder of autosomal dominant transmission with incomplete penetrance that is seen primarily in Ashkenazic Jews. Torsion dystonia or torsion spasm are synonyms for dystonia musculorum deformans

Like all movement disorders, dystonia is worse when the patient is anxious or upset and better when the patient is relaxed. Dystonic movements disappear when the patient is asleep. These characteristics, shared by virtually all movement disorders, have often misled clinicians to mistakenly diagnose dystonia as a conversion (somatiform) disorder. Purely psychogenic causes of dystonia are extremely rare. In the largest published series of patients with dystonia, only 24 of 932 cases were psychogenic (Fahn, 1988). Despite this, approximately about 40 percent of patients with dystonia are given a diagnosis of conversion or somatiform disorder at some point (Fahn et al., 1983) but not always by psychiatrists.

Lacking neuropathologic definition, dystonias have been classified by the age of onset, presumed cause, and by the distribution of symptoms. The age of onset is an important feature because of its prognostic implications. The younger the onset the more likely is dystonia to become generalized, spreading from the part of the body in which it commences to the spinal muscles and all extremities Generalization of dystonia is particularly likely when the onset of symptoms occurs before 10 years of age. In contrast, generalization is rare when dystonia begins after the age of 40.

There have been over 40 dystonia-associated disorders. Most of these disorders are within the neurological sphere and most are very rare. Dystonia is characteristic only of cerebral palsy and Wilson's disease. In cerebral palsy dystonia is associated with scarring in the basal ganglia (état marbré). In Wilson's disease, it has been correlated with cystic degeneration of the putamen.

Based on the distribution of symptoms, dystonia can be divided into five types: focal, segmental, multifocal, generalized, and hemidystonic. The focal symptoms affect only one body area. Blepharospasm, torticollis, and writer's cramp are examples. Segmental dystonia including Meige's syndrome affects two or more contiguous body areas. Multifocal dystonia affects two or more noncontiguous body areas. Generalized dystonia affects disparate body areas, and hemidystonia affects limbs, trunk, and/or face on the same side of the body.

In addition to their discussion in neurological texts, dystonic symptoms, like writer's cramp, also figure heavily in the pages of psychiatric textbooks as examples of conversion syndromes, illustrating the parallel but separate paths the two specialities have often taken in the twentieth-century. Writer's cramp was also considered a hysterical disorder in many leading text books as late as 1980.

Idiopathic dystonia is usually slow to develop and worsens over months or years. It is aggravated by voluntary activity and exercises generally make it worse.

Most patients learn some sensory tricks. These include the patient touching his chin, the vertex of his head, the back of his neck with his hand contralateral to the direction of rotation, placing his hand behind his back in a "hammerlock" position, yawning, reclining in a particular posture, listening to music, and looking intently at something. Each of these maneuvers, in an individual case, may lessen the severity of dystonia and contribute to the mistaken diagnosis of conversion disorder.

Focal dystonias may be quite task specific. A patient with writer's cramp, for instance, can drum his fingers well but cannot write. Another may be able to draw but cannot write. A patient who is unable to walk forward may be able to walk backward. One of our patients exercises by walking in a large, empty parking lot. He cannot walk counterclockwise around the lot at all. Yet he can walk around it clockwise, but only while he listens to music and reads to distract himself.

The treatment of idiopathic dystonia is generally unsatisfactory. Except in those few cases that are responsive to dopamine replacement therapy, symptoms are only slightly ameliorated by medication. Belladonna medications such as trihexyphenidyl and benztropine offer the best relief, but adults do not generally tolerate the doses that are effective in controlling dystonia. These range up to 100 mg per day of trihexyphenidyl (Artane). Children have a much lower incidence of the intolerable anticholinergic side effects of belladonnas (memory problems and hallucinations). Peripheral anticholinergic effects in both children and adults can be reversed with pyridostigmine. Less than half the children and somewhat fewer adults with idiopathic dystonia obtain at least moderate benefit from high-dose belladonnas, when they can tolerate them (Fahn, 1988). Focal and some segmental dystonias are best treated with injections of botulinus toxin (Botox). By injecting this into the muscles in spasm, the injected muscles are temporarily paralyzed or weakened. Symptomatic benefit can be achieved for 3 to 6 months at a time.

Any drug with dopaminergic blocking qualities can cause or worsen dystonia acutely. Drug-induced, acute dystonia in children is often severe and generalized, whereas in adults acute drug-induced dystonia is usually craniocervical. This parallels the situation in idiopathic dystonia where the illness tends to be generalized in children and focal or segmental in adults. Drug-induced dystonia develops suddenly, usually within 24 hours after treatment begins. Dystonia can be intermittent with minutes to hours between episodes. Other clinical features of acute, drug-induced dystonia are varied, bizarre, and often terrifying to the patient. They include all the manifestations of dystonia mentioned so far as well as finger and wrist posturing, hyperpronation, hyperextension of the spine (opisthotonos), jaw dislocation, and respiratory stridor. The treatment of acute, drug-induced dystonia is very simple. Belladonnas provide relief within minutes. Benztropine 0.5 mg intramuscularly is all that is usually needed. Barbiturates, benzodiazepines, and diphenhydramine have all been used successfully as well.

One of the most distressing features of dopamine-sensitive (Parkinsonian) dystonia is that it can be painful. It is a mercy that the severely deforming postures caused by idiopathic torsion dystonia are usually not painful, although they can be. When there is pain, muscle spasms are accompanied by cramps. The pain of curling toes may not look dramatic to the observer but is very real to the patient, interfering with gait. The painful postures associated with dopamine deficiency often bother the patient much more than the observer. (Dyskinesia, a painless condition, is more alarming to the onlooker than to the patient.) The treatment of Parkinsonian dystonia is dopamine replacement.

Tardive dystonia, which tends to begin in the muscles of the face and neck is usually of gradual onset after months or years of treatment with dopamine antagonists (Burke et al., 1982). The younger the patient the more likely it is to be generalized. In about half of the cases of Kang et al. (1986) dystonia was unassociated with other tardive movement problems like dyskinesia. Treatment consists of discontinuation of the offending drug and substitution of quetiapine or clozapine for other antipsychotics.

Dystonia and Mental Illness

Because of the uncertainty of the diagnosis and pathogenesis of dystonia, there have been very few detailed reports of psychiatric symptoms in patients with dystonia. It is our impression that in generalized dystonia there are often none. Comorbid depression has been described in a minority of patients with axial dystonia (Bhatia et al., 1997) but without controls. Depression in such patients may be secondary to the deforming movement disorder (Jahanshahi and Marsden, 1992) but this does not explain why most such patients are not depressed. Depression is common in Meige's syndrome, a segmental dystonia (Tolosa, 1981; Sharma et al., 1996) and in other segmental dystonias (Jahanshahi and Marsden, 1988, Wenzel et al., 1998). Subcortical lesions that cause dystonia can give rise to depression (Lauterbach et al., 1997) and dystonia has been associated with OCD (Bihari et al., 1992a, b). Focal dystonia (hand cramps) severe enough to require botulinus toxin injections are not associated with significant psychopathology (Grafman et al., 1991).

CHOREA

Chorea consists of involuntary, jerky movements of the face, tongue, extremities, the trunk, and respiratory muscles. Choreatic movements are rapid and irregular, and become more pronounced during voluntary movement and when patients try to maintain a posture. Patients with chorea may try to cover up their disability by blending the pseudopurposeful choreatic movements with normal voluntary movements. Sometimes a patient may demonstrate a slight lilt while walking. The gait may have the quality of a dance. Choreatic movements can sometimes be revealed by having a patient squeeze the examiner's fingers. The choreatic movements of the patient's fingers that this accentuates gives the examiner the sensation of being milked, hence the term, *milkmaid's sign.* Patients with chorea are often unable to maintain protrusion of the tongue, and when they put their hands above their heads, choreatic movements of the upper extremities are maximized and the hands tend to pronate (pronator's sign). Choreatic movements and paratonia superimposed on deep tendon reflexes cause the relaxation phase of the reflex to be discontinuous (*hung up reflexes*).

Chorea and the slower writhing movements of athetosis (with which it is often associated and from which it cannot always be clearly distinguished) may be manifestations of one of several diseases: perinatal brain injury, encephalitis, vascular disease, hypoparathyroidism, Wilson's disease, mitochondrial disorders, and, rarely, brain tumor. The only abnormalities on examination are likely to consist of chorea itself and behavioral–cognitive symptoms. Chorea imparts the appearance of anxiety, which, added to cognitive abnormalities, can easily be misdiagnosed as purely psychogenic.

Huntington's chorea (now called Huntington's disease [HD] as chorea occasionally may not develop) is a degenerative disease of the brain involving the frontal cortical mantle as well as the basal ganglia. Because of the prominent involvement of the caudate nucleus and putamen in this disease, it has been suggested that chorea may be related to pathology of striatum. It would, however, be a mistake to identify chorea with the pathology of the striatum solely. There are extensive striatal connections to the cortex, globus pallidus, and thalamus. Chorea may be the result of an interruption of or imbalance between other neural systems and the striatum. Unilateral lesions of the ventral-lateral thalamus and subthalamic nuclei in man and in monkeys sometimes produce choreatic movements. Chorea in such cases is believed to be the result of loss of inhibiting influences on the globus pallidus. Lesions in the dorsal caudate and putamen have been described in oral-facial dyskinesia, a localized chorea (Altrocchi and Formo, 1983).

Virtually all the diseases in which chorea occurs may be associated with severe emotional disturbance. Roughly half of the patients with HD present with psychiatric symptoms and half develop psychosis at some point in the illness. The mental symptoms of 25 percent are indistinguishable from the symptoms of schizophrenia (Heathfield, 1967).

A review of the behavioral changes associated with HD (Mendez, 1994) indicated that mood disorders are the most common behavioral disorders (23%, including mania in 4%), followed by personality changes (20%) and schizophrenia (8%). The main personality change is apathy; this is often manifested as withdrawal from activities and social relations. Disinhibited behavior has also been described where the patients become impulsive, erratic, and irritable with poor judgement and at times demonstrate explosive behavior. This often leads to antisocial behavior. Compulsive rituals and obsessive thinking are also manifestations of cognitive abnormalities in HD. The most common cognitive changes in HD are problems with attention, executive functions, memory, motor learning, and decreased verbal fluency; language is usually spared. Thus, the pattern of abnormality of the dementia is more frontal-subcortical than posterior parietal-temporal. In some cases the cognitive and behavioral changes occur long before the motor changes. In many cases, though, the degree of dementia correlates with the severity of the chorea (Webb and Trzepacz, 1987).

Emotional disturbances also frequently accompany Sydenham's chorea, a major manifestation of rheumatic fever (Goldenberg et al., 1992). The emotional instability that starts with Sydenham's chorea may persist for many years, long after the chorea has resolved (Freeman et al., 1965). Residual chorea also can persist for years, but in many Sydenham's patients, the use of stimulant drugs, such as amphetamines or, in female patients, pregnancy, can precipitate the recurrence of chorea. These induced recurrences of chorea can occur in patients who have enjoyed a total remission of all the motor symptoms of Sydenham's chorea for many years. Sydenham's survivors also show significant elevations in the psychotic tetrad on the MMPI, suggesting that they have a persistent dopaminergic sensitivity (Nauseida et al., 1983). Psychosis is a frequent, though not a constant, concomitant of chorea, irrespective of the cause of chorea.

Treatment

The drugs that help alleviate chorea can induce parkinsonism, that is, reserpine, phenothiazine, and the other D-2 receptor blockers as well as alpha-methyl dopa treatment (a-MPT, Aldomet). As noted above, all these drugs reduce dopamine concentrations: reserpine by releasing stored dopamine, phenothiazine and related compounds by competitively blocking dopamine at its receptor sites, and a-MPT by blocking dopamine synthesis. Amantadine is the most effective drug for suppressing chorea but the mechanism for this effect is not known.

Drugs that potentiate catecholamine activity increase choreatic activity. These include the belladonna compounds (Aquilonius and Sjöström, 1971; Klawans and Rubovits, 1972). Of the drugs that make chorea worse, L-dopa is by far the most important. About half of all patients receiving L-dopa in therapeutic doses for PD develop chorea (dyskinesia). L-dopa has been shown to worsen chorea in HD.

Though the effects of amphetamines or cocaine upon chorea have not been systematically studied, patients who have taken overdoses of amphetamines or cocaine, either acutely or chronically, may develop symptoms of restlessness, tremor, motor impersistence, and "jumpiness," which strongly resemble chorea. Motor signs of amphetamine and/or cocaine overdosage are minor in comparison with the abnormal mental state that they cause, however; paranoia and mania predominate among the symptoms of amphetamine toxicity. Depression ("the crash") can follow their discontinuation.

Since chorea is improved by drugs that have an antidopaminergic effect and is made worse or induced by drugs that augment catecholamine activity, chorea could be the result of excessive dopaminergic activity or sensitivity. Seeman and Van Tol (1994), Kanazawa et al. (1993), and Klawans (1970) summarized the pharmacological evidence that this could be true in HD.

When the brains of patients with HD are examined at autopsy, the basal ganglia, and especially the caudate and putamen, are characteristically depleted of neurons. Despite this serious loss of neurons, the dopamine content of the putamen and globus pallidus per gram of remaining tissue has been found to be normal and that of the caudate reduced to approximately 60 percent of normal. Since the number of neurons per gram is greatly reduced in HD in these regions, each remaining striatal neuron in this disease may be exposed to a relative excess of dopamine.

Imaging studies have revealed hypometabolism in the caudate in early cases of HD and caudate atrophy in moderate to advanced cases (Mendez, 1994). Using recombinant DNA techniques, Gusella and co-workers isolated fragments of chromosome 4 that transmit HD. The defective gene has subsequently been identified. (Huntington's Disease Collaborative Research Group, 1993). The severity of the genetic defect relates to the extent of repeats of the sequence: cytosine, arginine, and guanosine (CAG). Precise predictive testing for HD is now available. Some family members at risk for HD want to know whether they have the gene for the disease, which has 100 percent penetrance and expressivity. Others avoid this test, preferring not to know (Wiggins et al., 1992).

MOTOR TICS, TOURETTE'S SYNDROME, AND OBSESSIVE-COMPULSIVE DISORDER

Recent investigations link obsessive and compulsive symptoms with movement disorders and pathology of the basal ganglia (Berthier et al., 1996). Common features of Tourette's syndrome are multiple motor and vocal tics and obsessive-compulsive symptoms (OCD). Tourette's syndrome is a genetic condition in which neuropathologic changes have been described in the basal ganglia (Hyde and Weinberger, 1995a, b). The symptoms of Tourette's syndrome and OCD have been observed to develop following streptococcal infections (Swedo et al., 1997; Kurlan, 1998), which raises the question of whether both conditions are a sequelae of rheumatic fever and in this way similar to Sydenham's chorea. Minor distinctions have been made in the quality of OCD symptoms in patients who have both Tourette's syndrome and OCD, as compared with OCD alone (Cath et al., 2000).

Obsessions are recurrent and persistent thoughts (such as fear of contamination, or doubts about locking the house, turning off the stove, etc.), images, or impulsive thoughts that are intrusive, unpleasant, often violent. They are recognized by the patient as inappropriate. These thoughts cause marked anxiety and distress and can cripple the sufferer by producing an attention disturbance that prevents concentration on any matters besides the obsessive thoughts. Compulsions are repetitive behaviors or mental acts (hand washing, counting, praying, etc.) that are driven by obsessions and lead to rituals. Patients with OCD can be very irritable when their rituals are interrupted or the flow of life impinges on their obsessions. They are under constant stress from their own thoughts and engage in compulsive acts to relieve this feeling of stress. The obsessions and compulsions may become increasingly frequent, dominating the patient's life. The symptoms often begin in adolescence, and although there are no gender differences in the prevalence and severity, they occur earlier in males (6–15 years) than in females (20–29 years). The lifetime prevalence (approximately 2.3%) is similar in almost all countries (Weissman, 1994).

Functional imaging studies have shown hyperactivity of the orbitofrontal and cingulate cortex in OCD. With successful medical treatment, this hyperactivity diminishes. Structural imaging has shown reduced volume in the caudate nuclei of patients with OCD (Robinson et al., 1995; Rauch, 2000), and, oddly, focal brain lesions involving the frontal, temporal, or cingulate cortex and the basal ganglia can cause (as well as relieve) obsessive-compulsive behavior (Berthier et al., 1996).

Eighty-five percent of patients with OCD experience improvement when treated with SSRIs (Pigott and Seay, 1999). The symptoms of OCD are often quite dose responsive, especially to SSRIs. When the proper dose is achieved, the symptoms will resolve almost completely, and if the dose is lowered, the OCD symptoms will return. Of those patients who do not respond to medications, 25 percent will respond to surgical lesions placed in the cingulate gyrus or a portion of the orbital medial frontal lobes; sometimes both these areas are lesioned (Jenike et al., 1991; Baer et al., 1995). Other obsessive syndromes also respond to SSRIs. Trichotillomania (compulsive hair pulling) and some body dysmorphia, where the patient is obsessed with the idea that his body is malformed or ugly, respond to SSRIs (Phillips et al., 1998).

Some dogs will develop obsessive grooming to the point where the licking causes open wounds. Veterinarians call this animal model of compulsive behavior the acral lick syndrome. This condition also responds to SSRIs (Rapoport et al., 1992).

There is as yet little clarity concerning the specific neurotransmitter systems involved in OCD. Although the SSRIs are very effective for obsessive-compulsive behavior and implicate the serotonin system, other classes of antidepressants and even some anticonvulsants have also proved modestly effective for treating OCD. Dopamine antagonists have been useful in the treatment of chorea, psychosis, and manic-like symptoms in HD and for the tics in Tourette's syndrome, but their effectiveness in the treatment of OCD has been variable. There have been reports that high doses of the atypical neuroleptics improve the symptoms of OCD (Ramasubbu et al., 2000). In general, antipsychotics are more effective for the motor than the cognitive symptoms in HD and Tourette's syndrome. There has been no study of the differential effectiveness of atypical and older antipsychotics in Tourette's syndrome, HD, and OCD.

AFFECTIVE DISORDERS

The high comorbidity of movement disorders and affective disorders is intriguing. Not only are affective symptoms present in many of the disorders of movement but also significant psychomotor symptoms are present in the affective disorders. In affective disorders the motor dysfunctions can range from retardation to agitation. As the same neurotransmitters, particularly the catecholamines and serotonin are important to both motor and affective disorders it is fascinating to see how the same biologic systems can cause overlapping but different disorders.

Affective disorder is a ubiquitous condition and a frequent concomitant of many neurological and medical conditions. The major phenomenology of affective illness (depression or mania) is mood disturbance, usually accompanied by a disturbance of sleep, appetite, psychomotor agitation or retardation, and mood consonant thoughts. Depressed thoughts and feelings are usually described as sadness feeling "blue," "low," or "gloomy." Because of the ubiquity of these feelings, it is often not clear when they should be considered pathological. Usually, this judgment is made on clinical grounds by weighing such factors as the severity of the symptoms, the amount of interference with the functioning of the individual, the duration of the symptoms, the age at which they occur, the number of similar previous episodes, and a family history of the disorder.

In addition to changes in mood, there are alterations in the depressed patient's perception of self and the environment. The significance of a particular life event to which an individual is supposed to be reacting is determined only after he becomes depressed. Patients often perceive themselves as being worthless, hopeless, helpless, guilty, and even at times "evil." Frequently they view their accomplishments as meaningless and neither persuasion nor confrontation with reality can change their attitude. If they are delusional, the delusions usually relate to ideas of bodily illness, decay, or other dismal eventualities. Severe depression can be accompanied by paranoid delusions and even hallucinations. Differentiation from schizophrenia in such cases depends on the presence of depression, a relatively normal premorbid adjustment, and a family history of affective disorder. (In manic conditions, we see the obverse of depressive feelings: euphoria, grandiosity, and a heightened sense of one's abilities.) Sleep, appetite, digestion, sexual activity, and psychomotor activity may be disrupted. Sleep disturbances can vary from hyposomnia, difficulty in falling asleep, awakening frequently throughout the night, early morning awakening, or any combination of these, to excessive sleep (hypersomnia). Anorexia and weight loss or hyperphagia and weight gain are common. Decreased sexual interest and activity are the rule. Changes in psychomotor function, either agitation or retardation are frequently evident. Agitated patients seem anxious, wring their hands, pace about, and frequently sleep poorly. Psychomotor retardation is characterized by reduced physical and mental activity as well as hypersomnia. The slowing of thought processes in retarded depressions may suggest dementia (McAllister, 1983; Emery and Oxman, 1992). Suicidal ideation is common, and a very real risk, in severe depression.

If the symptoms of depression are present in mild form and transient (not lasting more than 1 to, at most, 6 months) and closely follow emotionally charged events (usually loss of job, health, or a loved one), the reaction may be considered to be grief or bereavement (Jacobs, 1993). If the symptoms are severe, regardless of the presence of precipitating factors, if they persist, and if they interfere with the patient's functioning from day to day, the condition should be regarded as depressive illness and should be treated. Summing up the symptoms rather than weighing individual symptoms best characterizes the severity of a depressive syndrome. Scales for quantifying the severity and variety of affective symptoms have been devised (Beck et al., 1961; Zung, 1965; Hamilton, 1969). We have found these scales that quantify the extent of depressive symptoms quite useful clinically. They are relatively reliable methods of judging the severity of depression, following the course of the disorder, and evaluating therapy.

The duration of an episode and the tendency of depression to recur, as well as the severity of symptoms, vary from patient to patient. In some patients, depression occurs as a single episode in an otherwise normal life. Most patients having their first depression have no family history of depression. When the family history is negative, there is no way of predicting the course of illness. The chances are that a remission will occur and that the symptoms will respond to antidepressant medication. Twenty-five percent of such patients will become depressed again in the future (Blazer, 1994).

Patients who have repeated episodes of affective disorder and their illnesses can be divided into two groups:

1. Unipolar-manifested by repeated depressive (or rarely manic) episodes, often also called Major Recurrent Depressive (or manic) episodes in DSM-IV.
2. Bipolar-characterized by repeated episodes of both mania and depression.

> In some bipolar patients, mania is more prevalent, almost to the exclusion of depression, though the opposite may occur.

The improved reliability of the diagnostic process using DSM-III (and it's successors), together with standardized interviewing methods, led to the NIMH-sponsored Epidemiologic Catchment Area Study (ECA) in which 18,000 community members from five different areas in the U.S. were interviewed. One of the more interesting aspects of this study was the finding that in both men and women the prevalence of mood disorder is higher in persons under the age of 45 years old than in those over 45 years old. Mood disorder has a higher prevalence in women but does not vary by race. Its overall prevalence in the ECA study was 6 percent (Blazer et al., 1994).

In a review of follow-up studies of unipolar and bipolar affective disorders, Robins and Guze (1972) noted that the median duration of the first attack of a depressive illness varied. In unipolar depression, it was 13 months; in bipolar depression, 6 ½ months. The mean duration of manic attacks was 3 ½ months but relapse is less likely. Between episodes of illness, unipolar patients tend to be insecure, sensitive, or obsessional, whereas bipolar patients tend to be more active and sociable.

Affective disorder presents with a consistent and recognizable clinical picture. The symptoms represent disturbances of biologic functions controlled by the brain, e.g., mood, cognition, perception, motor, sexual, sleep, and appetite.

Biologic Changes in Affective Disorders

Perhaps because the psychopharmacological agents that treat affective disorder affect the catechol and indoleamine systems, we tend to think primarily of these neurotransmitters when discussing the biologic changes in depression. However, this ignores a large older and newly emerging literature that demonstrates the wide-ranging biologic changes that are present in affective disorder, e.g., the motor system, cognition, sleep, sexual function, the immune system, and arousal. (Bejjiani et al., 1999).

Structural changes. Minor soft signs of diffuse neurological dysfunction and even electroencephalographic abnormalities, so often present in schizophrenic patients, have also been reported in patients with affective disorder (McAllister, 1983; Emery and Oxman, 1992). Previously, patients with such features were diagnosed as having pseudodementia (see Chapter 4, pp. 160–161, 239–240). However, it is clear that many of these signs of central nervous system dysfunctions observed in affective disorders remit as the depressive illness abates.

Imaging studies of depressed patients have begun to contribute some information on structural and functional changes in depression. In the studies of major depressive episodes (MDE), structural MRI has shown fairly consistently decreased frontal lobe, hippocampal, and basal ganglia volumes. Whereas FMRI and PET have shown decreased activity in the dorsolateral prefrontal cortex and increased activity in the ventrolateral prefrontal cortex and the ventral paralimbic structures. The structural findings have been more equivocal in bipolar patients, whereas the functional changes are similar to MDE (Drevets, 1999; Brody et al., 2001). Interestingly many of the functional changes are reversible with antidepressant treatment and sleep deprivation (Brody et al., 2001). Studies using tryptophan depletion and induced sadness cause the same functional changes as noted in depression (Brody et al., 2001). Magnetic resonance imaging signal hyperintensities in the deep and periventricular white matter, have been noted to occur significantly more frequently in elderly depressives. This finding has been reported less consistently in bipolar patients. These deep white matter hyperintensities have also been described in patients with dementia and cerebrovascular disease so their meaning and specificity is as yet unclear. These findings in the frontal and temporal lobes and the basal ganglia provide an anatomical basis for the mood, motor, cognitive, and perceptual symptoms observed in patients with affective disorders (Sobin and Sackheim, 1997). McHugh (1989) described a triad of symptoms in patients with basal ganglia disorders of depression, dyskinesias, and dementia. He noted that motor and sensory pathways, tracts from the cortical association regions, and the limbic system all funnel through the basal ganglia.

Hypothalamic changes. Many of the long observed sexual, appetite, and sleep disturbances (vegetative changes) in depressed patients can be related to neuroendocrine and hypothalamic changes. Sacher (1967) found that depressed patients have elevated blood and urine levels of corticosteroids. There has been a flood of investigations of neuroendocrine factors in affective illness. After many years of study, Carroll and colleagues (1981) published a paper with a definitive title “A Specific Laboratory Test for the Diagnosis of Melancholia.” This paper demonstrated that many patients with affective disorders fail to suppress cortisol excretion, as a normal person would when given dexamethasone. Thus, it not only confirmed Sacher’s original findings but also pointed to some defect in the hypothalamic-pituitary axis (HPA). As with many studies of psychopathologic conditions, when the control group was extended to other types of psychiatric patients rather than just to normals, the positive findings became less definitive. Cortisol nonsuppression after dexamethasone has now been noted in a wide range of conditions, including normal health, old age, dementia, OCDs, alcoholism, and weight loss (Amsterdam et al., 1982; Insel et al., 1982; Spar and Grener, 1982; American College of Physicians, 1984). The test may correlate with therapeutic outcome in that patients with affective disorder who still fail to suppress after treatment have a poorer prognosis (Nemeroff and Evans, 1984). Although it is clear that the dexamethasone suppression test (DST) is not a specific biologic test of depression, it is also clear that in affective illness there is often a disturbance of cortisol metabolism. This metabolic disturbance often returns to normal with remission of the affective symptoms. Corticotropin releasing factor (CRF) levels in depressed patients are consistently elevated (Schatzberg and Nemeroff, 1998). Kurlan et al. (1988) found elevated levels of CRF in the spinal fluid of Huntington's disease patients, correlated with the severity of their depression but there were no significant differences in CSF 5-HIAA levels between the HD patients and controls. There are several studies that now show that elevated cortisol levels are related to childhood abuse and may serve as predisposing factors to depression (Heim et al., 2000; Kaufman et al., 2000).

Hypothalamic dysfunction in depression is further suggested by sleep disturbances, slowed heart rate, lowered body temperature, loss of weight and appetite, disturbances of the menstrual cycle, and impotence and frigidity (Hill, 1968). Diminished secretion of gastric juice and saliva, reduced peristalsis, and a lower basal metabolic rate have also been noted in affective disorders.

Hypothalamic disturbance is also reflected in the extensive studies of thyroid stimulating hormone (TSH) to a dose of thyrotropin-releasing hormone (TRH), which has consistently shown aberrant responses in 20%–30% of depressed patients. Depressed patients may have normal T3 and T4 blood levels but will have diminished or blunted TSH response to TRH stimulation (Loosen and Prange, 1982). Other studies have shown diminished responses of growth hormone, prolactin, gonadol hormones, CRF, and melatonin in patients with affective disorders (Lewy et al., 1982a, b; Kupfer and Thase, 1983; Gold et al., 1984; Bauer and Whybrow, 1988).

Anxiety and arousal. Affective disorder has always presented with a mixture of depressive and anxiety symptoms (Maras et al., 1996). Consequently, it is not surprising that many depressives manifest a general state of hyperarousal. Both elevated galvanic skin responses and muscle tension have been observed in depressed patients (Whatmore and Ellis, 1962; Whybrow and Mendels, 1969). Buchsbaum and colleagues (1971) noted that depressed patients tended to augment the intensity of incoming stimuli.

Sleep. Sleep disturbance is one of the most consistent features of depressive illness. In general, it parallels depression in severity. There is little diagnostic specificity as to the type of sleep disturbance e.g., early morning awakening or difficulty in falling asleep (Hawkins and Mendels, 1966). Hyposomnia is characteristic of most depressive illness. This can be manifested as early morning wakefulness, a longer latency of sleep onset, and a decrease in non–rapid-eye-movement sleep, both absolute and relative to total sleep. In contrast to other forms of depressive illness, the depressive phase of bipolar depressive illness is often characterized by increased total sleep and increased relative and total time spent in the rapid-eye-movement (REM) stage of sleep. There is shortened latency (appearance) of the first REM sleep period in 60 to 90 percent of moderately to severely depressed patients. Conditions such as narcolepsy, drug and alcohol withdrawal, and dementia show a similar pattern (Kupfer, 1983; Nofzinger et al., 1999).

An interesting variant of affective disorder, seasonal affective disorder, reflects a disturbance of circadian rhythms. Longitudinal studies have confirmed that there are a group of patients who are sensitive to the light changes in fall and early winter that lead to depression. Many of these patients can be treated by early morning or evening artificial light that shifts their circadian rhythms (Sakamoto et al., 1995; Schwartz et al., 1996).

Neurotransmitter changes. No single neurotransmitter deficiency has been consistently associated with depression. No single defect, such as the lack of dopamine, as in PD, has as yet been found in any affective disorders. As most of the effective medications affect either norepinephrine or serotonin or both, these two neurotransmitters have been studied extensively. To date neither norepinephrine nor serotonin has been found to be exclusively defective in depressed patients. Defects in both pre- and postsynaptic receptors, and reuptake of norepinephrine and serotonin have been found variously in groups of depressed patients. Such findings are often not replicated (Schatzberg and Schildraut, 1995; Maes and Meltzer, 1995). Some of the deficiencies in both neurotransmitters are corrected by antidepressant treatment. Compounds that interfere with the metabolism of norepinephrine and serotonin do not cause depression in normals, but surprisingly will cause relapse in patients treated with antidepressants (Miller et al., 1996; Smith et al., 1997). Dopamine is also reduced in some depressive patients (Wilner, 1995). Decreased serotonergic function has been fairly consistently found in patients at high risk for suicide and those who have actually committed suicide (Mann and Arango, 1999). Although it is clear that these key neurotransmitters are often disturbed in depression, it is not clear if these are causal or epiphenomenona of another process. There is increasing evidence that the antidepressants function at the intracellular level to produce their therapeutic effect. Duman has postulated that chronic antidepressant treatment increases cyclic-adenosine monophosphate (AMP) formation, which in turn regulates monoamine function (Duman et al., 1997). Also neurotrophic factors such as brain-derived neurotrophic factor (BDNF) is up-regulated by either antidepressant or ECT treatment in the hippocampal regions of depressed patients, in a time frame that is also more consistent with the clinical response to antidepressants (Nibuya et al., 1995).

Immune responses. One of the more exciting areas of research in psychobiology is the increasing amount of data demonstrating that stress and depression diminish the responsivity of the immune system (Ader, 1983; Dubovsky, 1997; McEwen, 1998). Although the results are often conflicting, a significant number of studies show that in depression, natural killer (NK) cells, mitogen-induced T cell activity, and certain lymphocytes are reduced (Herbert and Cohen, 1993). The possibility of a relationship between disturbed immune function and affective disorder is also suggested by the increasing number of reports of major affective and cognitive symptoms in patients with multiple sclerosis (Klonoff et al., 1990; Nyenhuis et al., 1995; Sadovnick et al., 1996).

The cognitive changes in MS are similar to those found in PD and HD patients. However, they represent changes in the efficiency of mental functioning more than an actual loss of function (Caine et al., 1986). Multiple sclerosis patients also have significant elevations in cortisol and CRF, just as has been noted in depressed patients who do not have MS (Fassbender et al., 1998).

Genetics. A recent meta-analysis of the genetic etiology of major depressive disorders concludes that major depression results from both genetic and environmental factors, that major depression is heterogeneous, and that there are many pathways leading to depression (Sullivan et al., 2000). These authors also note that few of the many genetic studies met their criteria for inclusion in the meta-analysis (clear diagnostic criteria, actual interviews, distinctions made between bipolar and unipolar depressions, etc.), but of the six twin studies that did so the heritability of major depression in the monozygotic twins was 31%–42% and of bipolar disorder approximately 70 percent. There was no evidence for gender differences in heritability even though the incidence of depression is greater in women. Sullivan and his collegues also found that major depression runs in families (15%–21% risk in first-degree relatives of patients with major depression); however, they could not distinguish genetic from enviromental influences. There is evidence of specificity in the transmission of both bipolar and unipolar depression as the rate of bipolar disorder in the offspring of unipolar depressives is about half that of bipolar probands. The best estimates of risk for offspring of bipolar probands is 12 percent and for major depressive offspring approximately 7 percent (Merikangas and Kupfer, 1995).

Most recent molecular genetic studies have involved bipolar patients, and to date there has been replication of linkage studies for sites on chromosomes 18 (Berrettini et al., 1994; Stine et al., 1995) and 21 (Straub et al., 1994; Gurling et al., 1995; Detera-Wadleigh et al., 1996). Many other sites have been identified but not replicated, and some studies have not confirmed the chromosome 18 and 21 findings (Sanders et al., 1999).

Stress and negative life events. In most affective disorders, stress and negative life events are as critical as a hereditary predisposition. The evaluation of negative life events in patients with affective disorder is often difficult, as depressed patients tend to recall mood consonant events. Depressed patients frequently distort life events or overemphasize their unfavorable aspects; these allegedly causal events may actually be a product of the depressive feelings themselves. Fogarty and Hensley (1983) demonstrated that mood influences the retrieval of memories that were encoded during similar mood states; thus, the depressed patient is more likely to recall events from periods of depression. However, negative life events are more frequent in patients with affective disorder. Negative life events, particularly in a person with a family history of depression, are critical to the onset of affective disorder (Cui and Vaillant, 1996; Harkness et al., 1999; Kohn et al., 2001). An intriguing question is whether or not the presence of depression also tends to create negative life events. Cui and Vaillant (1997) assessed 113 normal college men for negative life events. These men were followed for 35 years and given systematic psychological assessments. The authors divided negative life events into dependent (self-imposed, e.g., marital separation) and independent (not self-imposed, e.g., death of a relative, illness in a child) and found that the depressed group, compared to a control group, had a higher density of dependent negative life events after the first episode of depression. They concluded that affectively disordered patients apparently do generate negative life events.

Whether self-imposed or imposed on them from the outside, it is clear that the person with depression often experiences considerable stress. Possibly as a reflection of this stress, there is an increased mortality in depressed populations (Harris and Barraclough, 1998). This increased mortality is not just as a result of suicide. The suicide rate accounted for less than 20 percent of the depressed patients' deaths (still very high when compared to a 1 percent suicide rate in control samples). The increased mortality rate was caused by cardiovascular disease (but not cancer) (Wulsin et al., 1999).

Is it possible that depression in many instances is a failed generalized response to stress, that after a prolonged period of stress (either psychological or physical) the clinical picture we call depression is really the end result of a failure of adaptive mechanisms to stress. In 1973, Akiskal and McKinney (further elaborated in 1984 with Whybrow and recently by McKinney, 2001) postulated that depressive disorders were a general failure of adaptation to chronic stress. They proposed that depression was the result of environmentally induced endogenous factors that caused reversible deficits in the diencephalic structures related to pleasure and reward. Interestingly, most animal models of depression rely on creating continual stress in the animal (Holsboer, 1999). There is considerable biologic evidence the depressed patient's body is responding to great stress. As we have noted, the HPA is altered in depression; both cortisol and CRF are consistently elevated in the CSF of depressed patients. New research has shown that chronic hypercortisolemia alters brain structure, particularly in the hippocampal regions (Newport and Nemeroff, 2002). Lesions in the hippocampus could explain the chronicity of depressive reactions, some of the imaging findings, and perhaps even the memory and cognitive changes observed in depressed patients (Lupien et al., 1998). There is increasing evidence that our treatments for depression decrease the activity of the hypothalamic-pituitary axis and thus decrease the amount of circulating steroids (Romeo et al., 1998). The treatments increase BDNF in the hippocampus and this might repair the steroid-induced damage (Nibuya et al., 1996; Duman et al., 1997). The time frame of these reactions coincides with the 10-day to 2-week time frame for the therapeutic response to antidepressants better then their biochemical effect on neurotransmitter systems, which are complete usually in minutes to hours.

The depression of immune functions in affective disorder could also be related to stress. We now know that stress depresses immune functions significantly (McEwen, 1998). Perhaps the depressed immune function and the added stress of a medical illness in depression increase the morbidity, mortality, and cost of the care of patients with medical and surgical disorders (Kayton, 1998). The incidence of depression in most hospitalized medical and surgical patients is four- to fivefold greater (20%–30%) then the general population (6%).

In summary, then, depressed patients commonly undergo changes in many physiological systems. No single etiological mechanism causing these changes has yet been defined. However, it is clear that depression relates to a genetic predisposition, environmental stressful events, and a cascade of biologic changes. Although DSM-IV has made the diagnosis of affective disorders more reliable, the categorization of affective disorders is still descriptive. Affective illnesses are probably very heterogeneous with regard to etiology. For example, a unipolar depression and the depressive phase of bipolar illness are phenomenologically indistinguishable, but their chains of causation are probably quite different, the similarity may represent the limited number of responses of the central nervous system to different etiologies.

Treatment. Depression is a common concomittant of neurologial disease. As we note in Chapter 7, depression can be an emotional reaction to the disease; it can be caused by the neurologic disorder; or it can be a recurrent primary psychiatric disorder. The clinical history is one of the key methods of categorizing these. It is also important to examine the medications the person is taking before attempting to treat the depression; many of the medications used to treat neurologic conditions can cause depression, particularly anticonvulsants, antiparkinsonian agents, anticholinergics, and muscle relaxants. Medications used for general medical disorders can also cause depression, e.g., antihypertensives, antiarrhythmics, steroids, oral contraceptives, antiemetics and antihistamines (Tucker et al., 1997). There is little difference in efficacy among the older tricyclic antidepressants (TCAs), the selective serotonin reuptake inhibitors

(SSRIs), and the newer mixed-effect antidepressants (Table 5–2); 60%–70% of depressed patients will respond to any of these drugs. One of the best indicators of which drug to select is whether the patient has responded well to a particular drug in the past. With so many antidepressants now available however the choice is often related to potential side effects that one wishes to avoid. Although similar in efficacy, the new antidepressants have supplanted the TCAs for several reasons: *(1)* they have fewer anticholinergic and cardiac side effects and *(2)* overdoses of the new drugs are less dangerous (Hirschfeld, 1999). Many pain syndromes and peripheral neuropathies still seem to respond better to the TCAs (Stahl, 1998). Each of the new drugs has a very different chemical structure, so there is a real advantage in changing medications if one does not work (this was not the case with many of the TCAs). For instance, going from fluoxetine to venlafaxine, mirtazapine, or sertraline, etc. can often improve the clinical effect (Thase, 1995). Perhaps the two most common reasons for the antidepressant failure are using too low a dose and not treating the patient for a long enough period. Whichever antidepressant is chosen, the dose should be gradually built up to maximum (if there is no clinical response) and the patient kept at a maximum dose for 4–8 weeks A major problem with the SSRIs and the other new drugs is that they inhibit the cytochrome P450 system and thus can seriously affect the metabolism and subsequent blood levels of medications used for neurologic disorders such as anticonvulsants, benzodiaepines, tacrine, coumadin, beta blockers, etc. Consequently, any time one of these new antidpressants is used, a check should be made for potential drug interactions with other drugs the patient is currently taking (Nemeroff et al., 1996). The primary side effects of the SSRIs and the newer antidepressants are gastrointestinal (nausea and vomiting, flatulence), CNS (headache, nervousness, tremor, sleep disurbance), and sexual dysfunction (decreased libido, arousal and delayed ejaculation or orgasm). Bupropion, nefazodone, and mirtazapine have the least effects on sexual function (Dewan and Annand, 1999). Cognitive psychotherapy has proven to be quite effective as both an adjunct and a primary treatment for depression, and has replaced many of the more insight-oriented therapies (Horton et al., 1992).

CONCLUSION

Parkinson's disease is the model for disorders of the catecholamine systems because its pathogenesis is best understood. The primary symptoms of dopamine deficiency (resting tremor, bradykinesia, and postural instability) can be reversed with dopamine replacement; hence the primary treatment is with L-dopa. Some patients with dopamine deficiency also have symptoms that derive from dysfunction of other portions of the nervous system outside the dopamine system.

Table 5–2 Antidepressant Drugs

DRUG TYPE	COMMENT
Tricyclic Antidepressant (TCAs)	
Desimpramine (Norpramin)	Primarily noradreneric, anticholinergic, hypotension, QRS, blood levels useful
Nortrityline (Pamelor)	
Serotonin Reuptake Inhibitors	
Fluoxetine (Prozac) Sertraline (Zoloft) Paroxetine (Paxil) Fluvoxamine (Luvox) Citalopram (Celexia)	Metabolites present for 6 weeks (fluoxetine) All inhibit P450 system = many drug interactions, GI symptoms, sex dysfunction, weight or, tremor, sedation, or agitation
Antidepressants with Varied Actions	
Bupropion (Wellbutrin)	Norepinephrine and dopamine by reuptake inhibition, seizures, few drug interactions
Velafaxine (Effexor)	Serotonin and norepinephrine uptake inhibitor, drowsiness, tremor, sex dysfunction, risk of hypertension More like SSRI at low dose
Nefazodone (Serzone)	Serotonin antagonist and reuptake inhibitor, hypotension, tremor, paraesthesias
Mirtazapine (Remeron)	Alpha adrenergic blockade and serotonin post synaptically, sedating at low dose but not at high, may decrease sexual dysfunction of SSRIs
Reboxetine	Norepinephrine inhibitor, fewer anticholinergic effects than TCAs, tremors, hypotension
Trazodone (Desyrel)	Primarily weak serotonin reuptake inhibition, few anticholinergic effects, hypotension, sedation (often used for sleep), some help with agitation in dementia, priapism
Monoamine Oxidase Inhibitors	
Phenelzine (Nardil) Tranylcypromine (Parnate)	Serotonin and norepinephrine, hypotension, severe food and TCAs interactions
Psychostimulants	
Dextroamphetamine (Dexadrine) Methylphenidate (Ritalin)	Norepinephrine, rapid action, useful in patients with apathy related to brain damage

These symptoms do not resolve with dopamine replacement. As the degeneration of the dopaminergic cells advances, changes must be made in the schedule of L-dopa administration and the diet to maintain a smooth response. All the drugs that relieve the symptoms of PD are believed to potentiate the concentration of dopamine at its receptors.

Clinicians frequently misattribute certain symptoms of dopamine deficiency to psychological reactions, chiefly depression. There is probably some increase in the prevalence of depression in PD but a kind of pseudodepression is very common as well. The overlapping characteristics of depression and PD may explain the confusion. If such symptoms as decreased energy, motivation, and initiative, increased sleeping and contentment at doing nothing do not respond to dopamine replacement or antidepressants, they probably derive from degenaration of the frontal-thalamic projections that pass through the corpus striatum. As such, these symptoms constitute not the well-known pseudodementia of depression but the pseudodepression of frontal dementia.

Another easily misdiagnosed symptom of dopamine deficiency is akasthisia. This presents as panic attacks that are associated with "restless legs." Along with painful, dystonic cramps, akasthisia tends to occur as the preceeding dose of L-dopa has worn off. For this reason, both akasthisia and dystonic cramps are more common in the evening and at night. Neither responds to antidepressants; both respond to dopamine replacement therapy, to benzodiazepines, and to sleep.

Psychosis, confusion, and visual hallucinations can be the result of neuronal degeneration outside the dopamine system and are encountered in patients who also have dopamine deficiency. Psychosis with visual hallucinations, for example, characteristically occurs early in the course of Lewy body dementia. Usually, however, psychosis in PD patients reflects the toxicity of anti-Parkinson medications, all of which can cause psychosis and all of which probably potentiate the concentration of dopamine at dopamine receptor sites. Only two atypical antipsychotic drugs (clozapine and quetiapine) can control the toxic psychosis of anti-Parkinson drugs without exacerbating the symptoms of dopamine deficiency. Presumably these two drugs control psychosis in some other way than by blocking D-2 receptors. D-2 recptor bockade is the leading mechanism of antipsychotic action of most neuroleptic drugs most of which can induce parkinsonism and acute dystonic reactions. Because they block dopamine uptake (inactivation), belladonna compounds and diphenhydramine can reverse such acute reactions.

Almost all the anti-Parkinson medications can cause or exacerbate chorea. This form of acute dyskinesia is usually of more concern to the care giver than to the patient. It is not painful and is the worst when the previous dose of L-dopa is at peak levels. The one exception to the rule is amantadine, a weak anti-Parkinson drug, which currently has as its main clinical role the control of chorea. It effectively ameliorates the acute dyskinesia caused by L-dopa, the tardive dyskinesias caused by prolonged treatment with antipsychotic drugs, and the chorea of Huntington's disease. Its mechanism of action is not known. Chorea, whether drug induced or the result of intrinsic brain disease, is often associated with psychic symptoms: loose associations, difficulty concentrating, inability to stay on target mentally, impulsivity, hypomania, paranoia, and sometimes frank psychosis. In some sense, chorea and psychosis are the opposites of PD as both chorea and psychosis can be the result of too much dopamine or too great a sensitivity to dopamine. This is an oversimplification but it explains much phenomenology. It is a form of the catecholeamine hypothesis.

Like Parkinson's disease, many dementing disorders can be inherited as autosomal dominants. This list includes Alzheimer's, Pick's, Creutzfeldt-Jakob, Huntington's, and some nondementing genetic diseases (spinocerebellar degenerations). Some nongenetic degenerative diseases (Lewy body dementia, multisystem atrophy) share with the aforementioned conditions the intraneuronal accumulation of a protein, different in composition and/or distribution in each disease. The protein is usually a portion of, or closely related to, a normal cellular constituent. Evidence has been gathering that indicates that these conditions may be caused by improper genetic instructions for synthesizing the protein or disordered enzymes that normally catabolize it.

Idiopathic dystonia, often inherited as an autosomal dominant, is a disabling, chronic movement disorder of unknown etiology. It has no known neuropathology; no abnormal protein has yet been found within the brain associated with it, and no test other than history and physical examination can confirm the diagnosis. Unlike the dystonia of dopamine deficiency, it is usually painless. Symptoms are often bizarre and psychiatric diagnoses are almost always considered early in its course. It can involve the entire body or it can be restricted to one side, one body segment, or can even be focal. It is typically unassociated with psychic symptoms, except in one focal form, Meig's syndrome, that has been said to be associated with depression. The medications that relieve it are the belladonna compounds in very high doses and benzodiazepines. The mechanism through which they provide a measure of symptomatic relief is unknown.

Another autosomal dominant condition of unknown pathophysiology is Tourette's syndrome's motor tics and vocalizations. This is often associated with OCD, another genetic disorder of unknown cause. Within living memory both were regarded as unrelated purely psychological disorders. Their association, genetic determination, and response to medication has changed this perception. Tourette's syndrome can be ameliorated by dopamine receptor blockers and OCD can be ameliorated by SSRIs in high doses. Some basal ganglia abnormalities have been described in Tourette's syndrome but these are not sufficiently characteristic that a neuropathologist could make the diagnosis without clinical data. Functional imaging in OCD has revealed hyperactivity in the orbitofrontal and cingulate cortex that diminishes with successful treatment. The response of

OCD to SSRIs, a new class of drugs that was introduced to treat depression, has raised the possibility that the pathogenesis of OCD and depression is similar. There is considerable comorbidity, though these disorders are clinically distinct.

According to the catecholamine hypothesis, depression is the result of insufficient serotonin and/or norepinephrine and mania is the result of too much of one or both of them. This theory explains many facts. In general, drugs that potentiate the concentration of norepinephrine and serotonin at their receptors relieve depression and precipitate mania, but the theory must be incorrect or at least a gross oversimplification as it does not explain all the facts, e.g., the effect of antidepressant medications on catecholamines is established within minutes but their clinical effect does not begin for weeks. No theory has fully replaced the catecholamine hyothesis. Bipolar affective disorder is probably transmitted as an autosomal dominant and other forms of depression may have genetic determinants. Though mood disorders affect the hyothalamic-pituitary axis and the immune system and can be triggered by physical illnesses and emotional stress, no confirmatory test has provided a reliable diagnosis.

REFERENCES

Aarsland, D. E. Tandberg, J. P. Larsen, J. L. Cummings. Frequency of dementia in Parkinson disease. *Arch Neurol* 53:538, 1996.

Ader, R. Developmental psychoneuroimmunology. *Dev Psychobiol* 16:251, 1983.

Agid, Y. Levodopa: is toxicity a myth. *Neurology* 50:858, 1998.

Akiskal, H., W. T. McKinney. Depressive disorders: toward a unified hypothesis. *Science* 182:20, 1973.

Altrocchi, P. U., L. S. Fomo. Spontaneous oral-facial dyskinesia: neuropathology of a case. *Neurology* 33:802, 1983.

American College of Physicians. The dexamethasone suppression test for the detection, diagnosis, and management of depression. *Ann Intern Med* 100:307, 1984.

Amsterdam, J., A. Winokur, S. Coroff, J. Conn. The dexamethasone suppression test in outpatients with primary affective disorder and healthy control subjects. *Am J Psychiatry*. 139:287, 1982.

Aquilonius, S. M., R. Sjorstrom. Cholinergic and dopaminergic mechanisms in Huntington's chorea. *Life Sci* 10:405, 1971.

Armon, C., C. Shin, P. Miller, et al. Reversible parkinsonism and cognitive impairment with chronic valproate use. *Neurology* 47:626, 1996.

Baer L., S. L. Rauch, H. T. Ballantine Jr., et al. Cingulotomy for intractable obsessive-compulsive disorder. *Arch Gen Psychiatry* 52:384, 1995.

Bauer, M., P. Whybrow. Thyroid hormone and the CNS in affective illness. *Integr Psychiatry* 6:75, 1988.

Beck, A. T., C. H. Ward, M. Mandelson, J. Mock, J. K. Erbaugh. An inventory for measuring depression. *Arch Gen Psychiatry*. 4:561, 1961.

Bejjani, B. P., P. Damier, I. Arnulf, et al. Transient acute depression induced by high-frequency deep-brain stimulation. *N Engl J Med* 340:1476, 1999.

Berrettini, W., T. Ferraro, L. Goldin, et al. Chromsome 18 DNA markers and manic depressive illness. *Proc Natl Acad Sci USA* 91:5918, 1994.

Berthier M. L., J. Kulisevsky, A. Gironell, et al. Obsessive-compulsive disorder associated with brain lesions: clinical phenomenology, cognitive function, and anatomic correlates. *Neurology* 47:353, 1996.

Bhatia, K. P., N. P. Quinn, C. D. Marsden. Clinical features and natural history of axial predominant, adult onset, primary dystonia. *J Neurol Neursurg Psychiatry* 63:788, 1997.

Bihari, K., J. L. Hill, D. L. Murphy Obsessive-compulsive characteristics in patients with idiopathic spasmodic torticollis. *Psychiatry Res* 42:267, 1992.

Bihari, K., T. A. Pigott, J. L. Hill, D. L. Murphy. Blepharospasm and obsessive-compulsive disorder. *J Nerv Ment Dis* 180:130, 1992.

Blazer, D. G., R. C. Kessler, K. A. McGonagle, et al. The prevalence and distribution of major depression in a national community sample: the National Comorbidity Survey. *Am J Psychiatry* 151:979, 1994.

Bracco, F., R. Malesani, M. Saladini, et al. Protein redistribution diet and antiparkinsonian response to levodopa. *Eur Neurol* 31:68, 1991.

Brody, A., M. Barsom, R. Bota, et al. Prefrontal-subcortical and limbic circuit mediation of major depressive disorder. *Semi Clin Neuropsychiatry* 6:102, 2001.

Brown, F., P. H. Redfern. Studies on the mechanism of action of amantadine. *Br J Pharmacol* 58:561, 1976.

Buchsbaum, M., F. Goodwin, D. Murphy, G. Borge. AET in affective disorders. *Am J Psychiatry* 128:19, 1971.

Burke, R. E., S. Fahn, J. Jankovic, et al. Tardive dystonia: late onset and persistent dystonia caused by antipsychotic drugs. *Neurology* 32:1335, 1982.

Caine, E. D., K. A. Bamfor, R. B. Schiffer, et al. A controlled neuropsychological comparison of Hungtington's disease and multiple sclerosis. *Arch Neurol* 43:249, 1986.

Caligiuri, M. P., J. P. Lacro, E. Rockwell, et al. Incidence and risk factors for severe tardive dyskinesia in older patients. *Br J Psychiatry* 171:148, 1997.

Carroll, B., M. Feinberg, J. Greden, et al. A specific test for the diagnosis of melancholia: standardization, validation, and clinical utility. *Arch Gen Psychiatry* 3 8: 15, 1981.

Cath, D. C., P. Spinhoven, B. J. van de Wetering, et al. The relationship between types and severity of repetitive behaviors in Gilles de la Tourette's disorder and obsessive-compulsive disorder. *J* Clin Psychiatry 61:505, 2000.

Coyle, J. T., S. H. Synder. Antiparkinsonian drugs: inhibition of dopamine uptake in the corpus striatum as a possible mechanism of action. *Science* 166:899, 1969.

Crowther, R. A., S. E. Daniel, M. Goedert. Characterisation of isolated alpha-synuclein filaments from substantia nigra of Parkinson's disease brain. *Neurosci Lett* 292:128, 2000.

Cui, X., G. Vaillant. Antecedents and consequences of negative life events in adulthood. *Am J Psychiatry* 153:21, 1996.

Cui, X., G. Vaillant. Does depression generate negative life events? *J Nerv Ment Dis* 185:145, 1997.

Cummings, J. L. Behavioral complications of drug treatment of Parkinson's disease. *J Am Geriatr Soc* 39(7):708, 1991.

Cummings, J. L. Depression and Parkinson's disease: a review. *Am J Psychiatry* 149(4): 443, 1992.

Cunningham-Owens, D. G. Dystonia-A potential psychiatric pitfall. *Br J Psychiatry* 156: 620, 1990.

Davies, S. W., M. Turmaine, B. A. Cozens, et al. From neuronal inclusions to neurodegeneration: neuropathological investigation of a transgenic mouse model of Huntington's disease. *Philos Trans R Soc Lond Biol Sci* 354(1386):981, 1999.

Detera-Wadleigh, S., J. Badner, J. Goldin, et al. Affected-sib-pair analyses revel support of prior evidence for a susceptibility locus for bipolar disorder, on 21Q. *Am J Hum Genet* 58:1279, 1996.

Dewan, M., V. Anand. Evaluating the tolerability of the newer antidepressants. *J Nerv Ment Dis* 187:96, 1999.

Dewan, M. J., V. S. Anand. Evaluating the tolerability of the newer antidepressants. *J Nerv Ment Dis* 187:96, 1999.

Diamond, S. G., C. H. Markham, M. M. Hoehn, F. H. McDowell, M. D. Muenter Multicenter study of Parkinson mortality with early versus later dopa treatment. *Ann Neurol* 22:8, 1987.

Doraiswamy, M. W. Martin, A. Metz, et al. Psychosis in Parkinson's disease: diagnosis and treatment. *Biol Psychiatry* 19:835, 1995.

Drevets, W., K. Gadde, K. Ranga, et al. Neuroimaging studies of mood disorders. In: *Neurobiology of Mental Illness*, D. Charney, E. Nestler, B. Bunney, eds. Oxford University Press, New York, 1999, pp. 394–418.

Drevets, W. C. Prefrontal cortical-amygdalar metabolism in major depression. *Ann NY Acad Sci* 877:614, 1999.

Dubovsky, S. *Mind Body Deceptions*, Norton, New York, 1997 pp. 309–339.

Duda, J. E., V. M. Lee, J. Q. Trojanowski Neuropathology of synuclein aggregates. *J Neurosci Res* 61:121, 2000.

Duman, R. S., G. R. Heninger, E. J. Nestler. A molecular and cellular theory of depression. *Arch Gen Psychiatry* 54:597, 1997.

Durif, F., M. Vidailhet, A. M. Bonnet. Levodopa-induced dyskinesias are improved by fluoxetine. *Neurology* 45:1855, 1995.

Emery, O., T. Oxman. Update on the dementia spectrum of depression. *Am J Psychiatry* 149:305, 1992.

Eriksson, T,. A. K. Granerus, A. Linde, A. Carlsson. 'On-off' phenomenon in Parkinson's disease: relationship between dopa and other large neutral amino acids in plasma. *Neurology* 38:1245, 1988.

Fabbrini, G., M. M. Mouradian, J. L. Juncos, et al. Motor fluctuations in Parkinson's disease: central pathophysiological mechanisms, Part I. *Ann Neurol* 24:366,1988.

Fahn, S. The varied clinical expressions of dystonia. *Neurol Clin* 2:554, 1984.

Fahn, S., Is levodopa toxic? *Neurology* 47 (Suppl 3):S184, 1996.

Fahn, S. Concept and classification of dystonias. In: *Advances in Neurology*, S. Fahn, D. Marsden, D., eds. Calnevol. Dystonia, Raven Press, New York 1988 pp. 1–9.

Fahn, S., Generalized dystonia: concepts and treatment. *Clin Neuropharmacol* 9: (Suppl 2) S37, 1986.

Fahn, S., D. Williams, A. Reches, et al. Hysterical dystonia, a rare disorder: report of five documented cases. *Neurology* 33 (Suppl 2)161, 1983.

Fassbender, K., R. Schmidt, R. Mossner, et al. Mood disorders and dysfunction of the hypothalamic-pituitary-adrenal axis in multiple sclerosis. *Arch Neurol* 55:66, 1998.

Fenton, W. S., C. R. Blyler, R. J. Wyatt, T. H. McGlashan. Prevalence of spontaneous dyskinesia in schizophrenic and non-schizophrenic psychiatric patients. *Br J Psychiatry* 171:265, 1997.

Fogarty, S. J., D. R. Hemsley. Depression and the accessibility of memories. *Br J Psychiatry*. 142:232, 1983.

Freeman, J. M., A. M. Aron, J. E. Collard, et al. The emotional correlates of Syderham's chorea. *Pediatrics* 35:42, 1965.

Frucht, S., J. D. Rogers, P. E. Greene, et al. Falling asleep at the wheel: motor vehicle mishaps in persons taking pramipexole and ropinirole. *Neurology* 52:1908, 1999.

Gibb, W. R., A. J. Lees, C. D. Marsden, Pathological report of four patients presenting with cranial dystonias. *Mov Disord* 3:211, 1988.

Glazer, W. M., H. Morgenstern, N. Schooler, et al. Predictors of improvement in tardive dyskinesia following discontinuation of neuroleptic medication. *Br J Psych* 157:585, 1990.

Goedert, M. Filamentous nerve cell inclusions in neurodegenerative diseases: tauopathies and alpha-synucleinopathies. *Philos Trans R Soc Lond B Biol Sci* 354(1386):1101, 1999.

Goedert, M., M. G. Spillantini. Tau mutations in frontotemporal dementia FTDP-17 and their relevance for Alzheimer's disease. *Biochim Biophys Acta* 502:110, 2000.

Goedert, M., M. G. Spillantini, S. W. Davies, Filamentous nerve cell inclusions in neurodegenerative diseases, *Curr Opin Neurobiol* 8:619, 1998.

Gold, P., O. Chrousos, C. Kellner, et al. Psychiatric implications of basic and clinical studies with corticotropin-releasing factor. *Amer J Psychiatry* 141:619, 1984.

Golden, W. E., R. C. Lavender, W. S. Metzer. Acute postoperative confusion and hallucinations in Parkinson disease. *Ann Intern Med* 111:218, 1989.

Goldenberg, J., M. B. Ferraz, A. S. Fonseca, et al. Sydenham chorea: clinical and laboratory findings. Analysis of 187 cases. *Rev Paul Med* 110:152, 1992.

Gomez-Tortosa, E., A. O. Ingraham, M. C. Irizarry, et al. Dementia with Lewy bodies. *J Am Geriatr Soc* 46:1449, 1998.

Gorell, J. M., C. C. Johnson, B. A. Rybicki, et al. The risk of Parkinson's disease with exposure to pesticides, farming, well water, and rural living. *Neurology* 50:1346, 1998.

Grafman, J., L. G. Cohen, M. Hallett. Is focal hand dystonia associated with psychopathology? *Mov Disord* 6:29, 1991.

Granacher, R. P. Differential diagnosis of tardive dyskinesia: an overview. *Am J Psychiatry* 138:1288, 1981.

Greene, P., H., Shale, S. Fahn. Experience with high dosages of anticholinergic and other drugs in the treatment of torsion dystonias. In: *Advances in Neurology*, S. Fahn, D. Marsden, D., eds. Calnevol. Dystonia, Raven Press, New York, 1988, pp. 547–556.

Gurling, H., C. Smyth, G. Kalsi, et al. Linkage findings in bipolar disorder. *Nat Gen* 10: 8, 1995.

Guttman, M., P. Seeman, G. P. Reynolds, et al. Dopamine D2 receptor density remains constant in treated Parkinson's disease. *Ann Neurol* 19:487, 1986.

Hamilton, M. Standardized assessment and recording of depressive symptoms. *Psychiatr Neurol Neuroclin* 72:201, 1969.

Harkness, K., S. Monroe, A. Simons, et al. The generation of life events in recurrent and non-recurrent depression. *Psychol Med* 1:135, 1999.

Harris, E. C., B. Barraclough. Excess mortality of mental disorder. *Br J Psychiatry* 173: 11, 1998.

Hawkins, D. R., J. Mendels. Sleep disturbance in depressive syndromes. *Am J Psychiatry* 123:682, 1966.

Heathfield, KWC. Huntington's chorea: investigation into the prevalence of this disease in the area covered by the North East Metropolitan Regional Hospital Board. *Brain* 90:203, 1967.

Heim, C., D. Neuport, S. Heit, et al. Pituitary-adrenal and autonomic responses to stress in women after sexual and physical abuse in childhood. *JAMA* 284:592, 2000.

Herbert, T, S. Cohen. Depression and immunity. *Psychol Bull* 1133:472, 1993.

Hill, D. Depression: disease, reaction or posture. *Am J Psychiatry* 125:445, 1968.

Hirschfeld, R. Efficacy of SSRIs and newer antidepressants in severe depression: comparison with TCAs. *J Clin Psychiatry* 60:326, 1999.

Horton, S., R. DeRubeis, M. Evans, et al. Cognitive therapy and pharmacotherapy for depression. *Arch Gen Psychiatry* 49:774, 1992.

Holsboer, E. The rationale for cortiotropin releasing hormone receptor antagonists to treat depression and anxiety. *J Psychiatr Res* 33:181, 1999.

Hornykiewicz, O. The mechanisms of action of L-dopa in Parkinson's disease. *Life Sci* 15:1249, 1974.

Huntington's Disease Collaborative Research Group. A novel gene containing a trinucleotide repeat that is expanded and unstable on Huntington's disease chromosomes *Cell* 72:971, 1993.

Hyde, T. M., D. R. Weinberger. Tourette's syndrome. *JAMA* 273(6):496, 1995a.

Hyde, T. M., D. R. Weinberger. Tourette's syndrome: a model neuropsychiatric disorder. *JAMA* 273(6): 498, 1995a.

Insel, T. R., N. H. Kalin, L. B. Guttmacher, et al. The dexamethasone suppression test in patients with obsessive compulsive disorder. *Psychiatry Res* 6:153, 1982.

Jacobs, S. *Pathologic Grief.* American Psychiatric Press, Washington, DC, 1993.

Jahanshahi, M., C. D. Marsden. Depression in torticollis: a controlled study. *Psychol Med* 18:925, 1988.

Jahanshahi, M., C. D. Marsden. Psychological functioning before and after treatment of torticollis with botulinum toxin. *J Neurol Neurosurg Psychiatry* 55:229, 1992.

Jellinger, K. A. Post mortem studies in Parkinson's disease—is it possible to determine brain areas for specific symptoms? *J Neural Transm Suppl* 56:1, 1999.

Jenike, M. A., L., Baer H. T., Ballantine et al. Cingulotomy for refractory obsessive-compulsive disorder. *Arch Gen Psychiatry* 48:548, 1991.

Johnson, W. G. Late-onset neurodegenerative diseases—the role of protein insolubility. *J Anat* 196(Pt 4):609, 2000.

Juncos, J. L., G. Fabbrini, M. M. Mouradian, et al. Dietary influences on the antiparkinsonian response to levodopa. *Arch Neurol* 44:1003, 1987.

Junque, C., M. Alegret, F. A. Nobbe, et al. Cognitive and behavioral changes after unilateral posterventral pallidotomy: relations with lesional data from MRI. *Mov Disord* 14:780, 1999.

Kanazawa, I., M. Murata, M. Kimura. Roles of dopamine and its receptors in generation of choreic movements. *Adv Neurol* 60:107, 1993.

Kang, U. J., R. E. Burke, S. Fahn. Natural history and treatment of tardive dystonia. *Move Dis* 1: 193, 1986.

Kane, J. M., M. Woerner, M. Borenstein, et al. Integrating incidence and prevalence of tardive dyskinesia. *Psychopharmacol Bull* 22(1):254, 1986.

Karstaedt, P. J., J. H. Pincus. Protein redistribution diet remains effective in patients with fluctuating parkinsonism. *Arch Neurol* 49:149, 1992.

Kayton, W. Major depression and chronic medical illness. *Sem Clin Neuropsychiatry* 3: 81, 1998.

Kaufman, J. P. Plotsky, C. Nemeroff, et al. Effects of early adverse experience on brain structure and function. *Biol Psychiatry* 48:778, 2000.

Klatka, L., E. Louis, R. Schiffer. Psychiatric features of Lewy Body dementia, *Neurology* 47:1148, 1996.

Klawans, H. L., Jr. A pharmacologic analysis of Huntington's chorea. *Eur Neurol* 4:148, 1970.

Klawans, H. L., R. Rubovits. Central cholinergic-anticholinergic antagonism in Huntington's chorea. *Neurology* 2 2:107, 1972.

Klawans, H. L., A. Barr. Prevalence of spontaneous lingual-facial-buccal dyskinesia in the elderly. *Neurology* 32:558, 1982.

Klonoff, H., C., Clark, J. Oger, et al. Neuropsychological performance in patients with mild multiple sclerosis. *J Nerv Ment Dis* 179(3):127, 1990.

Kohn, Y., J. Zislin, O. Agid, et al. Increased prevalence of negative life events in subtypes of major depressive disorder. *Comp Psychiatry* 42:57, 2001.

Koller, W. C. Edentulous orodyskinesia. *Ann Neurol* 13:97, 1983.

Kornhuber, J., G. Quack, W. Danysz, et al. Therapeutic brain concentration of the NMDA receptor antagonist amantadine. *Neuropharmacology* 34:713, 1995.

Koshino, Y., Y. Wada, K. Isaki, K. Kurat. A long-term outcome of tardive dyskinesia in patients on antipsychotic medication. *Clin Neuropharmacol* 14(6):537, 1991.

Kupfer, D. J., M. E. Thase. The use of the sleep laboratory in the diagnosis of affective disorder. *Psychiatr Clin N Am* 5:3, 1983.

Kurlan, R., E., Caine, A. Rubin, et al. Cerebrospinal fluid correlates of depression in Huntington's disease. *Arch Neurol* 45:881, 1988.

Kurlan, R. Tourette's syndrome and 'PANDAS": will the relation bear out? *Neurology* 50:1530, 1998.

Kuzis, G., L., Sabe, Tiberti, et al. Cognitive functions in major depression and Parkinson. *Arch Neurol* 54:982, 1997.

Lachenmayer, L. Parkinson's disease and the ability to drive. *J Neurol* 247 (suppl 4): 28, 2000.

Landau, W. M. Clinical neuromythology IX. Pyramid sale in the bucket shop: DATATOP bottoms out. *Neurology* 40:1337, 1990.

Lauterbach, E. C., J. G., Jackson, S. T. Price, et al. Clinical, motor, and biological correlates of depressive disorders after focal subcortical lesions. *J Neuropsychiatry Clin Neurosci* 9:259, 1997.

Leenders, K. L., A. J., Palmer, N. Quinn, et al Brain dopamine metabolism in patients with Parkinson's disease measured with positron emission tomography. *J Neurol Neurosurg Psychiatry* 49:853, 1986a.

Leenders, K. I., W. H. Poewe, A. J., Palmer, et al Inhibition of L-[18F]fluorodopa uptake into human brain by amino acids demonstrated by positron emission tomography. *Ann Neurol* 20:258, 1986b.

Lees, A. J. The concept of bradyphrenia *Rev Neurologique* 150:823, 1994.

Lewy, A. J., T. A. Wehr, F. K. Goodwin, et al. Manic-depressive patients may be sensitive to light. *Lancet* 1: 383, 1982a.

Lewy, A. J., T. A. Wehr, N. E. Rosenthal et al. Melatonin secretion as a neurobiological marker and effects of light in humans. *Psychopharmacol Bull* 18:127, 1982b.

Lieberman, A., Managing the neuropsychiatric symptoms of Parkinson's disease. *Neurology* 50(Suppl 6):S33–S38, 1998.

Loosen, P. T., A. J. Prange. Serum thyrotropin response to thyrotropin releasing hormone in psychiatric patients: a review. *Am J Psychiatry* 139:405, 1982.

Lorenzo, A., M. Yuan, Z. Zhang, et al. Amyloid beta interacts with the amyloid precursor protein: a potential toxic mechanism in Alzheimer's disease. *Nat Neurosci* 3:460, 2000.

Lupien, S. J., M. deLeon, S. DeSanti, et al. Cortisol levels during human aging predict hippocampal atrophy and memory deficits. *Nat Neurosci* 1:69, 1998.

Maes, M., H. Meltzer. The serotonin hypothesis of major depression. In *Psychopharmacology*, F. Bloom, D. Kupfer, eds. Raven Press, New York, 1995, pp. 933–944.

Mann, J., V. Arango. Abnormalities of brain structure and function in mood disorders. In: *Neurobiology of Mental Illness*, D. Charney, E. Nestler, B. Bunney, eds. Oxford University Press, New York, 1999, pp. 385

Maras, K., L. Clark, W. Katon, et al. Mixed anxiety-depression. *DSM IV Sourcebook*. American Psychiatric Press, Washington, DC, 1996, p. 623.

Marder, K., M. X. Tang, L. Cote, et al. The frequency and associated risk factors for dementia in patients with Parkinson's disease. *Arch Neurol* 52:695, 1995.

Maricle, R. A., J. G. Nutt, R. J. Valentine, J. H. Carter. Dose-response relationship of levodopa with mood and anxiety in fluctuating Parkinson's disease: a double-blind, placebo-controlled study. *Neurology* 45:1757, 1995.

Martinez-Martin, P., C. F. O'Brien. Extending levodopa action: COMT inhibition. *Neurology* 50(Suppl 6):S27–S32, 1998.

McAllister, T. Pseudodementia. *Am J Psychiatry* 140:52:81, 1983.

McEwen, B. S. Protective and damaging effects of stress mediators, *N Engl J Med* 338: 171, 1998.

McHugh, P. R. The neuropsychiatry of basal ganglia disorders: a triadic syndrome and its explanation. *Neuropsychiatry, Neuropsychol Behav Neuro* 2:239–247, 1989.

McKinney, W. Stress adaption and affective disorders. *Sem Clin Neuropsychiatry* 6:1, 2001.

Melamed, E., F. Hefti, R. J. Wurtman. Nonaminergic striatal neurons convert exogenous L-dopa to dopamine in parkinsonism. *Ann Neurol* 8:558, 1980.

Mena, I., G. C. Cotzias. Protein intake and treatment of Parkinson's disease with levodopa. *N Engl J Med* 292:181, 1975.

Mendez, M. F. Huntington's disease: update and review of neuropsychiatric aspects. *Intl J Psychiatry Med* 24:189, 1994.

Menza, M. A., L. I. Golbe, R. A. Cody, et al. Dopamine-related personality traits in Parkinson's disease. *Neurology* 43:505, 1993. a

Menza, M. A., D. E. Robertson-Hoffman, A. S. Bonapace. Parkinson's disease and anxiety: comorbidity with depression. *Biol Psychiatry* 34:465, 1993. b

Menza M. A., M. H. Mark, D. J. Burn, D. J. Brooks. Personality correlates of [^{18}F] dopa striatal uptake: results of positron-emission tomography in Parkinson's disease. *J Neuropsychiatry Clini Neurosci* 7:176, 1995.

Merikangas, K., D. Kupfer. Mood disorders: genetic aspects. In: *Comprehensive Textbook of Psychiatry/VI,* H. Kaplan, B. Sadock, eds. Williams and Wilkins, Baltimore, 1995, pp. 1102.

Metman, L. V., P. Del Dotto, P. van den Munckhof Fang, et al. Amantadine as treatment for dyskinesias and motor fluctuations in Parkinson's disease. *Neurology* 50:1323, 1998.

Metman, C. V, P. Del Dotto K. LePoole, et al. Amantadine for levodopa-induced dyskinesias: a 1-year follow-up study. *Arch Neurol* 56:1383, 1999.

Miller, H., P. Delgado, R. Salomon, et al. Effects of alpha-mehyl-paratyrosine (AMPT) in drug-free depressed patients. *Neuropsychopharmacol* 14:151, 1996.

Mouradian, M. M., I. J. Heuser, F. Baronti, et al. Pathogenesis of dyskinesias in Parkinson's disease *Ann Neurol* 25:523, 1989.

Mouradian, M. M., J. L. Juncos, G. Fabbrini, et al. Motor fluctuations in Parkinson's disease: central pathophysiological mechanisms, Part II. *Ann Neurol* 24:372, 1988.

Murphy, D. L., H. K. Brodie, F. K. Goodwin. Regular induction of hypomania by L-DOPA in "bipolar" manic-depressive patients. *Nature* 229:135, 1971.

Nauseida, P. A., L. A. Bieliauskas, L. D. Bacon, et al. Chronic dopaminergic sensitivity after Sydenbam's chorea. *Neurology* 33:750, 1983.

Nemeroff, C., Evans, D. Correlation between the dexamethasone suppression test in depressed patients and clinical response. *Am J Psychiatry* 141:247, 1984.

Nemeroff, C., L. DeVane, B. Pollock. Newer antidepressants and the cytochrome P450 system, *Am J Psychiatry* 153:311, 1996.

Newport, J., C. Nemeroff. Childhood trauma: psychiatric and neurobiologic consequences. *Sem Clin Neuropsychiatry* (7), 2002.

Nibuya, M., S. Morinobu, R. Duman. Regulation of BDNF and trkB mRNA in rat brain by chronic electroconvulsive seizure and antidepressant drug treatment. *J Neurosci* 15: 7539, 1995.

Nibuya, M., E. J. Nestler, R. S. Duman. Chronic antidepressant administration increases the expression of cAMP response element binding protein (CREB) in rat hippocampus. *J Neurosci* 16: 2365, 1996.

Nofzinger, E., M. Keshavan, D. Buysse, et al. The neurobiology of sleep in relation to mental Illness. In: *Neurobiology of Mental Illness,* D. Charney, E. Nestler, B. Bunney, eds. Oxford University Press, New York, 1999, pp. 915.

Nyenhuis, D. L., S. M. Rao, J. M. Zajecka, et al. Mood disturbance versus other symptoms of depression in multiple sclerosis. *JINS* 1:291, 1995.

Nutt, J. G., W. R. Woodward, J. P. Hammerstad, et al The "on-off" phenomenon in Parkinson's disease. relation to levodopa absorption and transport.*N Engl J Med* 23;310, 1984.

Olanow, C. W., P. Jenner, D. Brooks. Dopamine agonists and neuroprotection in Parkinson's disease. *Ann Neurol* 44(3 Suppl 1):S167, 1998.

Olanow, R. Watts, W. Koller. An algorithm (decision tree) for the management of Parkinson's disease (2001): treatment guidelines. *Neurology* 56 (Suppl 5): S1, 2001.

Olanow, T. Freeman, J. Kordowes. Transplantation of embryonic dopamine neurons for severe Parkinson's disease. *N Engl J Med* 345:146, 2001.

Parkinsonism Study Group. Pramipexole vs levodopa as initial treatment for parkinson disease: a randomized controlled trial. *JAMA* 284:1931, 2000.

Phillips, K., M. Dwight, S. McElroy, Efficacy and safety of fluvoxamine in body dysmorphic disorder. *J Clin Psychiatry* 59:165, 1998.

Piggott, T., S. Seay. A review of the efficacy of selective serotonin reuptake inhibitors in obsessive-compulsive disorder. *J Clin Psychiatry* 60:101, 1999.

Pincus, J. H., K. M. Barry. Dietary method for reducing fluctuations in Parkinson's disease. *Yale J Biol Med* 60:133, 1987.

Pincus, J. H., Plasma levels of amino acids correlate with motor fluctuations in parkinsonism. *Arch Neurol* 44:1006, 1987.

Pincus, J. H., Influence of dietary protein on motor fluctuations in Parkinson's disease. *Arch Neurol* 44:270, 1987.

Pincus, J. H., Protein redistribution diet restores motor function in patients with dopa-resistant "off" periods. *Neurology* 38:481, 1988.

Post, R., S. R,. Weiss. A speculative model of affective illness cyclicity based on patterns of drug tolerance observed in amygdala-kindled seizures. *Mol Neurobiol.* 13:33, 1996.

Price, D. L., S. S. Sisadia, D. R. Borchelt. Genetic neurodegenerative diseases: the human illness and transgenic models. *Science* 282:1079, 1998.

Rabey, J. M., T. A. Treves, M. Y. Neufeld, et al. Low-dose clozapine in the treatment of levodopa-induced mental disturbances in Parkinsion's disease. *Neurology* 45:432, 1995.

Rajput, A. H., R. Pahwa, P. Pahwa, A. Rajput. Prognostic significance of the onset mode in parkinsonism. *Neurology* 3:829, 1993.

Ramasubbu, R. A. Ravindran, Y. Lapierre. Serotonin and dopamine in obsessive-compulsive disorder. *Phamacopsychiatry* 33:236, 2000.

Rapoport, J. L., D. H. Ryland, M. Kriete. Drug treatment of canine acral lick: an animal model of obsessive-compulsive disorder. *Arch Gen Psychiatry* 49:517, 1992.

Rascol, O., D. J. Brooks, A. D. Korczyn, et al. A five-year study of the incidence of dyskinesia in patients with early Parkinson's disease who were treated with ropinirole or levodopa. 056 Study Group. *N Engl J Med* 342:1484, 2000.

Rauch, S. Neuroimaging research and the neruobilogy of obsessive compulsive disorder. *Biol Psychiatry* 47:174, 2000.

Riley, D., A. E. Lang. Practical application of a low-protein diet for Parkinson's disease. *Neurology* 38:1026, 1988.

Robinson, D., H. Wu, R. A. Munne, et al. Reduced caudate nucleus volume in obsessive-compulsive disorder. *Arch Gen Psychiatry* 52:393, 1995.

Romeo, E., et al. Effects of antidepressant treatment on neuroactive steroids in major depression. *Am J Psychiatry* 155:910, 1998.

Sacher, E. J. Corticosteroids in depressive illness. *Arch Gen Psychiatry* 17:544, 1967.

Sadovnick, A. D., R. A. Remick, J. Allen, et al. Depression and multiple sclerosis. *Neurology* 46:628–632, 1996.

Sage, J. I., M. H. Mark. Basic mechanisms of motor fluctuations. *Neurology* 44(Suppl 6):S10, 1994.

Sage, H., S. Trooskin, P. K. Sonsalla, et al. Experience with continuous enteral levodopa infusions in the treatment of 9 patients with advanced Parkinson's disease. *Neurology* 39(Suppl 2): 60, 1989.

Sage, J. I., M. H. Mark. Basic mechanisms of motor fluctuations. *Neurology* 44 (7Suppl 6):S10, 1994.

Sajatovic, M., L. Ramirez. Clozapine therapy in patients with neurologic illness. *Intl J Psychiatry Med* 25(4):331, 1995.

Sakamoto, K., S. Nakadaira, K. Kamo, et al. A longitudinal follow-up study of seasonal affective disorder. *Am J Psychiatry* 152:862, 1995.

Sanchez-Ramos, J. R., R. Ortoll, G. W. Paulson. Visual hallucinations associated with Parkinson disease. *Arch Neurol* 53:1265, 1996.

Sanders, A., S. Detera-Woodleigh, E. Gershon. Molecular genetics of mood disorders, In: *Neurobiology of Mental Illness* D. Charney, E. Nestler, B. Bunney, eds. Oxford University Press, New York, 1999.

Schatzberg, A., J. Schildkraut. Recent studies on norepinephrine systems in mood disorders. In: *Psychopharmacology*, F. Bloom, D. Kupfer, eds. Raven Press, New York, 1995.

Schatzberg, A., C. Nemeroff. *APPI Textbook of Psychopharmacology*, 2nd Edition, American Psychiatic Press, Washington DC, 1998.

Schwartz, P., C. Brown, T. Wher, et al. Winter seasonal affective disorder. *Am J Psychiatry* 153:1028, 1996.

Seeman, P., H. H. Van Tol. Dopamine receptor pharmacology. *Trends Pharmacol Sci* 15: 264, 1994.

Shannon, K. M., R. D. Penn, J. S. Croin, et. al. Stereotactic pallidotomy for the treatment of Parkinson's disease. Efficacy and adverse effects at 6 months in 26 patients. *Neurology* 50:434, 1998.

Sharma, A. K., M. Behari, G. K. Ahuja. Clinical and demographic features of Meige's syndrome. *J Assoc Phy Ind.* 44:645, 1996.

Smith, K., G. Fairburn, P. Cowen. Relapse of depression after rapid depletion of tryptophan, *Lancet* 349:915–919, 1997.

Sobin, C., H. A. Sackeim. Psychomotor symptoms of depression. *Am J Psychiatry* 154:4, 1997.

Spars, J. E., R. Grener. Does the dexametbasone suppression test distinguish dementia from depression? *Am J Psychiatry.* 139:238, 1982.

Spencer, S. E., G. F. Wooten. Altered pharmacokinetics of L-dopa metabolism in rat striatum deprived of dopaminergic innervation. *Neurology* 34:1105, 1984.

Spillantini, M. G., M. Goedert. The alpha-synucleinopathies: Parkinson's disease, dementia with Lewy bodies, and multiple system atrophy. *Ann NY Acad Sci* 920: 16, 2000.

Stahl, S. Selecting an antidepressant by using mechanism of action to enhance efficacy and avoid side effects. *J Clin Psychiatry* 59(Suppl 18):23, 1998.

Stein, M. B., I. J. Heuser, J. L. Juncos, et al. Anxiety disorders in patients with Parkinson's disease. *Am J Psychiatry* 147 2:217, 1990.

Stern, Y., K. Marder, M. X. Tang, R. Mayeux. Antecedent clinical features associated with dementia in Parkinson's disease. *Neurology* 43:1690, 1993.

Stevens, J. R. Motor disorders in schizophrenia. *Engl. J Med* 290: 110, 1974.

Stibe, C. M., A. J. Lees, P. A. Kempster, et al Subcutaneous apomorphine in parkinsonian on-off oscillations.*Lancet* 1(8582):403, 1988.

Stine, O., J. Xu, R. Koskela, et al. Evidence for linkage of bipolar disorder to chromosome 18 with parent-of-origin effect. *Am J Hum Genet* 57:1384, 1995.

Straub, R., T. Lehner, Y. Luo, et al. A possible vulnerability locus for bipolar affective disorder on chromosome 21q22.3. *Nat Genet* 8:291, 1994.

Sullivan, P., M. Neale, K. Kendler. Genetic epidemiology of major depression. *Am J Psychiatry* 157:1552, 2000.

Swedo, S. E., H. L. Leonard, B. B. Mittleman, et al. Identification of children with pediatric autoimmune neuropsychiatric disorders associated with streptococcal infections by a marker associated with Rheumatic fever. *Am J Psychiatry* 154:110, 1997.

Tandberg, E., J. P. Larsen, D. Aarsland, K. Laake, J. L. Cummings, Risk factors for depression in Parkinson's disease, *Arch Neurol* 54:625, 1997.

Tandberg, E., J. P. Larsen, D. Aarsland, J. L. Cummings. The occurrence of Parkinson's disease. *Arch Neurol* 53:175, 1996.

Taylor, A. E., J. A. Saint-Cyr, A. E. Lang. Procedural learning and neostriatal dysfunction in man. *Brain* 111:941, 1988.

Taylor, A. E. Lang, J. A. Saint-Cyr, et al. Cognitive processes in idiopathic dystonia treated with high dose anticholinergic therapy: implications for treatment strategies *Clin Neuropharm* 14:62, 1991.

Thase, M. Treatment resistant depression. In: *Psychopharmacology*, F. Bloom, D. Kupfer, eds. Raven Press, New York, 1995, pp. 1081.

Tolosa, E. S. Clinical features of Meige's disease (idiopathic orofacial dystonia): a report of 17 cases. *Arch Neurol* 38:147, 1981.

Trendelenburg, U. Mechanisms of supersensitivity and subsensitivity to sympathomimetic amines. *Pharmacol Rev* 18:629, 1966.

Tsui, J. K., S. Ross, K. Poulin, et al. The effect of dietary protein on the efficacy of L-dopa: a double-blind study. *Neurology* 39:549, 1989.

Tucker, G., P. Roy-Byrne, J. Fann, et al. Psychiatry for the neurologist. *Continuum* 3: 3, 1997.

Vandel, P., B. Bonin, E. Leveque, et al. Tricyclic antidepressant-induced extrapyramidal side effects. *Eur Neuropsychopharmacol* 7:207, 1997.

van Harten, P. N., H. W. Hoek, G. E. Matroos, et al. Intermittent neuroleptic treatment risk for tardive dyskinesia: Curacao Extrapyramidal Syndromes Study III. *Am J Psychiatry* 155(4):565, 1998.

Verhagen Metman, L. P. Del Dotto, P. van der Munckhof, et al. Amantadine as treatment for dyskinesias and motor fluctuations in Parkinson's disease. *Neurology* 50:1323, 1998.

Webb, M., P. T. Trzepacz. Huntington's disease: correlations of mental status with chorea. *Biol Psychiatry* 22:751, 1987.

Weiner, W. J. Is levodopa toxic? *Arch Neurol* 57:408, 2000.

Weissman, M. M. Cross-national epidemiology of obsessive-compulsive disorder. The Cross National Collaborative Group *J Clin Psychiatry* 55(Suppl 3):5, 1994.

Wenzel, T. P. Schnider, A. Wimmer, et al. Psychiatric comorbidity in patients with spasmodic torticollis. *J Psychosom Res* 44: 687, 1998.

Whatmore, C. B., R. M. Ellis. Further neuropbysiologic aspects of depressed states. *Arch Gen Psychiatry* 6:243, 1962.

Whybrow, P, J. Mendels. Towards a biology of depression. *Am J Psychiatry* 125:1491, 1969.

Whybrow, P., H. S. Akiskal, W. T. McKinney, *Mood Disorders*, Plenum Press, New York, 1984.

Wiggins, S., P. Whyte, M. Huggins, et al. The psychological consequences of predictive testing for Huntington's disease. *N Engl J Med* 327:1401, 1992.

Wilner, P. Dopaminergic mechanisms in depression and mania. In: *Psychopharmacology*, F. Bloom, D. Kupfer, eds. Raven Press, New York, 1995, pp. 921.

Wooten, G. F., Progress in understanding the pathophysiology of treatment-related fluctuations in Parkinson's disease. *Ann Neurol* 24:363, 1988.

Wulsin, L., G. Vaillant, V. Wells. A systematic review of the mortality of depression. *Psychosom Med* 61:6, 1999.

Zeman, W. Pathology of the torsion dystonias (dystonia musculorum deformans). *Neurology* 20:79, 1970.

Zung, W.K.K. A self-rating depression scale. *Arch Gen Psychiatry* 12:63, 1965.

Chapter Six

DISTINGUISHING NEUROLOGICAL FROM PSYCHIATRIC SYMPTOMS

In the eighteenth century, hysteria was called the English malady, and although the various paralytic symptoms and unusual seizures were attributed to a disorder of the emotions, the biologic mechanism that mediated these symptoms remained a mystery. A prominent explanation relied on the newly discovered laws of gravity; it was postulated that the mind caused paralysis of an arm by an "action at a distance," just as gravity made the apple fall (Vieth, 1965). While medicine has made great advances since the eighteenth century and our understanding of the central nervous system has increased enormously, we still have trouble delineating the exact mechanisms that cause patients to express their emotional discomfort through somatic symptoms. We still do not have laboratory measures that will tell us whether an isolated neurological symptom is caused by a neurological illness or by a specific emotional state. Consequently, much of what is included in this chapter is the clinical lore that has been gathered since the time of Charcot about how to differentiate neurological disorders from psychiatric disorders.

COMMONALITY OF NEUROLOGICAL AND PSYCHIATRIC SYMPTOMS

A solitary neurological symptom can have many different etiologies. Headache can be caused by anxiety, brain tumor, or head trauma and it is the task of the physician to determine the correct etiology so that appropriate treatment can be instituted. Although there is some help from imaging and other laboratory measures, the correct etiology (or the inability to stipulate an etiology) is most often determined by the clinical examination and history. As both neurological and psychiatric disorders are related to dysfunctions of the central nervous system, it is not surprising that the major differential diagnosis is between a neurological or a psychiatric disorder.

Many general medicine patients suffer from symptoms that are frequently associated with disorders of the central nervous system. Kroenke and Mangelsdorf (1989) reviewed the records of 1000 patients followed in an internal medicine clinic. They found that 567 patients had at least one or more of the following possible neurological symptoms: fatigue, dizziness, headache, back pain, insomnia, numbness, impotence, as well as such general symptoms as chest pain, abdominal pain, dyspnea, edema, weight loss, cough, and constipation. A biologic etiology to the symptoms could be found in only 16 percent of the patients; 10 percent of the symptoms were classified as psychological (the authors speculated that many of the unexplained symptoms were probably related to undiagnosed psychiatric disorders). Several studies of neurology inpatient admissions show that 30%–40% of the patients were given a psychiatric diagnosis of somatization disorder, whereas no specific diagnosis could be made for approximately 30 percent (Creed et al., 1990; Ewald et al., 1994). Carson et al. (2000a) found that 47 percent of 300 referrals to a neurology outpatient clinic met the criteria for a DSM-IV anxiety or depressive disorder. Raja (1995) found that 13.5 percent of acute psychiatric inpatients and 68.1 percent of chronic psychiatric inpatients also had a neurological disorder. This enormous overlap of psychiatric and neurological disorders and unexplained symptoms is precisely what makes the clinical practice of psychiatry and neurology so intriguing.

Such symptoms as dizziness, headache, syncope, and motor problems, are common to all patients, and particularly to psychiatric and neurological patients (Kroenke et al., 1992, 1993; Kapoor et al., 1995; Crimlisk et al., 2000). In the past when no cause for such symptoms could be found, they were labeled hysterical. With the advent of DSM-III the term hysteria was banished from the psychiatric nomenclature. In large part this was caused by the fact that hysteria had taken on so many different and sometime pejorative meanings, e.g., a paralysis; a personality disorder, or simply a gross disorganized emotional discharge. Somatic symptoms of psychological origin are now grouped under the heading Somatoform Disorders, which in DSM-IV encompasses somatization, conversion, pain, and hypochondriasis disorders; all of these disorders manifest the presence of physical symptoms that suggest a general medical condition but are not fully explained by that condition. The somatoform disorders are descriptive categories and may represent one end of a continuum that ends with somatization disorder and begins with somatic symptoms related to anxiety and depressive disorders (Katon et al., 1991).

PANIC DISORDER/HYPERVENTILATION AS A CAUSE OF COMMON NEUROLOGICAL SYMPTOMS

The symptoms of a panic attack, e.g., palpitations, sweating, trembling, shortness of breath, feeling of choking, chest pain, nausea and abdominal distress, dizziness, feelings of unreality, fear of losing control or dying, paresthesias, and chills or hot flashes (DSM-IV, 1994) are very real and frightening to the patient. They are the symptoms that patients most frequently consult their physicians about. The question for the physician is do the symptoms represent a panic attack or do they represent some other medical disorder. Although panic attacks may occur spontaneously, most are precipitated by feelings of anxiety. There is a significant comorbidity between panic attacks and hyperventilation (Cowley and Roy-Byrne, 1989; Spinhoven et al., 1993). Hyperventilation usually causes any or all of the following symptoms: faintness, visual disturbances, inability to concentrate, nausea, vertigo, headache, a feeling of fullness in the head, chest, and/or epigastrium, breathlessness, palpitations, feelings of being hot or cold, sweating, paresthesias, and occasionally vomiting. The overlap of symptoms with a panic attack is evident.

Hyperventilation causes symptoms by lowering of PCO2. Two deep breaths produced by yawning or sighing are enough to alter PCO2 significantly and produce symptoms. The lowered PCO2 reduces cerebral blood flow, since there is a direct relation between PCO2 and the caliber of the cerebral blood vessels. In 240 seconds of over breathing, cerebral blood flow can be reduced by 40 percent (Plum and Posner, 1972) Thus, hyperventilation leads to cerebral hypoxia, and this is the cause of the EEG slowing so often seen with over breathing (Gotoh et al., 1965). Prolonged hyperventilation can produce respiratory alkalosis, which in turn can induce tetany. Hyperventilation can also precipitate panic attacks (Katon et al., 1991).

Hyperventilation is a routine part of electroencephalographic testing and may induce an epileptiform abnormality. Of course, it can also induce actual seizures. Hyperventilation in response to anxiety may, in fact, be a major mechanism by which emotional tension induces seizures in susceptible individuals (Mattson et al., 1970). The cerebral hypoxia caused by hyperventilation, when compounded by a mild degree of orthostatic hypotension and/or the Valsalva maneuver, may reduce cerebral blood flow to the degree that the patient faints or has a tonic convulsion. (Many young boys have learned to induce syncope by over breathing and then performing the Valsalva maneuver for the amusement of their friends.)

Hyperventilation can also cause nonspecific ST- and T-wave changes in the electrocardiogram (EKG) (Christensen, 1946), and many hyperventilation syndrome patients showing such EKG changes have been admitted to coronary care units. Hyperventilation is often associated with air swallowing and this, in turn, can lead to epigastric distress and gastrointestinal symptoms.

Hyperventilation is a very common response to anxiety. One might almost call it a universal human reaction to anxiety, since it is part of the autonomic response to threatening situations. The somatic symptoms it causes may often cause the unwary physician to pursue an extensive workup that only serves to convince the patient that something is physically wrong with him thus reinforcing the medical symptoms and ignoring source of the anxiety (Katon, 1991).

SOMATIZATION DISORDER

Somatization disorder as defined in DSM-IV encompasses what has been previously referred to as hysteria or Briquet's syndrome. DSM-IV defines somatization disorder as a polysymptomatic disorder that begins before the age of 30 and is characterized by at least four pain symptoms, two gastrointestinal symptoms, one sexual symptom, and one pseudoneurological symptom. This is a descriptive category and one can see why when a patient complains of many somatic symptoms he or she is likely to be assigned to the category of somatization rather than medical disorder (Katon et al., 2001). Historically, the DSM-IV criteria were developed from the work of Perley and Guze (1962). In their view the term hysteria had been used indiscriminately for any psychosomatic symptom so they developed an elaborate and restrictive system for diagnosing hysteria (Briquet's syndrome). They assigned the diagnosis if patients had *(1)* a dramatic or complicated medical history before age 35; *(2)* a minimum of 15 symptoms distributed in at least 9 of 10 organ systems and *(3)* no medical diagnosis that adequately explained their symptoms. For 6 to 8 years, Perley and Guze studied 39 patients who met these criteria. Ninety percent of the sample did not develop any other illness that might explain their symptoms, however, the patients tended to develop additional psychosomatic complaints over the years. Using the criteria first designed by Perley and Guze and incorporated in DSM-IV a patient so labeled usually has an almost lifelong history of unexplained somatic symptoms.

UNEXPLAINED SYMPTOMS

If a patient presents with a long history of many different unexplained somatic symptoms it should make one think immediately of a possible somatization disorder or other psychiatric illness. A large number of unexplained medical symptoms often indicates that the patient has an anxiety or depressive disorder (Katon et al., 1991d; 2001). In a recent study, Carson et al. (2000b) found a high incidence of unexplained symptoms and psychiatric disorders in neurology practice. They studied 300 new referrals to a neurology clinic at a general hospital who had unexplained symptoms. A third of these cases remained unexplained. Seventy percent of the patients in the unexplained group had anxiety and depressive disorders, whereas only 32 percent of the explained group had a psychiatric diagnosis. Interestingly this high number of unexplained symptoms is not much different than is found in other medical specialty clinics. Kroenke and Mangelsdorf (1989) reported that only 16 percent of unexplained physical complaints were explained by organic disease. Hamilton et al. (1996) found that the symptoms of 53 percent of the patients referred to a GI clinic and 32 percent of patients referred to a cardiac clinic could not be medically explained. They also noted that the patients with the unexplained symptoms complained of significantly more symptoms, more bodily pain, and had more impaired social functioning.

The most pressing clinical concern is whether the unexplained symptoms represent the early symptoms of a neurological disorder or instead are manifestations of a psychiatric disorder presenting with neurological symptoms. In a classic study Slater and Glithro (1965) attempted to answer this question. They evaluated 85 patients 10 years after they had received a diagnosis of hysteria (most would now be called conversion reactions). Of the 85 patients with a chart diagnosis of hysteria, they found on follow-up that 22 had later been given a diagnosis of an organic disease that could have explained their initial symptoms. At the time they were diagnosed as hysterical, 19 of the patients had medical illnesses that could have explained their symptoms. Eight had died of their medical conditions. Well over half the total population of "hysterics" had medical problems that were mistaken as psychogenic or that had precipitated emotional reactions. Four patients had committed suicide. In 1998 Crimlisk and colleagues published a paper entitled "Slater Revisited" reporting how they replicated, with modern research techniques, Slater and Glithro's study of 1965. Their paper highlights the changes in research methods that have taken place since 1965. They used clearly defined diagnostic criteria, standardized interviews, and rating scales to examine 73 consecutively admitted patients to a neurological clinic, who had unexplained motor symptoms. The patients were followed up 5–7 years after the initial visit. During the follow-up period only three subjects developed a neurological disorder that fully or partly explained their initial symptoms.

Seventy-five percent of the patients met criteria for a psychiatric diagnosis (45% had personality disorders) and in 75 percent of those given a psychiatric diagnosis; this diagnosis coincided with the onset of the motor symptoms. Only one patient developed a new psychiatric diagnosis that could have explained his symptoms. Interestingly, 42 percent had a history of neurological disorder. This study indicates that conversion disorder is not a benign condition in the sense that at follow-up only 33 percent of the patients were employed full time and the symptoms in 52 percent had remained the same or got worse.

CONVERSION DISORDERS

Conversion disorders can be a symptom of somatization disorder or a separate diagnostic category. Conversion disorders are defined in DSM-IV as unexplained symptoms or deficits affecting voluntary motor or sensory functions that suggest a medical or neurological condition. The differentiation of conversion symptoms from neurological disease is a frequent problem in neurological, medical, and psychiatric practice. Some physicians believe that somatization disorder, as defined above, can be differentiated from isolated conversion symptoms. In our experience, conversion symptoms rarely occur in isolation. When doctors label unexplained findings "conversion reaction" in patients lacking a history of hypochondriasis, the diagnosis is almost invariably wrong. We have found that two criteria are extremely important in making a positive diagnosis of conversion reaction. Unless both are present, the diagnosis should be held in doubt. These criteria are *(1)* that no medical diagnosis explains the patient's symptoms and *(2)* that there is, even in children, a past history of psychosomatic illness (conversion reaction, hypochondriasis, or psychophysiological reaction).

The two classic hallmarks of conversion, *la belle indifference* and secondary gain, have been, in our experience, more often misleading than helpful in establishing the diagnosis. Apparent indifference is often a sign of stoicism, and stoical hospitalized patients are often seriously ill. Indifference to illness is also a common sign of brain damage. This is the basis of the therapeutic effect of frontal lobotomy. Many patients with progressive brain disease are mercifully indifferent to their desperate condition. Conversely, individuals may be excited and anxious when they develop conversion symptoms, though it is true that some do manifest *la belle indifference*.

The secondary gain, which refers to the reward for the patient who develops a conversion disorder, is often difficult to identify. Sometimes it is no more than staying in the hospital and avoiding contact with the family, sometimes it may be a subtler or even a fantasized gain. On the other hand, patients who have been injured in automobile or industrial accidents often have lawsuits or compensation claims pending, which are justified but could be mistaken as secondary gain by their physicians. No one has ever put forward criteria by which one can distinguish a legitimate from a secondary gain. The secondary gain may be quite clear after the diagnosis is established, but as a diagnostic aid, it is almost useless.

It has been our experience that most medical doctors consider a patient a conversion disorder or somatizer either when the physician cannot imagine an organic lesion that could explain his symptoms or when a patient with a well-known history of psychosomatic illnesses presents himself for examination. Mistakes are made because the physician's diagnostic acumen is naturally a function of his previous experience and knowledge. No one can know everything, and peculiar facets of difficult cases of organic disease that even the most experienced clinician has not encountered before can appear. Also, the tendency toward psychosomatic illness does not confer immortality, and even hysterics can become sick and die.

Certain neurological diseases seem to predispose to conversion symptoms. Patients whose judgment is impaired by mental retardation, intoxications or other encephalopathies, encephalitis, brain tumor, or multiple sclerosis may elaborate symptoms and signs or exaggerate real symptoms. This may draw attention away from the real disease, sometimes with tragic results.

It may be worthwhile to consider some of the classic conversion symptoms that mimic neurological conditions. In doing so, we wish to demonstrate that symptoms that cannot be easily ascribed to an organic lesion constitute an inadequate basis for the diagnosis of conversion disorder or somatization. The diagnosis requires such symptoms in *addition* to a past history of psychosomatic illnesses. Both are necessary; neither is sufficient.

SPECIFIC CLASSICAL CONVERSION SYMPTOMS

Inability to swallow or feeling a lump in the throat is typical of globus hystericus. Normal results on direct examination of the nasal and oral pharynx and on barium swallow studies are sufficient to rule out most lesions that could cause similar symptoms. On the other hand, both myasthenia gravis and polymyositis may begin with intermittent weakness of the swallowing mechanism. At the time of examination, the patient may be able to swallow normally and appear to be well. Similarly, pseudobulbar palsy, which interferes with swallowing, may wax and wane in severity. When unassociated with other signs of neurological disease, such symptoms have been mistakenly considered hysterical.

Hemisensory loss conversions usually involve half the entire body from head to foot and from the extremities to the midline. A pinprick felt normally on one side of the linea alba will not be felt on the other side. Sensory splitting at the exact midline and a shift of perception toward the side of normal sensation are considered by many to be hard-and-fast signs of conversion; organic hemisensory deficits typically appear 1 or 2 cm toward the anesthetic side of the midline. This is because segmental sensory nerve fibers extend 1 or 2 cm across the midline from the "good" side into the anesthetic side. It is also said that the diagnosis of conversion can be confirmed by testing vibratory sensation. A tuning fork placed on the skull or the sternum to one side of midline should be felt by neurological patients no matter which side the hemisensory loss is on because the oscillations of the tuning fork are transmitted throughout the entire bone. If the patient claims not to feel vibrations on one side, he may have a conversion reaction.

Unfortunately, these sensory signs of conversion are rather unreliable because some patients with neurological diseases report what they think their examiner wishes them to report, claiming that a change in sensation occurs at the midline when in fact this may not be so. In addition, it is conceivable that minorities of patients have a physiologically variant pattern of sensory function in which the anesthesia caused by a brain lesion does, in fact, change at the midline or to the "wrong" side of midline. Patients who report absent vibratory sensation on the anesthesia side of their skull or sternum may in fact feel the vibrations less on that side but report to the examiner that they feel nothing to be consistent. Whatever the reason, it is an empirical fact that patients with lesions that are undeniably organic—strokes, tumors, demyelinating diseases—have reported sensory changes with characteristics that are considered typical of hysteria.

Hemiplegic conversions may be diagnosed in the following way: placing his hands underneath the patient's paralyzed heel while the patient is supine, the examiner asks the patient to raise his normal leg. The examiner can thereby determine whether or not the patient is able to move his paralyzed leg because the normal response while raising one leg is to push down with the other. If the patient pushes down with his paralyzed leg, the factitious nature of his paralysis should be clear. By reversing the process and asking the patient to raise the paralyzed leg, the examiner can determine whether or not the patient is actually trying to lift it. If the patient does not push down with the good leg, the examiner can conclude that he is not trying to raise the paralyzed leg. This test is only useful in complete hemiplegia, however, and will not help in distinguishing conversion hemiparesis (which is more common than conversion hemiplegia) from true hemiparesis. The presence of unilateral changes in deep tendon reflexes, spasticity, and Babinski's reflex provides objective evidence indicating neurological disease. The absence of these alterations, however, cannot establish the diagnosis of conversion.

Paralysis of the extraocular muscles, those of the face and the tongue, does not occur in conversion syndromes. Paresis of the cervical muscles, with difficulty elevating the head from a pillow or with drooping of the head onto the chest, is extremely rare. Paralysis of the trunk muscles is also rare. Thus, conversion paralysis or paresis usually involves one or more of the extremities. Conversion weakness of the leg is more frequently encountered than weakness of the arm.

If the patient is ambulatory, the manner in which he moves, dresses, undresses, and mounts an examining table should be noted; for conversion paralysis is, mainly one of paralysis of movement as opposed to paralysis of individual muscles. The patient with a conversion disorder may complain that all movements at one joint are affected, but the object of the examination is to note the distribution of the paralysis as well as the muscles affected and to determine if the patient can still use the affected muscles to perform movements that he does not realize entail their use. On examination, patients with conversion weakness may manifest simultaneous and equal contraction of agonistic and antagonistic muscles, hence "paralysis."

Hemiparesis conversion is characteristically associated with *give-way* weakness. This means discontinuous resistance during direct muscle testing. Give-way weakness is absolutely diagnostic of factitious weakness, but occasionally a patient will exaggerate mild, real weakness in order to convince the examiner that he is, in fact, weak. In such cases, the patient may feel that the examiner is going to miss the diagnosis and so he helps out. Reflex abnormalities, when present, can rule out conversion but the absence of such abnormalities will not establish the diagnosis.

Astasia-abasia, or gait conversion, can sometimes be extremely difficult to differentiate from movement disorders. Physicians routinely place emphasis on the following indications that a disordered gait is hysterical. The patient walks well, never falls, and does not injure himself when unaware that be is being observed. The conversions involving gait are usually recognized by their bizarre character and dissimilarity from any disorder of gait produced by organic disease. In hemiplegia, the affected leg may ostentatiously be dragged along the ground and not circumducted as in organic hemiplegia. When severe, astasia-abasia will be manifested by the patient's attempting to fall as opposed to the organic patient who does his best to support himself. Some patients, who walk with great difficulty, cling to walls and furniture and to the examiners, but manifest normal power and coordination while lying in bed. This kind of inconsistency suggests conversion.

Because almost all movement disorders are worsened by anxiety, it is not wise to accept without reservation reports by nurses and other staff to the effect that the patient is able to walk nearly normally when unaware that he is being observed. If the patient is made nervous by an examiner or a large group of physicians on rounds, his organic movement disorder may worsen. Sometimes patients with gait conversion problems do, in fact, fall and may accidentally hurt themselves, so a history of falls with occasional scrapes and bruises does not necessarily rule out conversion.

Inconsistency of gait disturbance is common in gait apraxias caused by frontal or subcortical cerebral disease. Peculiarities of affect in such patients and an absence of Babinski's sign may lead to an incorrect diagnosis of conversion. Formal mental status and examination (see Chapter 7) are helpful in identifying these patients.

Gait disorders, whether neurological or psychosomatic, often cause a certain amount of confusion among clinicians. It is not at all uncommon to find a minority of competent neurologists who will consider a patient to have either a neurological or a conversion disorder even in the face of an opposite majority view. Fortunately, there are relatively safe and fairly objective tests for conversion in such cases: amytal infusion and hypnosis. Amytal is infused intravenously at a rate of 50 mg per minute until nystagmus develops. This usually requires 250 to 500 mg. As soon as nystagmus develops, the infusion is stopped and the patient is asked to perform the motor task that he previously found difficult. If there is a substantial improvement in his movement disorder, the diagnosis of conversion is supported. If the gait deteriorates, the diagnosis of neurological disorder is supported. This test is often extremely helpful but it can be misinterpreted. When anxiety is responsible for marked worsening of an organic movement disorder, amytal or hypnosis might improve the gait by relieving anxiety. When neither deterioration nor improvement is clear-cut, no inference about the etiology of the gait disturbance can be made.

It is probably fair to say that conversion dystonia and/or chorea virtually never occur together. It is possible to be misled by certain inconsistencies. Some inconsistencies are diagnostic. For example, in torticollis the examiner may not be able to straighten the patient's head even by exerting maximal effort, and yet the patient can often straighten his own head by merely touching his forehead with an index finger on the side toward which his head is tilted. This inconsistency is unexplained but is characteristic of dystonia of neurologic origin.

Conversion rigidity increases in proportion to the effort made by the examiner to move the rigid extremity. This feature may also be present in the frontal lobe disorders that lead to gegenhalten or counterpull. *Gegenhalten* is a semivoluntary resistance the patient increasingly offers to passive movement of his limbs. When the examiner attempts to extend the patient's elbow, for example, the patient will resist, and his resistance will increase as the elbow is extended further. Forced grasping may be seen in response to tactile stimulation of the patient's palm by the examiner's fingers. In frontal lobe disorders, when the examiner attempts to extend the patient's fingers while disengaging his own from the patient's grip, he may encounter counterpull.

Visual conversion symptoms include monocular diplopia, triplopia, tunnel vision, and blindness. Though monocular diplopia is, in most cases, caused by hysteria, ocular pathology such as dislocated lenses, cataracts, and parietal lobe lesions can give rise to it (Kestenbaum, 1961). A patient under our care who was recovering from well-documented disseminated leukoencephalitis reported triplopia, which is theoretically a physiological impossibility.

A test for the psychological etiology of tunnel vision depends upon the fact that the normal visual field expands in a cone of vision as the distance from the target to the patient is increased. If the patient's field is identical at 2 meters from his eye to what it is at 1 meter from his eye, the inconsistency suggests conversion. Patients who are blind on the basis of neurological disease usually have no pupillary response to light. In disease of the parietal or occipital lobes, however, cortical blindness may be present and pupillary reflexes will remain normal. If a patient with blindness and normal pupillary responses is presented with a slowly rotating, vertically striped drum and develops involuntary tracking movements (optokinetic nystagmus), his blindness can be considered factitious.

There are two tests that can be useful in detecting unilateral conversion blindness. The patient is asked to read a line of alternating black and red letters while a red glass is held over the good eye. In conversion blindness the patient will be able to see the red letters with the bad eye and will read all the letters in the line. Also, a distorting prism can be placed over the good eye and the patient will still be able to perform tasks requiring intact vision. Convergence spasms and blepharospasm (the result of spasm of the orbicularis oculi) can be manifestations of hysterical disturbances of ocular movements. Defects in the lateral and vertical planes of gaze caused by hysteria may induce a kind of coarse nystagmus. However, blepharospasm can also be a sign of Meigs' syndrome, which is an involuntary, dystonic syndrome.

Conversion deafness can be easily demonstrated as the patient can be awakened from sleep by sound. A conversion reduction of hearing (as opposed to deafness) is difficult to distinguish from neurologic disease of the ears. Variability of responses to audiological tests can reflect a neurological syndrome as well as conversion.

Conversion amnesias, fugue states, and pseudodementia can also confound the diagnostician. In earlier chapters, particularly the one on epilepsy, we noted that transient fluctuations in consciousness can be associated with epileptic conditions and we suggested some guidelines for diagnosis. Conversion states may partially mimic epilepsy and can be confused with it. It is a rare psychiatrist or neurologist who has not been confronted with a patient who says he does not know who he is, or who he was at a particular time, or where he came from. Such conversions states are most often seen in times of stress, for instance, among soldiers during war or in individuals indicted for crimes. Characteristics that help to distinguish those with psychogenic amnesia or dissociative states from neurological patients include the following: *(1)* the patient is able to carry out complex functions during the time of amnesia. *(2)* Memory loss and shift of identity to another person or personality are usually sudden. *(3)* The patient's behavior is fairly well integrated in that he usually has enough money to get where he is going and takes time to eat and drink. *(4)* Loss of memory usually affects a specific section of life or ability, that is, arithmetic or recognition of certain relatives. *(5)* The transition to a normal state is abrupt. *(6)* There is no history or physical evidence of neurological disease.

Berrington et al. (1956) studied 37 cases of fugue state and noted that depression was a frequent concomitant. Interestingly, they noted that a high proportion of the patients had a history of head injury and they speculated that this may have precipitated the fugue state. They also observed that the patients were usually completely unaware of their identity and past life and acted as if they were in a dream. During the episodes, they could travel and seemed able to answer complex questions adequately. They had either partial or complete amnesia for the episodes.

Even if all of the characteristics of amnesia indicate hysteria, unless the past history indicates a psychosomatic tendency, the diagnosis should be held in doubt. Other conditions can cause dissociative states. For example, the clearly neurological syndrome of "transient global amnesia," described by Fisher and Adams (1964) and by Shuttleworth and Morris (1966) is marked by periods of confusion and disorientation to time and place that usually last a few hours. Patients in these two studies had no recollection of events and described themselves as feeling strange during the episodes of amnesia. In contrast to the above-mentioned syndromes of conversion amnesia and fugue state, which usually affect individuals in the third or fourth decade, these patients were all middle-aged or elderly and had a history of hypertension or atherosclerosis. Although they did not lose their identity, they could not retain new information during these episodes. It was hypothesized that the episodes resulted from transient ischemia, specifically ischemia of the mamillary–hippocampal complex.

Complaints of pain are rarely completely fabricated. Patients who are considered to have conversion pain syndromes complain of severe pain, but they exhibit none of the physical reactions that are expected to be associated with pain of neurologic origin and thus present an appearance that belies their allegations of intense suffering. The diagnosis of conversion pain may also be applied to patients who are unusually distressed and agitated by their pain. Some of the most common syndromes ascribed to conversion are headaches, low back pain, abdominal pain, and atypical facial pain.

Many physicians regard low back pain as a common syndrome that can result from conversion and are likely to consider the diagnosis if there is no muscle spasm, if the neurological examination is normal, and if the standard imaging studies are completely normal. Complete investigation might also include pelvic and rectal examinations, prostatic specific antigen and alkaline phosphatase determinations. An incomplete and negative evaluation can erroneously seem to support the diagnosis of conversion.

Undiagnosable abdominal pain is very often the result of aerophagia. The statements of many physicians who attend pain clinics to the effect that two-thirds to three-quarters of their patients have solely psychosomatic pain (i.e., conversion pain) are incorrect in our opinion. Though patients often exaggerate real pain, it is the responsibility of the physician to determine its underlying physical cause.

A variety of diagnostic myths that have been perpetuated with regard to pain: *(1) Continuing pain in patients who have under*gone multiple *surgical procedures for pain without improvement means the pain is either psychogenic or an undesirable side effect of surgery.* Often, all this may imply is that the original cause of the pain has not been diagnosed or treated. *(2) A high intake of analgesics, or patient requests for analgesics more often than every 4 hours, indicate that the patient's problem is not pain but addiction.* In fact, some analgesics have a duration of action that is shorter than 4 hours (Goodman and Gilman, 1990). *(3) A lawsuit combined with an undiagnosable pain problem is a sure sign of psychogenic origin. If the lawsuit is settled, the pain will disappear.* The data supporting this common assumption are lacking. Lawsuits are often justified and patients who settle them do not necessarily improve. *(4) Negative findings on repeated tests and bizarre complaints with no physical findings indicate that pain is psychogenic.* Some of the most bizarre head pains we have seen were easily diagnosed as temporomandibular joint (TMJ) syndromes. True, repeated CT scans, EEGS, and standard neurological examinations revealed no abnormalities in these cases, but few physicians routinely palpate the head and face in headache patients. This is essential for the diagnosis of TMJ syndrome. Pain syndromes in other parts of the body may also be diagnosed when the correct test is done.

What we have tried to demonstrate with these examples is that the diagnosis of conversion can be made in error, even when the conversion symptoms are classic. It is exceedingly rare for conversion disorder to be the first manifestation of a psychosomatic tendency. Conversion disorders are nearly always preceded, even in children, by other symptoms deemed psychosomatic, many of which have not resulted in a visit to the physician. Stomachaches and headaches with frequent school absences, sleep disturbances, and/or school phobia, precede conversion hysteria by many months or years in childhood. Unless there is a history of previous psychosomatic disorders, the diagnosis of conversion reaction should remain open to question. On the other hand, psychosomatic illness is so common that its presence should not blind the physician to the possibility of organic disease. Of patients referred for neurological examination, 25 to 40 percent have psychosomatic complaints (Creed et al., 1990; Ewald et al., 1994; Carson et al., 2000a).

HEADACHE

The cause of headache is one of the most critical determinations a physician has to make. Headache can be a symptom of anxiety or depression, or it can be the first symptom of a brain tumor. It is not our purpose to provide a comprehensive discussion of the disorder. For this the reader is referred to two excellent books, Diamond and Dalessio (1999) and Dalessio's and Silbersteins 7th edition of *Wolf's Headache* (2001). We will merely put forward the criteria from the patient's history that are helpful in distinguishing headaches of psychogenic origin from those of neurological origin.

In general, if the headache is the worst headache ever experienced by the patient, if it is a new headache, or if it is associated with neurological signs, the physician must assume that an acute or life-threatening situation may be present, and a full investigation should be promptly initiated. A CT scan should be the first test. If normal, lumbar puncture should follow. When this rule is followed, the diagnoses of subarachnoid hemorrhage, meningitis, encephalitis, or brain tumor will not often be missed. For teaching purposes, we advise medical students to fully investigate any headache that is "the worst, the first, or cursed (by neurologic abnormalities)." Conversely, any headache that has been present for more than a year, almost irrespective of its character, is rarely caused by a serious or progressive disorder. In general, one should not think of headaches as related to emotional factors if the headache is of sudden onset, is caused by reclining or by coughing, awakens the patient from sleep, or is unilateral, even if the headache persists for days, weeks, or months.

Headaches that are dull, generalized, and constant for many days in a row usually have no neurological cause. Patients with such headaches often describe, a pressure feeling, which is what they mean by headache. These patients almost always have an impressive past history of psychosomatic illness and are depressed. The unremitting character of the headaches and the patient's complaints of their severity usually contrast with the fact that the patient is nonetheless able to work. Analgesics, tranquilizers, and sedatives are usually ineffective, but antidepressants often help.

Tension headaches are presumably caused by muscle tension. When the muscles in the posterior neck and temples are under the stress of continuous contraction, they begin to ache just as muscles anywhere in the body do when they have been overworked. The pain reflection is then generalized over the head. Such headaches are dull and steady, though occasionally, a sustained muscle contraction headache is followed by a typical vascular (throbbing) headache, and the two types of headache will coexist in an attack. Tension headaches can usually be attributed to emotional tension, but sometimes cervical pathology, such as osteoarthritis or cervical disc disease, will cause headache by inducing cervical muscle contraction. Tension headaches characteristically occur in the morning on awakening or in the late afternoon. These headaches are worse during the work week and tend to be relieved on weekends and vacations. Aspirin and sedatives generally relieve them. Tension headaches are often mistakenly attributed to essential hypertension or chronic sinusitis. With few exceptions, by the time a patient comes to a doctor for treatment of tension headaches, they will have occurred for months or years. Surprisingly, this holds true for children too. Some patients who initially deny the long-standing nature of their headaches, when pressed will admit that they have had similar headaches in the past, though perhaps not so severe or so frequent. This point is important in distinguishing ordinary tension headaches from those caused by brain tumors.

Headaches are caused by brain tumors in two ways, by increased intracranial pressure and by traction of the mass on pain-sensitive structures within the skull. No single headache is characteristic of a brain tumor. Headaches caused by increased intracranial pressure are, if anything, remarkable for being nonspecific. They are mild, dull, aching, and very often bifrontal or bioccipital. They may be present in the morning on awakening, last a few hours, and get better as the day goes on. They may not occur every day. Thus, they may be quite similar to tension headaches. Headaches produced by increased intracranial pressure, however, are characteristically of recent onset, usually starting within a few weeks before the patient presents himself to the physician. We have found this to be the single most important feature in distinguishing tension headaches from those caused by increased intracranial pressure. When brain tumors cause headaches by traction on pain-sensitive structures, headaches are often lateralized or localized to one spot. Intraventricular tumors can cause headaches that may be exacerbated or relieved by changes in position. Thus, when a patient complains of a headache that is brought on by putting his head in one position and relieved by changing the position, a mechanical factor must be considered and the possibility of a tumor investigated thoroughly. It is an ominous sign if sitting up relieves headache.

Prostrating headaches that are relieved by sleep, whether they are throbbing and severe, lasting several hours, and associated with nausea, and/or vomiting, are usually migraines. This is so whether or not they are unilateral or preceded by typical ischemic symptoms such as flashing lights, scintillating scotomata, or sensory or motor symptoms. Migraine headaches begin with throbbing but when the pain reaches its zenith, the throbbing may stop. Usually the pain at this time is unbearable, prostrating, and associated with vomiting and photophobia. Curiously, at this point in the headache, many patients can fall asleep and if so, they awaken improved. The incidence of migraine is the same in men and women but, presumably because of hormonal factors, headaches are usually more severe and more frequent in women. Patients with such prostrating headaches usually have a positive family history of migraine, which suggests a hereditary basis. There is a familial comorbidity with anxiety and affective disorders (Merikangas et al., 1993). Migraine headaches occur primarily in the young, often begin in the first decade, and seldom develop for the first time after the age of 30 years. They may tend to occur more frequently on weekends and vacations and are not satisfactorily relieved by ordinary nonnarcotic, orally administered analgesics. Recent studies have found a strong association between migraine, with or without aura, and affective and panic disorders. Panic disorder was also comorbid with other types of severe headache; in most cases the headache syndrome preceded the onset of panic disorder but not in all cases (Breslau et al., 2001). There also is a significant comorbidity with epilepsy and stroke (Breslau and Rasmussen, 2001). Propranolol, and other beta-blockers, have become useful therapeutic agents in reducing the frequency and severity of attacks. Antidepressants, particularly the tricyclics and the SSRIs, are also widely used with good effect but one wonders if tension headaches associated with depression have been labeled migraine in many patients who have experienced relief from antidepressants (Merikangas, 1991). Ergot-containing preparations are usually effective in stopping such headaches if they are taken in the early stages of the attack, especially during the prodromal period. Sumatriptin and other serotonin agonists have become the first line of therapy for severe attacks.

The syndrome of TMJ is often misdiagnosed as atypical migraine, atypical facial pain, or a functional disorder. The steady, nonthrobbing nature of the pain at onset distinguishes it from migraine. The occasional very brief headache, lasting minutes, and the lack of throbbing at the onset are other helpful features in distinguishing the TMJ syndrome from migraine. The tenderness of affected muscles distinguishes it from atypical facial pain, and the unilateral nature of the pain should distinguish it from functional or ordinary tension headache.

Temporomandibular joint pain is characterized by a usually unilateral, deep-seated pain in the side of the face, which is brought on or exacerbated by movements of the lower jaw. The pain is related to spasm of the muscles that operate the jaw, mainly the temporalis and pterygoid, but rarely, the masseter. It is not usually associated with actual pathology of the temporomandibular joint so that the name is somewhat misleading. Radiographs of the joint are abnormal in only a minority of cases. The syndrome is most common in young women. The characteristics of the pain are typical of muscle pain: it is steady (nonthrobbing) and severe. After several hours, throbbing can develop. The pain is exacerbated by quick stretches of the muscle, as in mouth opening, and by more prolonged use of the painful muscle, as in chewing. It may follow visits to the dentist when prolonged opening of the mouth and stretching of the muscles of mastication are necessary. Bruxism, yawning, shouting, singing, fellatio, and direct trauma to the jaw are other contributing factors.

Given that TMJ pain is usually experienced around or behind the eye and along the temple, palpation of the temporalis muscle and attempted lateral movement of the jaw against pressure usually produces pain. When the body of the pterygoid muscle is palpated from inside the mouth, there is great tenderness, and the muscle itself often feels tense and hypertrophied to the examiner. Direct pressure over the temporomandibular joint may also cause pain. Many patients with this syndrome are depressed, do not sleep well, and awaken feeling tired. They often grind their teeth during sleep and yawn a great deal in the morning after awakening. Thus, bruxism and yawning seem to be the major contributing factors in many cases.

The syndrome is easier to diagnose than to treat. Conservative therapy consists of heat applied to the affected area, a diet of soft foods, limitation of mouth opening, and mild analgesics and muscle relaxants. Certain exercises and surgical interventions have been helpful, and antidepressants are appropriate in some cases in which depression has caused sleeplessness, bruxism, lassitude, and frequent yawning and these manifestations of depression have caused pain, but no one specific treatment has emerged (Gaudet and Brown, 2000).

Another form of headache that is common but perhaps little known to psychiatrists often follows minor or major head trauma. This occurs in the post-traumatic stress syndrome, which also involves giddiness, irritability, sensitivity to noise, and minor memory and concentration difficulties. Lishman (1968) noted that the symptoms were unrelated to either the extent or the location of brain damage. Jacobsen (1969), however, reported that the symptoms were more likely to occur if the patient had been rendered unconscious at the time of impact. He observed that the headaches usually stopped within 2 months of the iniury and that most patients were free of all symptoms within 4 years. This syndrome is not usually associated with radiographic or electroencephalographic changes and many have questioned its organic basis. The distinctiveness of the syndrome argues against this psychosomatic view of its etiology, in our opinion, as does the fact that it may occur in individuals with no history of psychosomatic disease or pending lawsuits. Recently McAllister et al. (1999) showed that patients 1 month after traumatic brain injury had FMRI evidence of significant differences in the right parietal and dorsolateral cortical regions when asked to do a working memory task, as compared to controls, thus lending some physiological basis to the symptoms of poor concentration following traumatic closed head injury. Arciniegas et al. (2000) has also shown impaired auditory gating manifested by nonsuppression of P50 evoked waveforms in patients with persistent symptoms following traumatic brain injury. He postulates that this defect may represent a persistent cholinergic dysfunction and has found that low-dose donepezil provides some symptomatic improvement (Arceniegas, 2002).

CONCLUSION

Conversion disorders and somatization have long perplexed physicians. The serious study of these syndromes was inaugurated by the neurologist, Jean Martin Charcot (1825–1893). His studies provided the springboard for modern psychiatry through the work of one of his most illustrious pupils, Sigmund Freud. Conversion and somatization have been designated variously as a neurological syndrome, a psychiatric syndrome, and a disease of society (Vieth, 1965). To a degree these disorders crystallized the dilemma we have had in writing this book: We have had to constantly check ourselves from referring to psychiatric illnesses as functional, thereby implying a separateness from neurological illnesses that do not exist. It should be apparent that one or more neurological syndromes could produce almost every abnormal emotional state. It is self-evident that all behavioral symptoms, whatever their etiology, are mediated by the central nervous system, a common pathway for many different pathological processes. Though most conversion syndromes exist in the absence of neurological disease, one wonders why one patient and not another develops conversion in response to apparently similar life stresses. There is no clear answer to this problem. Genetic aspects have been incompletely explored, and we have not been able to identify causative environmental influences. Though our knowledge of these conditions has increased considerably over the years (we no longer believe that the varied symptoms are related to a wandering uterus, and we have been able to formulate criteria for their diagnoses), our skills are still exercised fundamentally at a descriptive level. This is still true of many neurological and psychiatric conditions. Though we look to basic medical research for the full understanding of these diseases, it behooves us meanwhile to polish our clinical skills and learn what we can from observation and description.

REFERENCES

Arciniegas, D., A. Olincy, J. Topkoff, et al. Impaired auditory gating and P50 nonsuppression following traumatic brain injury. *J Neuropsychiatry* 12:77, 2000.

Arciniegas, D., J. Topkoff, C. Anderson, et al. Low-dose donepezil normalizes P50 physiology in traumatic brain injury patients. *J Neuropsychiatry* 14:115, 2002.

Berrington, W. P., D. W. Liddell, G. A. Foulds. A re-evaluation of the Fugue *J Ment Sci* 102:280, 1956.

Breslau, N., L. Schultz, W. Stewart, et al. Headache types and panic disorder. *Neurology* 56:350, 2001.

Breslau, N., B. Rasmussen. The impact of migraine. *Neurology* 56 (Suppl 1):S4, 2001.

Carson, A., B. Ringbauer, L. MacKenzie, et al. Neurological disease, emotional disorder, and disability. *J Neurol Neurosurg Psychiatry* 68:202, 2000.

Carson, A., B. Ringbauer, J. Stone, et al. Do medically unexplained symptoms matter? A cohort study of 300 new referrals to a Neurology outpatient clinic. *J Neurol Neurosurg Psychiatry* 68:207, 2000.

Christensen, B. Studics on hyperventilation. II. Electrocardiographic changes in normal man during voluntary hyperventilation. *J Clin Invest* 24:880, 1946.

Cowley, D., P. Roy-Byrne. Panic disorder and hyperventilation syndrome. In: *Anxiety New Findings For the Clinician,* P. Roy-Byrne, ed. American Psychiatric Press, Washington DC, 1989, p. 19.

Creed, F., D. Firth, M. Timol, et al. Somatization and illness behavior in a neurology ward. *J Psychosom Res* 34:427, 1990.

Crimlisk, H., Bhatia, H. Cope, et al. Slater revisited: 6-year follow-up study of patients with medically unexplained symptoms, *BMJ* 316:582, 1998.

Crimlisk, H., Bhatia, H. Cope, et al. Patterns of referral in patients with unexplained motor symptoms. *J Psychosom Res* 49:217, 2000.

Dalessio, D., J. Silberstein. *Wolfe's Headache and Other Head Pain*, 7th Ed. Oxford University Press, New York, 2001.

Diamond, S., D. Dalessio. *The Practcing Physicians Approach to Headache*, 6th Ed. Saunders, Philadelphia, 1999.

Ewald, H., T. Rogne, K. Ewald, et al. Somatization in patients newly admitted to a neurological department. *Acta Psychiatr Scand* 89:174, 1994.

Fisher, C. M., R. D. Adams. Transient global amnesia. *Acta Neurol Scand* 40 (Suppl. 9): 7, 1964.

Gaudet, E., D. Brown. Tempromandibular disorder treatment and outcomes. *Cranio* 18: 9, 2000.

Goodman, L. S., A. Gilmans. *The Pharmacological Basis of Therapeutics*, 8th Ed. A. G. Gilman, T. W. Rall, A. Nies, P. Taylor, eds. Pergamon, New York, 1990.

Gotoh, F., J. S. Meyer, Y. Takagi. Cerebral effects of hyperventilation in man. *Arch Neurol* 1 2:410, 1965.

Hamilton, J. et al. Anxiety, depression and the management of medically unexplained symptoms in medical clinics, *J R Coll Physicians Lond* 30:18, 1996.

Jacobson, S. A. Mechanisms of the sequellae of minor craniocervical trauma. In: *The Late Effects of Head Injury*, A. E. Walker, W. F. Caveness, M. Critchley, eds, CC Thomas, Springfield IL., 1969, p. 35.

Kapoor, W., M. Fortunato, B. Hanusa, et al. Psychiatric illnesses in patients with syncope. *Am J Med* 99:502, 1995.

Katon, W. *Panic Disorder in the Medical Setting*. American Psychiatric Press, Washington DC, 1991.

Katon, W., E. Lin, M. Von Korff, et al. *Somatization. Am J Psychiatry* 148:34, 1991.

Katon, W., M. Sullivan, E. Walker. Medical symptoms without identified pathology. *Ann Int Med* 134:917, 2001.

Kestenbaum, A. *Clinical Methods of Neuro-ophthalmologic Examination,* 2nd Ed. Crune and Stratton, New York, 1961.

Kroenke, K, D. Mangelsdorf. Common symptoms in ambulatory care. *Am J Med* 86: 262, 1989.

Kroenke, K., C. Lucas, M. Rosenberg, et al. Causes of persistent dizziness. *Ann Int Med* 117:898, 1992.

Kroenke, K., R. Price. Symptoms in the community. *Arch Intern Med* 153: 2474, 1993.

Lishman, W. A. Brain damage in relation to psychiatric disability after head injury. *Br J Psychiatry* 114:373, 1968.

Mattson, R. H., G. R. Heninger, B. B. Gallagher, et al. Psychophysiological precipitants of seizures in epileptics. *Neurology* 20:406, 1970.

Merikangas, J. Headache syndromes in *Medical Psychiatric Practice*, Vol 1. A. Stoudemire, B. Fogel, eds. American Psychiatric Press, Washington DC, 1991, p. 393.

Merikangas, K. J. Merikangas, J. Angst. Headache syndrome and psychiatric disorders. *J Psychiatry Res* 27:197, 1993.

McAllister, T. W., A. Saykin, L. Flashman, et. al. Brain activation during working memory one month after traumatic brain injury. *Neurology* 53:1300, 1999.

Mattson, R. H., G. R. Heninger, B. B. Gallagher, C. H. Glaser. Psycbophysiological precipitants of seizures in epileptics. *Neurology* 20:406, 1970.

Perley, M. J., S. B. Guze. Hysteria-the stability and usefulness of clinical criteria. A quantitative study based on a follow-up of six to eight years in 39 patients. *N Engl J Med* 266:421, 1962.

Plum, F., J. B. Posner. *Diagnosis of Stupor and Coma*, 2nd Ed. Contemporary Neurology Series. F. A. Davis, Philadelphia, 1972.

Raja, M. Neurological diagnosis in psychiatric patients. *Ital J Neurol Sci* 16:153, 1995.

Shuttleworth, E. C., C. E. Morris. The transient global amnesia syndrome. *Arch Neurol* 15:515, 1966.

Slater, E., E. Glithero. A follow-up of patients diagnosed as suffering from "hysteria." *J Psychosom Res* 9:9, 1965.

Spinhoven, P., E. Onstein, P. Stark, et al. Hyperventilation and panic attacks in general hospital patients. *Gen Hosp Psychiatry* 15:148, 1993.

Veith, I. *Hysteria*. University of Chicago Press, Chicago, 1965.

Chapter Seven

CLINICAL EVALUATION

The history and examination of patients suspected of having brain disease are not standard. They vary from patient to patient depending on the presenting complaint. If every function that could be assessed were examined in every patient, each evaluation would require at least a full day. Testing all sensory modalities, including olfaction, hearing, vision, taste, and somatosensory functions as well as the interpretation of and memory of sensory stimuli, speech, numerical calculation, cerebellar function, and each cranial nerve might be excessive in a young woman with many years of typical migraine headaches, for example.

The history, appearance, and behavior of the patient indicate which functions are appropriate to test. Patients with disorders of behavior and thought must have a thorough examination of the functions that are mediated in the cerebral hemispheres.

Neurology and psychiatry are medical specialties that deal with a single organ, the brain. This separation within the medical profession should not prevent us from evaluating our patients appropriately. Lesions of the brain that everyone agrees would be within the province of neurology (e.g., anoxic brain damage, encephalitis, lead poisoning) may cause mental symptoms or worsen and distort the symptoms of mania and schizophrenia. Patients with neurological diseases may have mental symptoms that are indistinguishable from those encountered in psychiatric disorders. The treatment of neurological diseases can produce cognitive and behavioral changes, and the treatment of mental illnesses can produce neurological symptoms. Fortunately, history-taking and neurological examination encompass bedside techniques that provide sensitive and specific reflections of the functioning of the brain, and that can lead to a diagnosis. Unfortunately, for all psychiatric disorders and many neurological disorders, the history and physical neurological examination are the *only* tools for diagnosis.

THE IMPORTANCE OF THE CLINICAL HISTORY

Psychiatrists and neurologists encounter some of their most difficult diagnostic problems in differentiating disorders that are properly within the province of neurology from those that are best dealt with by psychiatry. Many patients have both neurological and psychiatric disorders. For example, when a patient with multiple sclerosis (MS) becomes depressed, certain questions should come to the clinician's mind such as the following:

- Is the depressed mood a psychological reaction that was precipitated by an awareness that multiple sclerosis can cripple and kill?
- Does the demyelination of the brain that causes the symptoms of multiple sclerosis also cause the depressed mood?
- Is the depressed mood a recurrent depression that accidentally coincides with, but is actually unrelated to, the diagnosis of multiple sclerosis?

There are no specific clinical criteria that would clearly distinguish one of the above etiologies from the other. Regardless of the etiology of the depression, a depressed patient looks like a depressed patient. In fact, the similarity of the clinical picture of depression despite varying causes makes the diagnostic process in behavioral neurology intriguing and challenging. The fact that a diverse number of etiologies can cause the same symptoms is not surprising. The central nervous system, like other organ systems, has a limited repertoire of symptoms (Table 7–1).

The most important clues to the etiology of a patient's behavioral disturbances are past psychosocial and psychiatric history. Consider the depressed MS patient. If he or she has a history of excellent psychosocial functioning (e.g., good performance at work or school, the capacity to form friendships) and no history of psychiatric illness, we would be inclined to think that the depressive symptoms were probably caused by multiple sclerosis. If the patient has an extensive history of poor psychosocial functioning, a family history of psychiatric illness and of past psychiatric disorders (particularly if the past symptoms were similar

Table 7–1 Mental Symptoms Seen in Brain Disorders

Cognitive
Affect modulation
Intellectual function
Judgement
Memory
Orientation
Behavioral
Anxiety
Arousal
Mood
Motor
Personality
Perceptions
Somatosensory
Kinesthetic pain
Auditory
Olfactory
Taste
Visual

to the current depressive symptoms), then we would be more likely to view the depressive symptoms as only coincidentally related to multiple sclerosis.

The seeds of a patient's presenting mental illness can usually be seen in past behavior. The exceptions are mania and other affective disorders. These can occur in mid or late life for the first time without any significant history of psychosocial dysfunction and without a history of previous psychiatric illness, though that is rare. In most cases, when the first onset of mental symptoms occurs after age 30, there must be a strong suspicion of neurological disease. The presence of any neurological findings on the physical or laboratory examination also increases the suspicion that a neurological disorder may be involved. Also developmental landmarks should be assessed during the clinical interview, as this will give some indication of early neurological impairment. This information can also put the patients current symptoms into perspective. Also to be assessed are maternal alcohol consumption or exposure to other neonatal toxins, that could lead to the fetal alcohol syndrome or other developmental problems. The sequelae of childhood learning disabilities can lead to subtle adult cognitive and behavioral impairments (Townes and Slade, 2000). In particular, the syndrome of nonverbal learning difficulties can often present a picture that looks as if the patient's problems are characterological e.g., apathetic, unmotivated, and unable to detect social cues, with normal IQ (Dugbarty, 2000).

The course of the symptoms is also important. Abrupt changes in personality, mood, or ability to function are much more typical of neurologic diseases than of psychiatric disorders. Also, rapid fluctuations of behavior or mental status are more likely caused by neurological disorders such as seizures, toxic-metabolic encephalopathy, delirium, or infection. In fact, any change in personality should raise the clinician's index of suspicion (even if the change is for the better). If a characteristically irritable and obsessive individual suddenly becomes placid or loses his obsessive traits (or the opposite), the clinician should consider the possibility that some cerebral disturbance such as a tumor, hydrocephalus, or stroke has developed.

If symptoms are sudden in onset and gradually improve or stabilize, a stroke should be considered. If symptoms are asymmetrical and develop gradually, a tumor may be present. If symptoms are gradual in onset and diffuse, a degenerative disorder needs to be considered. Patients that have primarily behavioral symptoms that have been present for many years, most likely have a psychiatric disorder.

When a patient's symptoms do not quite fit the diagnostic criteria for the many disorders outlined in DSM-IV, a neurological disease may be the cause. Even though DSM-IV represents an arbitrary classification system, the classical descriptions of the major disorders such as mania, schizophrenia, etc, have been fairly consistent for over 100 years and when a patient fits the criteria for diagnosis outlined in DSM-IV perfectly, than one can have confidence in the diagnosis. It is when the patient's symptoms or clinical course do not fit or fit the diagnostic criteria poorly that we should become suspicious (Fig. 7–1).

Many clinicians invoke a psychiatric diagnosis when the patient's symptoms do not fit a neurological diagnostic category. The opposite also occurs. When a patient's behavior is abnormal but not typical of mental illnesses, one should think of neurological conditions that could cause it.

The duration of symptoms is an important criterion for diagnosing mental illnesses. Isolated or brief psychiatric symptoms may not signify a psychiatric disorder. Feeling sad following events that would make anyone sad is not a

Figure 7–1 Flowchart for differentiating psychiatric from neurological disorders. The starting point for differential diagnosis is the primary symptoms of central nervous system dysfunction (excluding a history of substance abuse). The primary symptoms of central nervous system dysfunction are also covered in Table 7–1. * Dementia is one of the main risk factors for delirium, so there may be an underlying dementia in delirious patients. ** Diagnostic evaluation must now include appropriate blood work, EEG, and imaging studies.

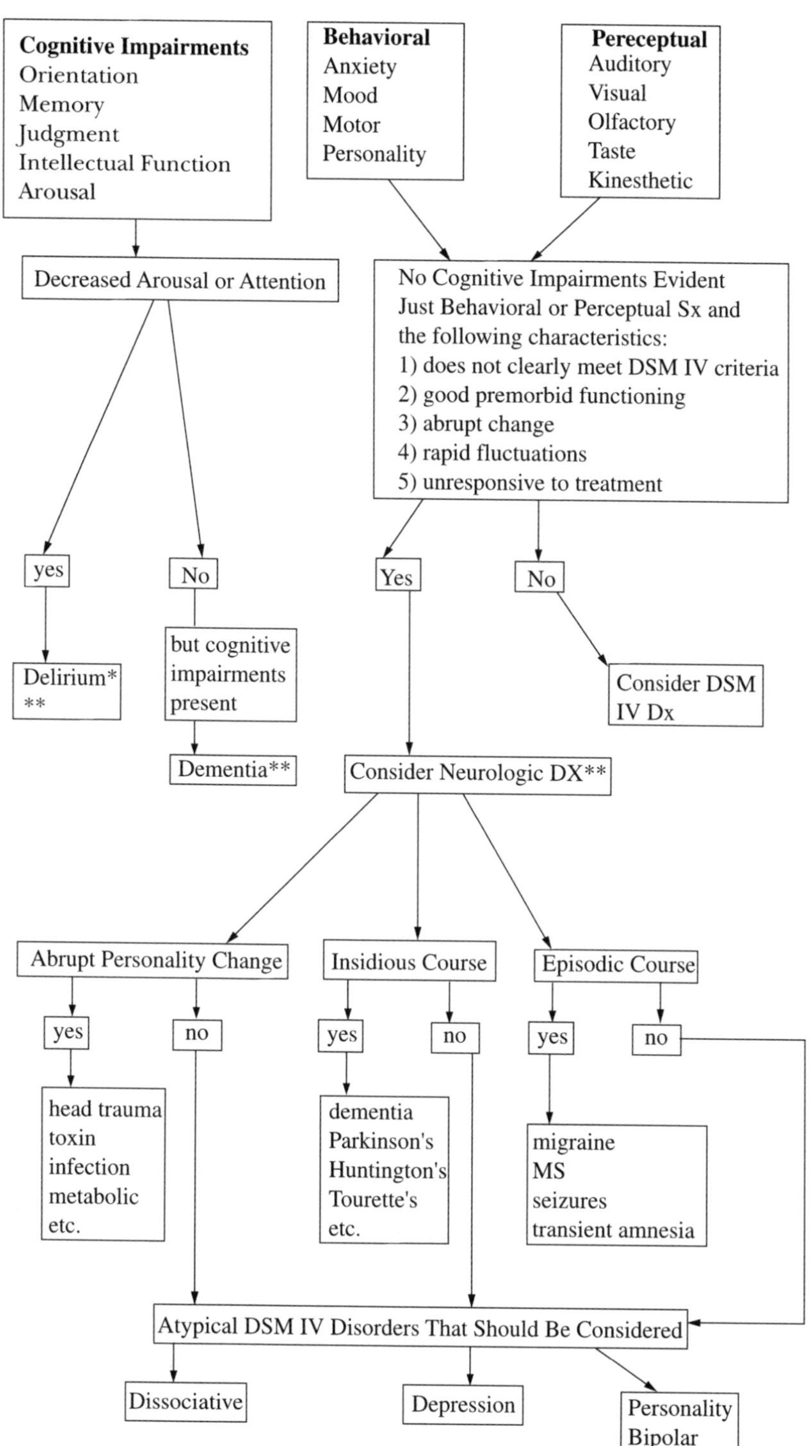

Cognitive Impairments
Orientation
Memory
Judgment
Intellectual Function
Arousal
Behavioral
Anxiety
Mood
Motor
Personality
Pereceptual
Auditory
Visual
Olfactory
Taste
Kinesthetic
Decreased Arousal or Attention
No Cognitive Impairments Evident
Just Behavioral or Perceptual Sx and
the following characteristics:
1) does not clearly meet DSM IV criteria
2) good premorbid functioning
3) abrupt change
4) rapid fluctuations
5) unresponsive to treatment
yes
No
Yes
No
Delirium*
**
but cognitive
impairments
present
Consider DSM
IV Dx
Dementia**
Consider Neurologic DX**
Abrupt Personality Change
Insidious Course
Episodic Course
yes
no
yes
no
yes
no
head trauma
toxin
infection
metabolic
etc.
dementia
Parkinson's
Huntington's
Tourette's
etc.
migraine
MS
seizures
transient amnesia
Atypical DSM IV Disorders That Should Be Considered
Dissociative
Depression
Personality
Bipolar

mental illness. The patient who is having trouble functioning and admits being sad and in a depressed mood nearly every day for at least several weeks, as well as having persistent sleep, appetite, and sexual disturbances, psychomotor slowing and feelings of worthlessness, guilt, or suicidal ideation, meets the full criteria for a major depressive disorder. Even if a patient does not meet the full DSM criteria for a major depressive reaction, however, it is still worth noting and following the depressive symptoms. For example, in a patient who has lost a spouse of many years, bereavement may last for 6 months to 1 year, but at times this normal process can become a major depressive reaction with many biologic symptoms such as sleep and appetite disturbances or psychomotor retardation. In the same way, a neurological patient can have mild depressive symptoms that may progress over time to a full major depressive disorder.

NEUROLOGICAL CONDITIONS COMMONLY ASSOCIATED WITH A HIGH INCIDENCE OF PSYCHIATRIC COMPLICATIONS

Many neurological conditions have an association with psychiatric disorders (Table 7–2), but it is often very difficult to separate preexisting psychopathology from current behavior (Popkin and Tucker, 1992; Brown et al., 1994). Still the origin of behavioral symptoms is the brain. If neurologic disease of the brain coexists, it is likely that the behavioral symptoms also arise from the same illness. The literature delineating associations between behavioral symptoms and neurological disorders consists mostly of case reports, where it is never clear whether the association is a chance occurrence or there is a strong relationship between the neurological disorder and a specific behavior. For example, Waxman and Geschwind (1975) reported three patients with seizure disorders who seemed to have specific interictal personality traits: hyposexuality, hypergraphia, and philosophical or religious interests. When large groups of patients with seizure disorders are studied, however, this constellation of symptoms is not prominent (Bear and Fedio, 1977; Mungas, 1982). Another problem is that the data often come from academic medical centers, which tend to serve skewed populations, e.g. atypical patients, treatment failures, or unusually complicated patients. The incidence of depression in patients with stroke (Robinson, 1998)) and Parkinson's disease (Mayeux et al., 1986) has usually been cited as 20 to 30 percent. These studies have come almost exclusively from university inpatient and outpatient services. When community surveys are carried out among patients with these conditions, the incidence and prevalence of depression is only slightly higher than in a normal population of comparable age (House et al., 1990; Tandberg et al., 1997).

Table 7–2 Common Behavioral Conditions Associated with Neurological Illness

SPECIFIC CONDITIONS	PSYCHOSIS	AFFECTIVE (MANIA/ DEPRESSION)	ANXIETY	DEMENTIA
Alzheimer's disease	X	XX	X	X
Epilepsy	XX	XX	X	
Huntington's disease	XX	X		X
HIV	X	X	X	XX
Multiple sclerosis	X	XX	X	X
Parkinson's disease	XX	X		X
Wilson's disease	XX	X		X
Categorical Conditions				
Affective disorders	XX	XX	XX	XX
CVAs	X	XX	X	X
Encephalitis	XX		XX	
Head trauma	X	XX	X	XX
Hypoxia		X	X	XX
Toxins	X	X	X	XX
Tumors	X	X	X	X
Vitamin deficiencies	XX	X		XX

X, reported.

XX, commonly reported.

CVA, cerebrovascular accident.

THE CLINICAL EXAMINATION OF THE BRAIN

In addition to the history, the physical neurological examination can be confirmatory. Often it provides guidelines for further laboratory and diagnostic testing. The clinical examination should be used to test hypotheses about anatomic aspects of the patient's disorder that the history generated. The examination can determine whether there is a diffuse or a focal process and whether there is peripheral nervous system and/or central nervous system involvement.

The neurological examination is a way of determining if various parts of the brain and spinal cord are functionally intact. It is easiest to test the lower, phylogenetically more primitive parts of the nervous system and then progress to more complex functions.

The human brain is organized in layers of interacting regions. At the base, just behind the mouth, is the brain stem, which controls most elemental functions such as breathing, blood pressure, and swallowing. It also controls the cranial nerves subserving eye movement, facial movement, and the muscles of the throat, mouth, and neck. The brain stem mediates sensation in the head, face, and neck and, through the cerebellum, general motor coordination. Above the brain stem, behind the nose and its sinuses, is the diencephalon. This controls body temperature, appetite, sleep, and wakefulness. Circling around that central region of the brain is the limbic system and amygdala-hippocampus complex, the seat of the primitive emotions involved in sexual behavior, fear, anger, and aggressive attack, as well as memory. Virtually all mammals share these features.

Cortical Functions

Covering the entire surface of the brain stem, and lying just below the skull, is the cerebral cortex, the thick layer of gray matter that is the source of intelligence. The cortex is anatomically and functionally distinct from the rest of the brain. Complex perceptual and cognitive functions take place in the cortex. Vision registers and is integrated at the back of the brain in the occipital lobes. Somatosensory information like touch, pain, and position in space is interpreted in the parietal lobes; smell and taste in the temporal lobes. Speech and the understanding of language are usually identified with the left posterior temporal lobe (Wernicke's area), and the actual expression of language comes from a posterior part of the left frontal lobe (Broca's area). Voluntary movement derives from the motor strip in the posterior part of the frontal lobes. Voluntary movement is modified by deep subcortical centers called the basal ganglia. Almost all mammals have well-developed occipital, parietal, and temporal lobes as well as motor control systems that are very similar to the human ones.

To determine if the brain is intact, the examiner must test reflexes and sensorimotor functions, comparing the patient's right and left sides and observing his stance and gait. The head circumference should be measured with a tape and compared with a table of normal standards. If the circumference is more than two standard deviations below the mean, the patient is microcephalic and will have a 95 percent chance of being cognitively impaired.

Tests of motor coordination include skipping, hopping, and walking a straight line forward and backward. The patient should be asked to spread his fingers apart and hold his hands apart while the examiner looks for discontinuous, involuntary, jerky movements of the fingers and arms, called choreiform movements. The patient should be tested to see if he is right handed and right footed. If dominance is mixed, it might mean that his nervous system has not developed the way that it should.

Abnormality on a single test usually does not mean that the person is brain damaged, but a pattern of abnormalities does indicate that the brain is malfunctioning. Asymmetrical (lateralized) abnormalities are likely to reflect structural abnormalities of the central nervous system, but severe damage to the brain can be present in patients whose sensorimotor functions, coordination, and reflexes are normal.

Many psychiatric disorders manifest clinical neurological signs. Although this is of clinical and theoretical interest, it can complicate the interpretation of the neurological findings. Neurological signs have been noted in 36 to 50 percent of schizophrenic patients. Some of these signs disappear when the patient's behavioral and cognitive symptoms have remitted (Tucker et al., 1974). Many of the neurological deficits observed in psychiatric patients relate to difficulties in sensory integrative functions, such as graphesthesia, stereognosis, and audiovisual integration; and to motor coordination, or movement sequencing, and patterning.

Regressive reflexes, e.g., snout, suck, or grasp, nuchocephalic reflex, etc. (Jenkyn et al., 1977) are associated with diffuse cerebral dysfunctions (e.g., delirium, dementia). These reflexes are called "regressive" because they are normally present in very young children and infants but not in adults. When regressive reflexes are observed in psychiatric patients one should investigate further and not attribute them to the psychiatric disorder. Aging (Jenkyn et al., 1985) and neuroleptic medications can cause regressive reflexes

Cognitive Functions

Given that the brain is the organ of cognition, cognitive functions must also be tested in the neurological exam. The Mini-Mental Status Examination (MMSE) is a standard tool for the screening of cognitive status (Task Force for the Handbook of Psychiatric Measures, 2000). Patients must be able to identify the day, date, time of day, and where they are. They should be asked to name several objects that have just been presented to them. Patients are given three words, asked to repeat the three words and to remember them; to subtract 7 from 100 and to perform 5 serial subtractions of 7; to spell the word "world" forward and backward, and to recall the three words they were instructed to remember earlier. Patients must be able to read, repeat, write a sentence, copy a standard diagram, and follow a three-step command.

Although the MMSE has gained wide acceptance as a clinical and research tool, other standardized evaluations have been developed for assessing cognitive dysfunction in specific neurological disorders e.g., The Dementia Rating Scale (DRS) and the Alzheimer's Disease Assessment Scale (ADAS) are widely used to quantify cognitive dysfunction in dementia patients; the Galveston Orientation and Amnesia Test (GOAT) for measuring amnesia and orientation; and the DRS for quantifying the degree of delirium (Task Force for the Handbook of Psychiatric Measures, 2000). Cummings et al. (1994) have developed the Neuropsychiatric Inventory (NPI) that assesses 10 behavioral domains (e.g., anxiety, agitation, depression, motor behavior, etc.) in patients with dementia.

Except for the behavioral measures, most of these tests assess similar functions of orientation, memory, calculation, reading, writing, and speaking. They are useful for uncovering evidence of damage to the posterior two-thirds of the brain, the parietal, temporal, and occipital lobes, and for quantifying changes in the patients' conditions, but are insensitive tools for detecting damage and dysfunction of the frontal lobes even when they are severely damaged.

Behaviors Associated with the Frontal Lobes

The most obvious difference between the brains of humans and other primates is the size of the frontal lobes. The frontal lobes of humans are massive in relation to the other parts of the cortex and account for about one third of the cortical mass. It is the job of the frontal lobes to organize motor and cognitive functions, to focus attention, to make decisions, and to modify and inhibit the behavioral impulses that surge up from the other parts of the brain. The frontal lobes permit us to check impulses, to say to ourselves, "No. Do not say or do that," in response to our urges. The frontal lobes allow us to anticipate adverse or favorable circumstances, to care about the results, to plan, invent, modify, and adapt in response to changes in our environment. The frontal lobes provide *social pragmatics*, a good term provided by Jean Fryer, an expert in the rehabilitation of patients with traumatic brain damage (personal communication, 1999). The frontal lobes subserve judgment.

The clinical history is the most important element in the assessment of the status of the frontal lobes. Frontally damaged individuals may not focus their attention for long periods of time and do not prioritize well. They are distractible. They may speak too loudly, stand too close, joke too much, and make others feel uncomfortable. They have difficulty in gauging the effect that they are having on observers and do not seem to care. This defect in social pragmatics can be a major impediment to obtaining and holding jobs, maintaining relationships, and succeeding in life. Patients with frontal lobe damage may be withdrawn, apathetic, and mute most of the time, they may also be unable to control the expression of emotions such as irritation and sexual attraction. They may express thoughts and desires that their intact frontal lobes would have controlled, spending too much money, driving at excessively high speeds, or fighting. They often cannot keep their behavior within the general bounds of society.

With frontal damage some people become boastful, others irritable and argumentative, and still others calm and apathetic. Some have no interest in sex, while others are hypersexual.

Wide fluctuations in mood and behavior can occur, erratically, in a short time unmodulated by the social brakes that the frontal lobes normally provide. When frontal injuries occur in persons with affective disorders, patients tend to have wider mood swings that occur more rapidly.

The frontal lobes can be damaged or even surgically removed without causing any abnormality in speech, arithmetic ability, reading, writing, or memory. Though these functions, tested by the MMSE and IQ tests, often remain intact after frontal lobe injury, profound and devastating changes can occur in the patient's social life.

The famous story of Phineas Gage exemplifies the kind of deficits that frontal lobe injury can produce. Gage was a hard-working, reliable, ethical foreman who supervised a crew laying railroad tracks in New England around 1850. Gage set up the gunpowder used for blasting. He was injured when a premature explosion blew an iron rod through his frontal lobes. He recovered from the injury and could walk, talk, read, write, calculate, and remember; however, he was a changed man. He could not hold a job because he lost his ambition and initiative and became unreliable. He began to drink, swear, fight, and carouse. He became a derelict. Because of the traumatic injury to the frontal lobes, he suddenly developed elements of what today would be called an antisocial personality disorder.

Evaluation of the Frontal Lobes

Fibers from the frontal lobes project to other regions of the brain such as the corpus striatum and the dorsomedial nucleus of the thalamus. Lesions in the dorsomedial thalamus can easily cause the kinds of abnormalities that frontal lesions can produce. For this reason it is a mistake to conceptualize the functions that are mediated by the frontal lobes as residing exclusively within this area of the brain, but for the sake of brevity, we will refer to them as frontal functions.

Judgment and the ability to deal with complexity are crucial functions of the frontal lobes. Unfortunately, there is no reliable, objective standard or test for measuring judgment that is sufficiently sensitive and specific. Asking a patient what he would do with a stamped addressed envelope he found lying in a street is not an adequate test of frontal lobe function. It is insensitive and nonspecific. There are, however, several simple physical tests of frontal lobe function.

The most useful of these tests evaluates the frontal eye fields, the portion of the frontal lobes that enables the eyes to track a moving object. The examiner asks the patient to follow the examiner's smoothly moving finger as it goes slowly from left to right horizontally in front of the patient. An abnormal response would be visual tracking in brief, staccato, discontinuous jerks (saccades) or inattentiveness with brief deviations of the patient's eyes from the examiner's finger rather than smooth movements. A normal response would be smooth visual tracking of the moving finger. The patient should also be able to stare for 30 seconds at the examiner's stationary finger without deviating his gaze. This helps demonstrate his ability to concentrate.

Tapping gently on the bridge of a patient's nose normally elicits blinking. If the blinking persists for more than three taps, it means that the patient cannot accommodate to a benign stimulus. After three taps it should be clear that there is no potential threat to his eyes. If the patient cannot suppress the urge to blink even though there is no threat, it shows that he cannot adapt to a new situation. This inflexibility reflects dysfunction in a frontally mediated pathway (Jenkyn et al., 1977)

Paying attention to two sensory stimuli simultaneously can be difficult for frontally damaged people. They tend to disregard the more distal of two unilaterally applied stimuli. For example, if the examiner touches the patient's right cheek and right hand simultaneously, while the patient's eyes are closed, the patient may report having been touched only on the cheek. This is called the face-hand test. If the patient extinguishes (pays no attention to) the more distal stimulus, it shows that his attention to somatosensory stimuli by the frontal lobes is attenuated.

To see if a patient can concentrate and suppress an urge, the examiner creates a visual urge and then asks the patient to ignore it. The examiner faces the patient, holds his hands to either sides of the patient's eyes, and asks the patient to look at the examiner's nose. He instructs the patient to deviate his eyes to the side of the examiner's briefly raised index finger and then return his gaze to the examiner's nose. Alternately, the examiner moves his right and then his left index fingers. The patient looks toward the moving finger and then back at the examiner's nose. Once it is clear to the examiner that the patient has mastered this and looks to the moving finger and then back to the examiner's nose, the examiner asks the patient to look toward the opposite side, toward the side that does not move. Patients with frontal damage have trouble suppressing the urge to look at the moving finger and first look there before correcting. This test uncovers impulsivity and inattentiveness. It is called the antisaccade test. It is performed five times, twice to the left, twice to the right, and then once to the left. More than one failure counts as an error.

Frontally damaged individuals often cannot perform two-and three-stepped motor sequences repetitively even though their strength and coordination are normal. This makes complex, repetitive motor tasks sensitive indicators of frontal function. The patient is asked to strike his thighs repeatedly, simultaneously, with the right palm and the left fist, then with the right fist and left palm, alternating with each blow. He should be able to perform three sets perfectly on his own after having been taught how to perform this by the examiner. This is the two-stepped Luria test. Then the examiner shows the patient how to strike his thigh successively with his right palm, fist, and the edge of his hand. The patient attempts this alone after he is shown how to do this by the examiner.

The patient is then asked to perform this task with his left hand, striking the palm, the fist, and the side of the hand in sequence. This is called the three-stepped Luria test. Frontal lesions often interfere with the proper sequencing of this task. Abnormality on either the two- or three-stepped Luria test indicates frontal dysfunction.

Patients with frontal disturbances often cannot relax their limbs when asked to do so and allow them to remain suspended in the air when one is raised and then dropped by the examiner. This is the placement test. Sometimes patients try to help by anticipating the position the examiner wishes them to assume after the examiner instructs them to be "limp as a rag doll." The abnormality is called paratonia. It represents perseveration of resting tone; it melds into perseveration of movement as the patient overcomes initial inertia and gets into rhythm with the examiner's testing movements. When the examiner releases the patient's arm or leg, instead of dropping, relaxed to the bed, the limb remains suspended or continues in perseverative fashion carrying out the supposedly passive movements for testing tone that the examiner was employing (Reeves, 2001). When this sign is severely abnormal, the limb will remain in any position in which it was placed. This phenomenon is called waxy flexibility or catatonia and can also be encountered in psychotic states of depression and schizophrenia.

Upward gaze is another frontally mediated function. When asked to look upward, the individual should be able to move the outer limbus of his iris upward at least 5 mm.

Testing the nuchocephalic reflex revels the patient's ability to adapt to postural change. It is often helpful in diagnosing frontal disease. With the patient's eyes closed, the examiner places his hands on the patient's shoulders and quickly turns him to the right or to the left. Normally, the head follows the shoulders but maintains its posture through looking straight ahead. Some frontally impaired individuals do not move their heads with their shoulders but maintain the posture of their heads as though they were looking straight ahead. They cannot adapt to this postural change.

The snout reflex is tested when the examiner uses the middle phalange of his flexed index finger and firmly presses the patient's relaxed lips and then draws his finger away. Any contraction of the orbicularis oris to this stimulus results in a puckering of the lips or the chin. The suck reflex is similar. The examiner firmly places the knuckle of his flexed index finger between the subject's lips. There should be no response from either stimuli. Any pursing or sucking motion by the subject's lips or movement of his chin is recorded as a disinhibited reflex and an abnormal response.

The grasp reflex is tested both with and without distraction. First the patient is told to relax his hand while the examiner uses his own finger to stroke its palmar surface of the patient's hand. Next the patient is distracted by being instructed to spell a simple word such as "fist" both forward and backward.

Each hand is stroked without distraction and then with distraction. The addition of a second task ("spell 'fist' backward") to the first task ("relax your hand") increases the stress on the person and allows a disinhibited reflex to become manifest in frontal lobe dysfunction. Absence of any flexion of the subject's fingers is normal. Any flexion of the fingers represents disinhibition and is abnormal.

The results of each of these tests are not abnormal in every case of frontal damage. A pattern of abnormality, i.e., three or more abnormal tests, sustains the conclusion that the frontal lobes are damaged. Three abnormal tests reliably correlate with abnormalities in both the MRI of the brain and neuropsychological testing with the Halstead-Reitan battery (Jenkyn et al., 1977; Jenkyn et al., 1985; Blake et al., 1995; Bae et al., 1998).

The correlation is significant but not absolute. We have found that the most sensitive and specific of these frontal neurological tests are the inability to perform smooth visual pursuit and the inability to perform accurately the three-step Luria test. Magnetic resonance imaging scans of patients who fail both of these tests are likely to be abnormal.

The abnormalities on these tests are age-dependent. They may not be abnormal if found in preschool children. Unfortunately, there are no studies of normal children that indicate at what age a "frontal sign" is abnormal.

Many of the frontal signs can be seen in older patients, and the signs accompany Parkinson's disease, chorea, and they can also be seen in patients who are receiving drugs that block dopamine receptors. Many of these signs may also be encountered in schizophrenics. Whether they reflect abnormalities of the brain that are induced by schizophrenia or are comorbid with the disease or caused by medication is uncertain. It is not known whether abnormalities on the frontal tests described above can distinguish a patient who has frontotemporal dementia from the pseudodementia of depression. The successful treatment of depression may reverse some frontal signs, but this has not been systematically studied.

Cognitive aspects of the frontal lobe evaluation. The word fluency test examines frontal function by testing the ability to generate words that are not in a context. In this test, the examiner asks the patient to name as many words as he can in 60 seconds that begin with either the letter "F" or "M." A normal score is 14 plus or minus 5. It is abnormal to name fewer than 9 words. This is not an intelligence test but a test of improvisation. A person with frontal damage might perform normally on an I.Q. test or MMSE. Because frontally damaged people have trouble improvising or in using old knowledge in a new way, the word fluency test provides an indication of frontal dysfunction.

The "king story" can be very useful in separating patients with attentional deficits from those with memory deficits. The story has a familiar sound but contains no familiar details:

> Once upon a time there lived a king who was very ill. His physicians could not help him so he sought the advice of his wise men. His wise men advised him to obtain the shirt of a happy man. The king sent out messengers who scoured the kingdom and finally found a happy man, but the happy man did not own a shirt.

Before this story is recited the patient is asked to pay close attention to the details and then to repeat the story, including as many details as possible. When patients are unable to provide all the details of this story, it indicates inattention. Sometimes the inattention is the result of frontal damage and sometimes it reflects nervousness, depression, mania, schizophrenia, obsessiveness, or intoxication. After the examination has been completed and 15 minutes have elapsed, the patient is asked to repeat the story. If the patient recalls 75 percent of the details that *he* included in his initial repetition of the story, the examiner can conclude that the patient's memory is intact. The combination of poor attention span and intact memory is frequently seen in patients with frontal dysfunction.

The psychological tests that most reliably reflect frontal dysfunction deal with executive functions that are mediated in large part through the frontal lobes. The most sensitive tests are the Wisconsin Card Sorting Test (WCST), Trail-Making Tests A and B, the Categories subtest of the Halstead-Reitan battery, and tests of continuous performance such as the Stroop Color and Word Test (Golden). None of these psychological tests is 100 percent predictive of the existence of frontal lobe damage as determined by MRI or the neurological examination, but a neuropsychological assessment for suspected frontal lobe damage that does not include the WCST, Trail-Making, Categories, and continuous motor performance is incomplete (Lezak, 1995).

MENTAL STATUS EXAMINATION

The mental status examination traditionally practiced by psychiatrists is little more than a way of organizing information. The traditional format (divided into appearance and behavior, mood and affect, language and thought, cognition, volition, suicide and homicide tendencies, and judgment) is the way an experienced psychiatrist will organize his or her observations of the patient's mental functions (Trzepacz and Baker, 1993). However, it often leaves one without knowledge of whether certain functions were assessed, or whether they were omitted because the patient could not perform them. The other major drawback of this type of examination is the lack of sufficient quantifiable data for comparing one patient to another, as well as the same patient's mental functions over time. Consequently many clinicians include standardized scales of cognitive function and behavior such as the MMSE and the NPI (see pp. 257–258) as part of their mental status examination.

IMAGING

With the data now available from the computerization of radiologic procedures and MRI, we are able to correlate observed behavior and performance on neuropsychological testing with the actual visualization of lesions in the central nervous system. The computerized axial tomography scan uses X-rays to produce excellent transverse images of the brain and is particularly useful for detecting meningeal and parenchymal abnormalities associated with metastatic neoplasia or inflammatory conditions as it measures tissue density. It is also very useful for finding calcified lesions, acute subarachnoid bleeding, and intracerebral hemorrhage. In general, however, MRI provides superior resolution. Though MRI is not sensitive to bone or to calcified lesions, it is particularly useful in detecting tumors, scars, and strokes as it delineates differences in the boundaries of tissue and fluid better than CT. Consequently it is superior to CT for evaluating the temporal lobes, the subcortical structures, the cerebellum, brain stem, and spinal cord. Magnetic resonance imaging is also much better in detecting white matter lesions, such as those associated with multiple sclerosis and microvascular disease (Hurley et al., 1997).

Another great advantage of MRI is the ability to obtain not only structural data but also functional data. During the MRI, a pulse of energy (a particular radio frequency) applied to the atomic nuclei in the brain (usually the hydrogen ion) generates a deflection pulse. From these pulses one can measure proton density, which in turn reflects the density of the hydrogen nuclei. Two measures give further information. The first, which is known as time constant one (T-1), is a measure of the relaxation of the hydrogen nuclei in a longitudinal plane. The second is spin relaxation (T-2), which is a measure in the transverse plane. These reflect in part the relationship of free water and lipids in the tissue. Magnetic resonance imaging series weighted between T-1 and T-2 can also be performed—and also reconstructed via computers retrospectively. This provides great detail, showing, for example, the anatomical boundaries of white and gray matter. It also has the potential for functional studies by demonstrating physiochemical differences in different brain regions.

With a variety of software programs, the MRI can provide arteriograms and venograms. It can detect edema and hemosiderin (evidence of past hemorrhage) within the brain, as well as indications of neural activity called functional MRI (FMRI). Most exciting has been the development of MR spectroscopy (MRS) to obtain assessment of various chemical structures within the working brain with great detail (Kortola, 1997).

The use of imaging technologies in psychiatric patients is certainly indicated when there are localizing neurological findings or a history suggesting neurologic causes like unexpected confusion, sudden cognitive decline, dementia, movement disorder, psychosis of abrupt onset, anorexia, catatonia, late onset affective or personality disturbances, and atypical symptoms in the course of chronic psychiatric illness (Weinberger, 1984; Hurley et al., 1997). Beresford et al. (1986) found high correlations, between positive findings on CT scan and abnormal cognitive examination. Often, patients with normal CT scans end up with an MRI of the head as the index of suspicion warrants further confirmation of the absence of structural pathology. Except for emergency room screening and demonstrating hemorrhage or calcium, MRI (when available) has eclipsed CT in the practice of neurology and psychiatry.

Other dynamic measures—such as PET, SPECT—are valuable for defining the functional areas of either hyper- or hypoactivity as well as measuring regional cerebral blood flow and have been useful for the diagnosis of dementia (Charpentier et al., 2000). Position emission tomography also has the potential for localizing various neurotransmitter receptors. These techniques are being used in research and are not really in routine clinical use.

CLINICAL LABORATORY TESTS

The brain can be disordered by conditions whose presence can only be detected by examinations of body fluids—namely, endocrine, infectious, metabolic, and toxic disorders. These conditions generally require investigation by blood tests such as complete blood count, sedimentation rate, urea, electrolytes, glucose, syphilis, HIV, and endocrine functions. B_{12}, folate, calcium, phosphorus, magnesium, porphyrin screens, antinuclear antibodies, and other laboratory tests may be required as clinically indicated. Lumbar punctures have become less necessary as imaging has improved, but suspected inflammatory conditions still require cerebrospinal fluid examination for diagnosis.

ELECTROENCEPHALOGRAPHY

The electroencephalogram (EEG) has been used widely in both neurology and psychiatry in disorders with an episodic course. Patients who have repeated episodes of disturbed behaviors who have paroxysmal spikes or spikes and waves on the electroencephalogram often have epileptic seizures. However mentally ill patients rarely manifest paroxysmal episodes of spikes. When they do, it often reflects a medication effect. However, if the patient with these paroxysmal spikes "due to medication effects," does not respond well to psychopharmacological management then a trial of anticonvulsants maybe in order. The EEG is also useful for detecting focal abnormalities, particularly when they occur in the temporal lobes (Tucker, 1998). Such abnormalities are most often dysrhythmic, slowed, nonparoxysmal, i.e., nonspecific, patterns. Again if a patient is not responding to treatment with standard antipsychotic or antidepressant drugs, a trial of anticonvulsants may be usefully tried, especially if the EEG is abnormal.

Normal EEG results do not exclude the existence of a brain disorder. Scalp electrodes may make it difficult to localize symptoms because symptoms originating from deep structures such as the mesial temporal areas may not be identified by surface electrodes. Even with depth electrodes, recording may be falsely negative because the placements have to be in exactly the areas associated with firing. Sleep EEG records significantly increase the likelihood of finding EEG abnormalities, particularly focal lesions such as temporal lobe lesions.

CONCLUSION

The most powerful diagnostic instrument in the evaluation of the patient with possible brain damage is a detailed history of the presenting symptoms and the patient's developmental history. The clinical evaluation should include a full physical, a comprehensive neurological, and a detailed evaluation of cognitive and cortical functions. The history and examinations will usually allow a preliminary diagnosis or at least point the way toward further evaluations necessary to make a diagnosis. After a detailed clinical examination one usually has a good idea about the nature of the problem. Usually blood and urine tests, waking and sleep EEGs, imaging studies, and neuropsychological assessment consolidate the clinical impression. Rarely are all tests abnormal. The abnormal, not the normal, test is definitive. No single test can reliably identify normal brain function. The patient who presents with a mixture of behavioral and neurological symptoms is a challenging clinical problem. Often the diagnosis does not fit into neat categorization. Sometimes the diagnosis will only become clear over time. The borderland between neurology and psychiatry remains, even in this era of high technology, a place where a knowledgeable and careful physician is still the crucial diagnostic instrument.

REFERENCES

Bae, C., J. H. Pincus, M. E. Quig, et al. Neurologic signs predict periventricular white matter lesions on MRI. *Neurology* 50:A448, 1998.

Bear, D., P. Fedio. Quantitative analysis of interictal behavior in temporal lobe epilepsy. *Arch Neurol* 34:454, 1977.

Beresford, T. P., F. Blow, R. Hall, et al. CT scanning in psychiatric inpatients. *Psychosomatics* 27:105, 1986.

Blake, P., J. Pincus, C. Buckner. Neurologic abnormalities in murderers. *Neurology* 45: 1641, 1995.

Brown, S., J. Fann, I. Grant. Post-concussional disorder. *J Neurpsychiatry* 6:15, 1994.

Charpentier, P., T. Lavenu, L. Defebvre, et al. Alzheimer's disease and frontotemporal dementia are differentiated by discriminate analysis applied to (99m) HmPAO SPECT data. *J Neurol Neurosurg Psychiatry* 69:1661, 2000.

Cummings, J. L., M. Mega, K. Gray, et al. The neuropsychiatric inventory. *Neurology,* 44:2308, 1994.

Dugbarty, A. T. Nonverbal learning disabilities. *Sem Clin Neuropsychiatry* 5:205, 2000.

House, A., M. Dennis, C. Warlow, et al. Mood disorders after stroke and their relation to lesion location. *Brain* 113:1113, 1990.

Hurley, R., R. Herrick, L. Hoffman. Clinical imaging in neuropsychiatry. In: *The American Psychiatric Press Textbook of Neuropsychiatry*, 3rd Ed. S. Yudofsky, R. Hales, eds. American Psychiatric Press, Washington, DC, 1997, p. 205.

Jenkyn, L. R., D. Walsh, C. Culver et al. Clinical signs in diffuse cerebral dysfunction. *J Neurol Neurosurg Psychiat* 40:256 1977.

Jenkyn, L. R., A. Reeves, T. Warren, et al. Neurologic signs in senescence. *Arch Neurol* 42:1154, 1985.

Kortola, K. Functional neuroimaging in neuropsychiatry. In: *The American Psychiatric Press Textbook of Neuropsychiatry*, 3rd Ed. S. Yudofsky, R. Hales, eds. American Psychiatric Press, Washington, DC, 1997, p. 239.

Lezak, M. *Neuropsychological Assessment.* Oxford University Press, New York, 1995.

Mayeux, R., Stern, Y., Williams, J. B. Clinical and biochemical features of depression in Parkinson's disease. *Amer J Psychiatry* 143:756, 1986.

Mungas, D. Interictal behavior abnormality in temporal lobe epilepsy. *Arch Gen Psychiatry* 39:108, 1982.

Popkin, M. K., G. J. Tucker. "Secondary" and drug induced mood, anxiety, psychotic, catatonic, and personality disorders: a review of the literature. *J Neuropsychiatry* 4: 369, 1992.

Reeves, A. G. *Disorders of the Nervous System—A Primer*, 4th Ed. Imperial Printers, New York, 2001.

Robinson, R. G. *The Clinical Neuropsychiatry of Stroke.* Cambridge University Press, Cambridge, 1998.

Tandberg, E., J. Larsen, D. Aarsland, et al. Risk factors for depression in Parkinson's disease. *Arch Neurol* 54:625, 1997.

Task Force for the Handbook of Psychiatric Measures. *Handbook of Psyschiatric Measures* 2000, American Psychiatric Press, Washington DC, p. 393.

Townes, B. D., P. D., Slade, eds. Psychological expression of early learning disabilities in adults, *Sem Clin Neuropsychiatry* 5:155, 2000.

Trzepacz, P., R. Baker. *The Psychiatric Mental Status Examination.* Oxford University Press, New York, 1993.

Tucker, G. J., E. Campion, P. Kelleher, et al. The relationship of subtle neurological impairments to disturbances of thinking. *Psychother Psychosom* 24:165 1974.

Tucker, G., Seizure disorders presenting with psychiatric symptomatology. *Psychiatr Clin North Am* 21:625, 1998.

Waxman, S. G., N. Geschwind. The interictal behavior syndrome of temporal lobe epilepsy. *Arch Gen Psychiatry* 32:1580, 1975.

Weinberger, D. R. Brain disease and psychiatric illness: when should a psychiatrist order a CAT scan? *Am J Psychiatry* 141:1521, 1984.

INDEX

Abuse in childhood, 14–16, 63–65, 70–76, 209
  and brain damage, 68–69
  and violence, 67–72
Acalculia, 141, 145
Acetazolamide (diamox), 19
Acetylcholine, 1
  in Alzheimer's disease, 155
  in Parkinson's disease, 187
  in schizophrenia, 105
Acquired brain damage, 4
Adenocorticotopic homone (ACTH), 19, 42
Affective disorders, 205–218
  anxiety and arousal in, 209
  biological changes in, 207–211
    brain structural changes, 207
    hypothalamic functions, 208
    imaging changes, 208
    immune responses, 211
    neurotansmitter changes, 210
    sleep, 209–210
    thyroid function, 209
  bipolar, 206–207
  course, 206–207
  circadian rhythms, 210
  dementia and, 160–161
  dexamethazone suppression test, 209
  differential diagnosis, 250–251
  genetics, 211–214
  and Parkinson's disease, 189–190, 216
  and seizures, 23, 32–34
  sleep, 209–210
  stress and life events, 211–213
  symptoms, 205–210, 250–251
  treatment of, 213–215
  unipolar, 206–207
  and violence, 66
Aggression, 43–45. *See also* Violence
Agnosia, 139–141, 145–146
Agnosognosia, 144
Agraphia, 139–141, 145, 146–147
Akathisia, 190–191, 216
Akinetic mutism, 136
Akinetic rigidity in Parkinsosn's disease, 181
Alexia, 145–147
Alpha-methyldopa (Aldomet), 202
Alzheimer's disease. *See* Cognitive disorders in adults
Amantadine, 187, 195, 202
Ammon's horn, 26, 39
Amnesia, 15, 69, 141–142, 239–240, 259

Amphetamines, 64, 100, 202
Amygdala, 4, 22, 37, 39, 42–43, 65, 104, 141, 256
Amytal (amobarbital) for diagnostic infusion, 23, 143, 238
Anticholinergic effects, 150–151, 166, 199, 213–214
  drugs in Parkinson's disease, 188–189
Antiepileptic drugs (AEDs), 1, 4, 7, 8, 28–29, 32–35, 37, 45, 46, 265
  in affective and bipolar disorders, 213–214
  blood levels of, 17–22
  in obsessive-compulsive disorder, 204
Antidepressants, 213–215
Antisocial personality, 64–65
Anxiety disorders and panic attacks, 231–232
  in affective disorder, 209
  in Alzheimer's disorder, 156
  in attention deficit hyperactivity disorder, 165
  in migraine, 243
  in movement disorders, 237
  in neurological patients, 230
  in vascular dementia, 156
Aphasia, 142–146
  in schizophrenia, 91
ApoE (apolipoprotein E), 155
Apraxia, 139–141, 146
Arousal
  in depression, 209
  in schizophrenia, 118
Aspergers, 162. *See also* autisim
Astasia-abasia, 237–238
Asterixis, 99, 150
Ataxia, 138
Attention deficit hyperactivity disorder (ADHD). *See* Cognitive disorders in adults and children
Atypical antipsychotics, 119, 204
Autism, *See also* Cognitive disorders in children
  aspergers, 162
  MRI in, 164
  neurotransmitters in, 164
  in schizophrenia, 92
Automatisms, 6–8, 15

Basal ganglia
  in frontotemporal dementia, 157
  in schizophrenia, 113–114, 116
  in speech, 143
Belladonna, 195, 202. *See also* Anticholinergic effects
Benztropine (Cogentin), 187
Bipolar disorder, 32, 66, 71, 74, 94–95, 97, 103, 109, 206, 213, 218
Bleuler, 89–82
Blindness, 139–141
Body dysmorphic disorder, 204
Botulism toxin (Botox), 199
Bradykinesia, 178. *See also* Motor and movement dysfunction
Brain damage
  in abuse, 67–69
  acquired, 4
  and trauma, 245
  in violence, 61–64
Brain derived neurotrophic growth factor (BDNF), 210, 213
Brain tumor, 242–243
Briquet's syndrome, 232
Broca's aphasia, 142, 256
Bromocriptine (Parlodel), 187
Buproprion, 167

CAG repeats, 194–195, 203
Carbamazepine(Tegretol), 16–22
Catecholamine metabolism, 177, 190, 202, 205, 214
Catechol-o-methyltransferase inhibitors (COMT), 188
Catastrophic reaction, 136
Caudate nucleus, 104
  in attention deficit hyperactivity disorder, 165
  in Huntington's disease, 201, 203
  in obsessive-compulsive disorder, 204
  in Parkinson's disease, 181
  in schizophrenia, 115
Cerebellar stimulation, 24
Cholorpromazine, 187, 195
Chorea, 193, 195–197, 200–203, 209, 216, 262
  differential diagnosis of, 201
  psychosis and, 216
  symptoms, 200–201
  treatment, 202–203
Clinical evaluation, 249–266
  of brain functions, 255–264
  clinical history, 250–254
  cortical functions, 135–136, 256–257
    symptoms of frontal lobe dysfunction, 136–138
    symptoms of parietal lobe dysfunction, 139–141
    symptoms of temporal lobe dysfunction, 141–142

differentiating neurological from psychiatric symptoms, 250–254
mental status, 257–258, 263
neurological disorders with a high incidence of psychiatric symptoms, 254–255
Cognitive disorders in adults, 153–161
attention deficit hyperactivity disorder, 167
dementia 152–154
Alzheimer's, 154–157, 193, 216
imaging in, 155
neurotransmitters in, 155
Creutzfeldt-Jakob, 193, 217
depression and, 152–154, 160
frontotemporal (Pick's), 153, 193, 217
HIV, 158
Lewy body, 153, 157, 178, 192–194, 217
multi-infarct, 153, 179
occult hydrocephalus, 158–159
psuedodementia, 160–161
vascular, 157
delirium, 150–152
EEG in 151
Cognitive disorders in children, 161–167
autism, 162–164
Asperger's syndrome, 162
Heller's syndrome, 162
MRI in, 164
neurotransmitters in, 164
attention deficit hyperactivity disorder (ADHD), 164–167
differential diagnosis, 165–166
imaging in, 165
treatment, 166–167
Clonazepam, 17–22
Clonidine, 167
Clozapine, 216
Cocaine, 100, 202
Commissurotomy. *See* Split brains
Complex partial seizures. *See* Seizure disorders
Computerized tomography. *See* Imaging
Conversion disorders, 234–242, 245–246
amnesia, 239–240
amytal test, 238
deafness, 239
differential diagnosis of, 234–235, 241
fugue states in, 239–240
gait (astasia-abasia) in, 237–238
hemiparesis in, 236–237
hemiplegia in, 236–237
hemisensory loss in, 235–236
la belle indifference, 234
movement disorders (dystonias, rigidity, chorea), 238
paralysis, 236–237
pain, 240–241
pseudoseizures, 13–16
and secondary gain, 234
sensory signs of, 235–236
swallowing inability, 235
visual, 238–239
Corpus callosum, 147–150. *See also* Split brains
Corticotrophin releasing factor (CRF), 69, 160, 208–209, 212
Cortisol, 161, 208, 212

Delirium. *See* Cognitive disorders in adults
Dementia. *See* Cognitive disorders in adults
Depression. *See* Affective disorders
Depersonalization, 5
Diazepam (Valium), 19
Diphenylhydantoin (Dilantin, Phenytoin), 16–22
Diphenylhydramine (Benadryl), 195
Dissociation, 15–16
and abuse, 15–16, 69
Disturbance of thinking
in autism, 163
in cognitive disorders, 133
differential diagnosis of, 98–99
in epilepsy, 2
in Parkinson's disease, 181
in schizophrenia, 89–92, 107, 118
Dizziness, 230–231
Dominance, 144–145
in aphasia, 144
Dopamine (DOPA), 12–13
agonists, 187–188
in attention deficit hyperactivity disorder, 166
Parkinson's disease 181–186, 216
in schizophrenia, 103, 104, 114
in tardive dyskinesias, 196
Dopamine receptor blockers, 202, 216
Dyskinesia, 195, 216
Dystonia, 195, 197–200
focal, 198–200
and mental illness, 200
painful, 191
Dyslexia, 12–13

Electrocardiogram (EKG), 232
Electroconvulsive therapy
and brain damage, 28
in depression, 210

Electroconvulsive therapy (*continued*)
  effect on EEG, 28
  and seizures, 24–29
Electroencephalogram (EEG), 265–266. *See also specific disorders*
  abnormalities in the absence of epilepsy, 13
  in abuse, 68
  in delirium, 151
  in dystonia, 197
  in epilepsy, 1–5, 7, 9–12, 46, 62
  in epilepsy surgery, 22
  in hemispheric dominance, 149
  in hyperventilation, 231
  nasopharyngeal leads, 10
  in neuroleptic malignant syndrome, 137
  in pseudodementia, 161
  in psuedoseizures, 14–15
  in psychosis associated with seizures, 29–34
    forced normalization, 30–31
  in schizophrenia, 13, 106–107, 111–112, 118
  sleep activation, 10–11
  sphenoidal leads, 10
  in violence, 38, 43–44
Encephalitis 2, 28, 32, 67, 85, 98, 137, 201, 235, 242, 249
Epilepsy. *See also* Seizures
  idiopathic, 2–3
  schizophrenic, like psychosis in, 4, 29–34
  symptomatic, 2–3
Episodic dyscontrol, 45–46
Ethosuccimide (Zarontin), 16–22
Excitatory amino acids, 69
Extrapyramidal disorders. *See* Chorea; Parkinson's disease
Eye movements
  in dominance, 149
  in frontal lobe lesions, 138, 259–260
  rapid (REM) in sleep, 159, 210
  in schizophrenia, 109

Febrile seizures, 24–26
Felbamate (Felbatol), 17–22
Focal seizures. *See* Seizures
Forced normalization (see EEGs)
Frontal lobe
  role in fugue and confusional states, 15, 237–240
  relation to temporal lobe, 40–42
  symptoms of frontal lobe leisons– 136–138, 235, 258–263
  in schizophrenia, 114–115
  in seizures, 8
Frontotemporal dementia. *See* Cognitive disorders in adults
Functional magnetic resonance imaging (fMRI). *See* Imaging
Fuge states, 239–240

GABA, 105–106, 150
Gabapentin (Neurontin), 17–22
Gegenhalten, 137, 238
Genetics. *See specific disorders*
Gerstmann syndrome, 139, 147
Glucocorticoids. *See cortisol*
Glutamate, 105
Grand mal seizures, 6, 13, 17, 27, 29, 31, 43. *See also* Seizure disorders

Hallucinogenic drugs, 100
Haloperidol (Haldol), 195
Headache, 230–231, 242–245
  in brain tumor, 242–243
  differential diagnosis of, 242–245
  migraine, 243–244
  posttraumatic, 245
  temporomandibular joint syndrome (TMJ), 241, 244–245
  tension, 242
Heller's syndrome, 162
Hippocampus, 4, 22, 37, 39–43, 65, 104, 141, 256
  in depression, 210, 213
  in schizophrenia, 115
Huntington's disease, 201–203, 209, 216. *See also* Chorea
  behavioral changes in, 201–202
Hydrocephalus (occult, low pressure, normal pressure), 4, 109, 111, 158–159, 252
Hyperventilation, 231–232
  EEG in, 231
  EKG in, 232
Hypochondriasis, 234
Hypothalamus, 208
Hysteria. *See* Conversion disorders
Hysterical psychosis, 97–98

Imaging (CT, MRI, PET, SPECT), 264–265
  in abuse, 608–609
  in Alzheimer's disease, 155
  in aphasia, 142–143
  in attention deficit hyperactivity disorder, 165
  in autism, 162
  in brain injury, 245
  in depression, 208

in dyslexia, 12–13
in Huntington's disease, 203
in obsessive-compulsive disorder, 204
in Parkinson's disease, 184
in schizophrenia, 112–115
in seizures, 11–12
in violence, 61–63, 65
Imipramine. *See* Tricyclic antidepressants
Infantile spasms, 163

Juvenile delinquents, 45, 62, 70–71

Kindling, 25
Kraeplin, 87, 95

Laboratory tests in differential diagnosis, 265
Lamotrigine (Lamictal), 17–22
Language, 143–144
function in parietal lobe syndromes, 139–141
Lesch-Nyhan, 65
Lewy body dementia (LBD). *See* Cognitive disorders in adults
L-dopa, 179–180, 181–186, 202, 216
Limbic system, 38–46
anatomy of, 39–41
and epilepsy, 4
physiological psychology of, 40–43
in schizophrenia, 115
and violent behavior, 43–45
Lithium, 19
Loose associations, 89

Magnetic resonance imaging and spectroscopy (MRI, MRS). *See* Imaging
Mania, 74, 205–207, 251, 263
and attention deficit hyperactivity disorder in children, 165
and dopamine, 181, 191–192
and Huntington's disease, 201–202
Marche a' petit pas, 138, 178
Meig's syndrome, 239
Memory, 134, 148, 156, 159–160. *See also* amnesia
and ECT, 28
and the hippocampus, 42, 69
and the limbic system, 39, 42
memory impairment as the only symptom, 153
and schizophrenia, 109, 115–117
and seizures, 6, 23, 26
and the temporal lobes, 141–142
Mesocortical tract, 104
Mesolimbic tract, 104
Methylphenidate (Ritalin), 161
Migraine, 6. *See also* Headache
Minimal brain damage (MBD). *See* Attention deficit hyperactivity disorder
Minor neurological signs
in attention hyperactivity deficit disorder, 165
in depression, 207
in schizophrenia, 106–111
in violent delinquents, 62
Monoamine oxidase inhibitors (MAOI), 188
Mood stabilizers. *See also* Antiepileptic drugs, 18–19
Motor and movement dysfunction
in chorea. *See* Chorea
drug induced, 195–197, 199–200. *See also* Tardive movement disorders
in frontal lobe lesions, 137–138, 258–261
in hysteria. *See* Conversion disorders
in parietal lobe lesions, 139–141
in Parkinson's disease. *See also* Parkinson's disease
in schizophrenia, 106–108
Multi-infarct dementia. *See* Cognitive disorders in adults
Multiple personality, 15
Multiple sclerosis (MS), 160, 250–251
Multisystem atrophy (MSA), 179, 194

Narcolepsy, 6, 98, 210
Neuroleptic malignant syndrome, 137
Nigrostriatal tract, 104
N-methyl-D-Aspartate (NMDA), 105
Neuropsychological tests, 161
in dementia, 161
in ECT, 28
in Parkinson's and Huntington's disease, 160
in schizophrenia, 116–117
in seizure disorders, 26–27
and soft neurological signs, 262
in white matter disorders, 160
Neurotensin, 105
Norepinephrine, 218
in Alzheimer's disease, 165
in depression, 259
DOPA and in Parkinson's disease, 190
in schizophrenia, 105
tricyclics and, 187
Normal pressure hydrocephalus, 158–159. *See also* Occult hydrocephalus
Nucleus accumbens, 104, 111, 252

Obsessive-compulsive disorder (OCD), 65, 203–205
  treatment of, 204, 217–218
Occipital seizures, 8. *See* Seizure disorders
Occult hydrocephalus. *See* Hydrocephalus
Olivoponto-cerebellar atrophy (OPCA), 179

Pallidotomy/thalamatomy, 188–189
Panic disorder, 6, 231–232
Paraldehyde, 19
Paranoia and violence, 66–67
Paranoid thinking, 67, 71
Parietal lobe, 139–141
  symptoms of parietal lobe dysfunction, 139–141
Parkinson's disease, 177–195, 262
  dementia in, 192–193
  dopamine deficiency in, 179–181, 182–186
  etiology, 193
  L-dopa in, 181–182
  painful dystonias (cramps), 191
  pathogenesis,181
  psychiatric, symptoms in
    anxiety, 190
    depression, 189–190, 216
    psychosis, 191–192, 216
  stages of, 182–186
  symptoms of, 197–179
  treatment
    brain stimulation, 189
    pharmacological treatment, 186–188
    protein restriction diet/large neutral amino acids (LNAA), 185–186
    surgical, 188–189
  "wearing off" and "on/off" phenomena, 183–185
Pavor nocturne, 6
Pergolide (Permax), 187
Perinatal trauma, 70, 106, 108
Petit mal seizures. *See* Seizure disorders, absence
Phenobarbital, 16–22
Phenothiazines, 202
  and dystonias, 216
  and tardive dyskinesias, 195–197, 199–200
  use in seizure disorders, 32–33. *See also* Atypical antipsychotics
Phenylketonuria, 163
Posttraumatic stress disorder (PTSD), 69
Prader-Willi syndrome, 66
Pramipexole (Mirapex), 187
Presenile degeneration. *See* Alzheimer's disease
Primidone (Mysoline), 16–22
Progressive supranuclear palsy (PSP), 179
Prolactin, 11
Pseudodementia, 160–161, 239–240
Pseudoseizures, 13–16
Psvchological tests. *See* neuropsychological tests
Psychomotor epilepsy. *See* Complex partial seizures, in Seizure disorders)
Psychosis
  in chorea, 216
  hysterical, 97–98
  in Parkinson's disease, 191–192, 216
  and seizures, 5, 29–34
  and the temporal lobe, 29–34, 141–142

Rapid eye movement (REM). *See* Eye movements
Reflexes, 261
  grasp, 261
  nuchocephalic, 261
  snout, 261
Reserpine, 202
Rigidity. *See* Parkinson's disease
Ropinerole (Requipp), 187

Schizoaffective disorder, 94–95
Schizophrenia, 85–120
  age of onset, 92–93
  arousal, 118
  biochemical aspects of, 103–106
  in childhood, 92–93, 162
  cognitive functions, 117
  course and natural history, 95–97
  diagnostic classification, 85–92, 93–94
  differential diagnosis, 97–100
    from drug reactions, 100
    from neurological conditions, 98–100
    from seizure disorders, 30
    from sleep disorders, 100
  and early childhood autism, 92–93, 162
  EEG in, 106–107, 111–112, 118
  and epilepsy, 29–34
  genetics of, 100–103,
  imaging in, 112–115
  neurological factors in, 106–111, 257
    minor nonlocalizing neurological abnormalities, 106–108
  neuropathological findings, 115–116
  obstetric complications and, 108–109
  personality disorder, 95
  process, 93–94
  prognosis, 93–94
  psychological testing in, 116–117
  reactive, 93–94

schizoaffective, 94–95
subtypes, 92–93
symptoms of, 86–92
thought patterns in, 89–92
treatment of, 118–119
vestibular function, 109
Schizophrenia-like psychosis. *See* Seizure disorders
Selegiline (Deprenyl, Eldepryl), 188
Seizure disorders, 1–47. *See also* Epilepsy
absence, 9
and antidepressants, 35
and anxiety, 35–36
brain damage in, 2, 4, 13, 15, 24–26
cognitive changes, 24–29
IQ, 26
complex partial seizures
differential diagnosis, 6–8
extratemporal origin, 8–9
frontal, 8
temporal origin, 4–8
depression in, 23, 34–35
EEG and diagnosis, 1–4, 7–8, 30–31
febrile, 24–25
focal, 2–4, 7, 12, 24–25, 36, 265–266
genetics of, 3–4
hysterical vs. complex partial seizures, 13–16
idiopathic vs. symptomatic, 2–3
imaging in, 11–12
kindling, 25–26
occipital, 8
and personality disturbance, 37–38
postictal depression, 8–9
prolactin and, 11
pseudoseizures, 13–16
versus complex partial seizures, 13–16
psychosis and schizophrenia, 5, 29–34
and sexual behavior, 36–37
and suicide, 15, 34, 44
surgery for, 22–24
thalamic nuclei stimulation, 24
treatment of, 16–24
and violence, 38–39
vagal nerve stimulation, 24
Selective serotonin reuptake inhibitors (SSRIs), 196, 204, 213–215, 217–218
Sensory deprivation, 110–111
Serotonin, 218
in autisim, 162
in schizophrenia, 104, 105, 114
in violence, 65
Sleep deprivation
in depression, 209–210
in schizophrenia, 98, 100
and seizures, 10–11
Split brain. *See also* corpus callosum, 147–150
Stress and depression, 161, 211–213
Striatonigral degeneration, 179
Syncope, 230–231
Sydenham's chorea. *See* Chorea

Tardive movement disorder, 195–197, 199–200, 216
Temporal lobe
anatomy, 39–40
and epilepsy, 4–8
lobectomy, 23
and memory, 141–142
and mood, 208
physiological psychology, 40–43
and psychosis, 29–34, 141–142
in schizophrenia, 113
and sexual behavior, 36–37, 141–142
smell and taste, 256
and speech, 256
symptoms associated with dysfunction, 141–142
and violence, 38–39
Temporal lobe epilepsy. *See* Complex partial seizures in Seizure disorders
Temporomandibular joint syndrome (TMJ), 241, 244–245
Testosterone, 65
Tics, 203–205,
Thalamus, 104, 113–114, 141, 146, 177
and chorea, 201
and frontal lobes, 259
limbic system, 38–39, 46, 65
and memory, 141–142
and Parkinson's disease, 177
and speech, 143
Thought disorder. *See* Disturbances of thinking
Thyroid, 209
Tiagabine (Gabatril), 17–22
Topiramate (Topamax), 17–22
Tourette's syndrome, 65, 203–205, 217–218
Transient global amnesia, 6, 240
Traumatic brain injury, 245
Treatment. *See specific disorders*
Tremor
in NMS, 137
in Parkinson's disease, 177–179, 181, 186, 187, 189, 195

Tricyclic antidepressants (TCAs), 196, 213–215
  in autism, 167
  in epileptics, 35
  in Parkinson's disease, 190
Trichotillomania, 204
Trihexyphendyl (Artane)
Trimethadione (Tridione), 19
  in dystonias, 199
  in Parkinson's disease, 186–187
Tryptophan
  in autism, 164
  in depression, 208
Tuberous sclerosis, 163
Tumor, 242–243

Unexplained symptoms, 233–234
Unipolar depression, 206–207

Valproic acid (Depakene, Depakote), 16–22
Vigabatrin (Sabril), 21
Violence, 43–44, 61–76
  and abuse, 67–69
  antisocial personality, 64–65
  brain damage in, 61–64, 69–72
  as a complex psychosocial–biologic interaction, 69–72
  EEG in, 43–47
  episodic dyscontrol, 45–46
  and frontal lobes, 64–65
  genetics, 66
  and limbic system, 43–45
  and mental illness, 66–69, 69–72
  and neurotransmitters, 65–66
  sociologic aspects, 72–76

Wada test, 23
Wernicke's aphasia, 142, 256
  encephalopathy, 142
Wilson's disease, 201
Witzelsucht, 136